Contents

About the authors

Monica Kesson Grad Dip Phys MCSP SRP Cert Ed
Elaine Atkins MA Grad Dip Phys MCSP SRP

The authors studied physiotherapy together at St Thomas' Hospital, London where the methods of Dr James Cyriax were taught. From that original inspiration they developed their clinical practice encompassing a wider scope of physiotherapy skills, but always building on the solid, logical base provided by orthopaedic medicine.

Both now work in private practice and combine this with a teaching commitment to the Society of Orthopaedic Medicine. As course principals they are involved in teaching orthopaedic medicine and are particularly interested in empowering students to learn.

Orthopaedic Medicine

A Practical Approach

Monica Kesson
Elaine Atkins

With a Foreword by

Nigel Palastanga MA, BA, MCSP, DMS, DipTP.
Dean, School of Healthcare Studies, University of Wales College of Medicine, Cardiff, UK

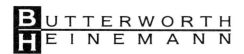

Butterworth-Heinemann
Linacre House, Jordan Hill, Oxford OX2 8DP
225 Wildwood Avenue, Woburn, MA 01801-2041
A division of Reed Educational and Professional Publishing Ltd

ℜ   A member of the Reed Elsevier plc group

OXFORD   AUCKLAND   BOSTON
JOHANNESBURG   MELBOURNE   NEW DELHI

First published 1998
Reprinted 1999

British Library Cataloguing in Publication Data
Kesson, Monica
  Orthopaedic medicine: a practical approach
  1 Orthopedics
  I Title   II Atkins, Elaine
  616.7

ISBN 0 7506 2543 0

Library of Congress Cataloguing in Publication Data
Kesson, Monica.
  Orthopaedic medicine: a practical approach / Monica Kesson, Elaine Atkins.
  p.   cm.
  Includes bibliographical references and index.
  ISBN 0 7506 2543 0
  1 Musculoskeletal system–Wounds and injuries–Physical therapy.
  2 Orthopedics.   3 Anatomy, Surgical and topographic.   I Atkins,
  Elaine.   II Title.
  [DNLM: 1 Musculoskeletal Diseases–diagnosis.   2 Musculoskeletal
  Diseases–therapy.   WE 140 K422o]
  RD736.P47K47
  616.7–dc21   97–26142
                                                                      CIP

Typeset by Latimer Trend & Company Ltd, Plymouth
Printed and bound in Great Britain by The Bath Press, Somerset

Foreword

Orthopaedic medicine has been a well established part of Physiotherapy for many years. Dr James Cyriax was a lifelong advocate of the treatment of musculoskeletal lesions using a variety of interventions and techniques which he always generously shared with physiotherapy colleagues. There was a danger with his death in 1985 that the approach would fossilize and not progress, but it is pleasing to see that his philosophy has been taken up enthusiastically by two skilled physiotherapists who trained at St Thomas' Hospital where Dr Cyriax was based. Monica Kesson and Elaine Atkins have taken up the baton left by Dr Cyriax and have produced a book which will be of immense use to the orthopaedic physician and physiotherapist, and keeps the 'Cyriax approach' alive. The book is divided into two sections, the first dealing with the principles of orthopaedic medicine and the second with the practice. In the second section various regions of the body are taken in turn and a comprehensive coverage of the relevant anatomy, examination, common lesions, and treatment is given for each. What makes this text really different is that the description of the technique of injection is as applicable to the physiotherapist as to the doctor, now that this is considered within the scope of physiotherapy practice for those suitably trained. This book must complement, not replace, those produced by Dr Cyriax, but the approach is new and refreshing.

I congratulate both authors on the job they have done. It would have been easy to shy away from the task as the standing of Dr Cyriax was such that the prospect must have been daunting. I am sure that all physiotherapists interested in orthopaedic medicine will find this a useful and interesting book. It has been well written and well produced and I congratulate all those involved.

N.P.P.

Acknowledgements

The following anatomy texts were invaluable and deserve special mention:

Backhouse, K.M., Hutchings, R.T. (1986) *A Colour Atlas of Surface Anatomy*. Wolfe Medical Publications.
Keogh, B., Ebbs, S. (1984) *Normal Surface Anatomy*. William Heinemann Medical Books.
McMinn, R.M.H., Gaddum-Rosse, P., Hutchings, R.T., Logan, B.M. (1995) *McMinn's Functional and Clinical Anatomy*. Times Mirror International.
Palastanga, N., Field, D., Soames, R. (1994) *Anatomy and Human Movement*. Butterworth-Heinemann.
Williams, P.L., Warwick, R., Dyson, M., Bannister, L.H. (1989) *Gray's Anatomy*, 37th edn. Churchill Livingstone.

We are very grateful to the following people, all of whom have been unstinting in their support and patience: Dr Ian Davies, for his major contribution to the injections; Sue Thompson, for assuming the role of model for the photographs, with all the inconvenience involved; and the Society of Orthopaedic Medicine, for allowing us to use the photographs, generously supported by an educational grant from Pfizer Pharmaceuticals.

Caroline Makepeace from Butterworth-Heinemann remained enthusiastic throughout, and spurred us on with the encouraging comments of her mysterious 'professional adviser'. Thanks are also due to him or her.

Thank you, too, to the reviewers from the Council of the Society of Orthopaedic Medicine and particularly those who suggested changes: Marilou Argote, Dr Ian Davies, Dr Philip Knowles, José Marcelino, Margaret Rees and Dr Andrew Watson.

The brunt of the pressure has been borne by our colleagues in our respective practices, who have soldiered on without us, even when we've been physically there.

Stephanie Saunders made a large contribution in the preparation of the original Society of Orthopaedic Medicine course manual. She produced a number of modifications in the examination and treatment techniques and defined the mobilization and manipulation Grades A, B and C. In particular, she devised a method of examination and management of the sacroiliac joint which was designed to harmonize with Dr James Cyriax's original concepts (page 450). Special acknowledgement is given to the following techniques, originally published by Dr Cyriax (Cyriax and Cyriax, 1983; Cyriax, 1984), but modified and adapted by Stephanie to facilitate their practical application in clinical practice: loose body mobilization at the elbow (page 168), reduction of the capitate at the wrist (page 203), loose body mobilization at the knee (page 336) and the meniscal tests at the knee (page 331).

A poignant note of thanks is also due to those who have inspired us from the beginning, and who, to us, have epitomized orthopaedic medicine: Jackie Caldow, Anne Crofts, Liz Edwards, Jenny Hickling, Stephanie Saunders and, of course, Dr James Cyriax himself.

Our families have been paragons of strength throughout, and have gamely carried on as normal. Thank you Rod, Andrew, Denise and Clive, Kate and Tess.

References

Cyriax, J. (1984) *Textbook of Orthopaedic Medicine*, vol. 2, 11th edn. Baillière Tindall.
Cyriax, J., Cyriax, P. (1983) *Illustrated Manual of Orthopaedic Medicine*. Butterworths.

Section 1

Principles of orthopaedic medicine

Introduction to Section 1

The aim of this book is to provide principles of diagnosis and treatment that can be applied to any of the soft-tissue lesions encountered in clinical practice.

Section 1 presents the theory behind the principles and practice of orthopaedic medicine, beginning with the theory underpinning the assessment procedure towards clinical diagnosis. Clinical diagnosis involves the development of a hypothesis through the consideration of both subjective and objective findings and each is discussed.

The histology and biomechanics of the soft tissues follow, with a review of the healing process, towards an understanding of the effects of injury on the soft tissues. This should enable the application of appropriate treatment to the different phases of healing, in order to achieve the restoration of full painless function.

Building on the theory of the first chapters, the section ends with a presentation of the principles of treatment as applied in orthopaedic medicine and discusses the techniques of mobilization and injection, aims and application and indications for use.

Clinical tips are provided throughout Section 1 to emphasize clinical application and indications for use.

In December 1995, injections were declared to be within the scope of physiotherapy practice. At the time of writing, physiotherapists working as rheumatology or orthopaedic practitioners, as seniors in hospital clinics or in private practice have risen to the challenge, albeit cautiously, taking care to comply with stringent protocols. The Chartered Society of Physiotherapy has produced an interim guide for the use of injections by physiotherapists which outlines the requirements of courses towards the 'safe and efficacious' practice of injections.

Courses in orthopaedic medicine (see Appendix) provide an excellent grounding in the theory and practice of injections, consistent with guidelines, particularly since the modules are attended by both doctors and physiotherapists in an atmosphere of shared experience. Developments are underway to provide supervised practice in the clinical setting to allow the demonstration of competence. More relevant, however, is the development of confidence in performing the techniques; the inculcation of both these aspects in physiotherapists is at present undergoing scrutiny.

Issues also still exist as regards the prescribing of drugs and with whom the responsibility rests for the injection itself. Clearly a close relationship must be maintained with the medical profession, but preferably not at the expense of physiotherapy autonomy.

Within this text, injections must therefore be considered to be as pertinent to the physiotherapist reader as to the doctor. However, in view of the scant pharmacology taught at undergraduate level, the physiotherapist may find it beneficial to explore some additional reading in this area. A brief presentation of relevant pharmacology and general considerations is presented here.

1 Clinical diagnosis

Summary

Orthopaedic Medicine is based on the life's work of the late Dr James Cyriax (1900–1985). He developed a method of assessing the soft tissues of the musculoskeletal system, employing a process of diagnosis by selective tension, which uses passive movements to test the inert structures and resisted movements to test the contractile structures.

This chapter describes the theory behind his logical method of subjective and objective examination, which, by reasoned elimination, leads to the incrimination of the tissue in which the lesion lies.

Dr Cyriax's starting point in the development of orthopaedic medicine was the premise that all pain has a source. It was a simple extension of that logic that, to be effective, all treatment must reach the source and all treatment must benefit the lesion.

He was intrigued by the number of patients passing through orthopaedic clinics who presented with normal X-ray findings, and acknowledged the soft tissues as the source of the complaints. He devised a mechanism of clinical examination to establish the source of the pain which was logical and methodical, and was deliberately pared to the minimum procedure in order to discover in which tissue the lesion lay. His style of assessment conformed to the claim of Sir Robert Hutchinson in 1897, that 'every good method of case taking should be both comprehensive and concise' (Hunter and Bomford, 1963).

An important emphasis of his examination procedure is that the negative findings are as significant as the positive, eliminating from the enquiry those structures which are *not* at fault. The systematic approach devised by Cyriax produces a set of findings that can be interpreted through logical reasoning towards eventual clinical diagnosis. The term diagnosis at this stage implies the hypothesis against which we all work, which becomes proven or disproved in the light of the patient's subsequent response.

In recent years, much work has been produced in developing areas of specialist assessment. However, the orthopaedic medicine examination procedure gives clinicians a sound framework from which to start and any special examination techniques can be superimposed upon it.

For example, once a basic spinal assessment has been carried out, extra tests can be included to search for aspects of neural tension, repeated or combined movements can be included, or localized joint palpation can be applied.

A further aim of the examination is to establish whether or not the lesion is suitable for the treatments offered in orthopaedic medicine, or other allied treatment modalities, or whether the patient should be more suitably referred on for appropriate specialist opinion.

The orthopaedic medicine assessment procedure follows a set routine which is easy to apply in the clinical setting. It contains the elements of:

- Observation, noting face, gait and posture.
- A detailed history.
- Inspection for bony deformity, colour changes, wasting and swelling.
- Palpation for heat, swelling and synovial thickening.
- Examination by selective tension, assessing active, passive and resisted movements.
- Palpation for the site of the lesion, once the causative structure has been identified.

More detailed tests such as blood tests, X-rays, computerized tomography (CT) and magnetic resonance imaging (MRI) scans can be employed as necessary but do not form part of the basic examination procedure.

Observation

Observation
• Face
• Gait
• Posture

Note the patient's *face*, *gait* and *posture*.

A general observation is made as the patient is met, or even before, without the patient's knowledge, as in walking across the car park or approaching reception. Note the patient's face for signs of sleeplessness and pain. Serious disease accompanied by unrelenting pain is usually indicated in the patient's overall demeanour.

Certain postures indicate specific conditions. An antalgic posture – one assumed by the patient to avoid pain – is often adopted in neck pain as a wry neck, or as a lateral shift when associated with a lumbar disc lesion.

In the upper limb, note any apparent guarding, perhaps with an altered arm swing associated with a painful shoulder, elbow or even wrist.

The gait pattern may be altered, with a limp indicating pain or a leg length discrepancy. An altered stride may be due to limitation of movement at a joint, or protection from weight-bearing. The use of aids such as a stick or crutches provides an obvious clue to the need for extra support to avoid or to assist with weight-bearing. As part of the overall observation, a check may also be made on whether such aids are being used correctly.

History

A complete history is taken from the patient to ascertain as much information as possible about the condition. At some joints the history is more relevant than at others, with respect to diagnosis. The spinal joints and knee joint history may give many clues to diagnosis, whereas with many of the commonly encountered conditions of the shoulder or elbow, such as capsulitis or tennis elbow, the history gives almost no clues at all.

The term *history* implies a chronological account of how the condition has progressed but this forms part of a broader compass that includes other aspects, such as aggravating and alleviating factors or past medical history. The history-taking is really the subjective part of the examination procedure and it is traditional in medical and physiotherapy practice to use a model for the collection of clinical data from the patient (Beckman and Frankel, 1984).

Most models, including that used in orthopaedic medicine, involve the categorizing of the subjective examination under different headings to ensure that all information is collected. However, if this is adhered to too rigidly, it can be restricting for the patient. The use of closed questions to steer the patient's responses results in the interview being physician/physiotherapist-led, and the constant interruptions may restrict the fluency of the patient's account, such that he or she may be prevented from presenting the true nature of the problem (Beckman and Frankel, 1984; Blau, 1989).

Studies on the process of history-taking revealed that physicians interrupted and took control of the interview on average 18 s into the consultation, and that by asking specific closed questions they halted the spontaneous flow of information (Beckman and Frankel, 1984). However, if allowed to continue uninterrupted and with no specific guidance, patients talked on average for less than 2 min, during which time most of the information required by the physician was disclosed (Blau, 1989). This study was repeated by Wilkinson (1989) who found the time taken to be even shorter, with 89 of the 100 patients surveyed speaking for less than $1\frac{1}{2}$ min and 41 of those for less than 30 s.

Bearing the previous points in mind, whilst consideration of the various categories adopted in orthopaedic medicine is necessary, in clinical practice it is better to begin the patient interview with an open question such as 'What can I do for you?' or 'What brings you to me?' and then to allow the patient to express the history in his or her own words. Anything not mentioned can be searched for after the patient has finished speaking.

Of course, not all patients will obligingly reveal their history and some guidance will be required to keep to the relevant. None the less, a balance should still be sought between allowing the patient time to speak and controlling the interview to prevent irrelevant deviation (Blau, 1989).

The model for history-taking in orthopaedic medicine will now be described. The clinician should note the relevant details from the history on the patient's record card for subsequent interpretation,

---

History or subjective examination

- Age, occupation, sports, hobbies and lifestyle.
- Site and spread.
- Onset and duration.
- Symptoms and behaviour.
- Past medical history.
- Other joint involvement.
- Medications.

whilst accepting that the process of clinical reasoning continues throughout the interview and that the 'rambling thoughts of a clinician' cannot, and should not, be impeded.

Age, occupation, sports, hobbies and lifestyle

The age of the patient may be relevant as certain conditions particularly affect certain age groups. For example, children may suffer from Perthes disease or slipped epiphysis in the hip, pulled elbow, or loose bodies associated with osteochondritis dissecans in the knee. Adolescents may suffer from Osgood–Schlatter's disease, chondromalacia patellae or maltracking problems in the knee. Mechanical lumbar lesions, ligament or tendon injuries are common in the middle-aged group and degenerative osteoarthrosis is usually suffered by the elderly.

Occupation may be relevant in terms of the postures adopted whilst at work and the activities involved in the patient's job. In this respect, it is important to explore the job's requirements rather than merely to note the job title.

An overview of the patient's general lifestyle may give clues to the cause of the problem and, relating to treatment, can provide an indication of the requirements for rehabilitation back to full activity. For example, tendon or muscle belly lesions frequently occur in sports requiring explosive activity, as in tennis and squash, and should not be placed back into training until the resisted tests and stretching are painfree.

Site and spread

Patients usually complain of pain but there may be other symptoms that cause them to seek advice, such as stiffness, weakness and pins and needles. Whatever the symptoms, much information can be gained towards diagnosis by establishing where the symptoms are and their overall spread. For instance, it is important not just to know where the symptoms are but where they have been. A low back pain often travels into the leg but usually becomes less apparent in the back as it does so – a typical presentation of a lumbar disc lesion. A low back pain moving into the leg without remission in the back implies a spreading lesion and requires a different interpretation.

Since pain is the most usual complaint, it will form the main basis of the discussion in this section. Whether right or wrong in their assessment, patients usually localize their pain as coming from a certain point and can describe the area of its spread, although sometimes only vaguely. Cyriax considered that all pain is referred (Cyriax and Cyriax, 1983) and explored the pattern of referred pain to try and establish some rules which would help in its interpretation towards establishing the true source of the pain.

The study of pain itself is a vast topic, most of which is outside the scope of this book, and the reader is referred to the many other sources which confine themselves to the indepth study of this field. However, pain and its behaviour are relevant to orthopaedic medicine, particularly in the assessment procedures, both towards the achievement of an accurate clinical diagnosis and as a guide to effectiveness of the treatment techniques applied.

To be able to identify the source of the pain, a thorough knowledge of applied and functional anatomy is essential, but coupled with an understanding of the behaviour of pain, particularly in relation to its ability to be referred to areas other than the causative site. It is acknowledged that other influences can affect the perception of pain and within this chapter *referred pain* will be discussed, with a brief consideration of *psychogenic pain*.

It is commonly found in clinical practice that pain of visceral origin can mimic that of somatic origin and vice versa. Pain arising from pathology in the heart, for example, will produce a spread of pain into the arm imitating the pain of nerve root sleeve compression from a cervical disc lesion. Similarly, mid thoracic back pain may arise from a stomach lesion.

There have been several suggestions put forward for the mechanism of referred pain and the more significant ones are discussed here. McMahon *et al.* (1995) cite Sinclair who suggested that primary sensory neurons have bifurcating axons which innervate both somatic and visceral structures. Some evidence was found for this theory, but some of the findings were challenged, particularly as such axons had failed to be demonstrated in appreciable numbers. Whilst unable to find neurons with visceral and somatic fields, McMahon *et al.* mention that Mense and colleagues did find a few single sensory neurons with receptive fields in two tissues, in both skin and muscle in the tail of a cat, but overall there was scant support for Sinclair's suggestion.

More evidence has been provided for the mechanism that visceral and somatic primary sensory neurons converge on to common spinal neurons, causing a confusion in the ascending spinal pathways and leading to misinterpretation of the origin of the pain. This was dubbed the convergence–projection theory.

A side-track from the convergence–projection theory, attributed to McKenzie, claimed that the viscera were insensitive and that visceral afferent activity did not directly give rise to pain. It was suggested that an irritable focus was produced within the spinal cord, where somatic inputs would take over to produce abnormal referred pain in appropriate segmental distribution. This was termed the convergence–facilitation theory but it was not generally accepted since it denied that true visceral pain could exist. However, it did provide an explanation for some delay in referred sensations, including that of hyperalgesia. Its basic concepts have also been developed in the early nineties under the descriptor of central sensitization that attempts to explain hyperalgesia and the prolongation of chronic pain.

Referred pain does not only present itself for misinterpretation between visceral and somatic structures but is also a phenom-enon which may prevent accurate localization amongst the musculoskeletal tissues. Cyriax and Cyriax (1983) suggested that the misinterpretation of pain occurs at cortical level where stimuli arriving at certain cortical cells from stimulation of the skin can be accurately localized to that area. When stimuli from other tissues of the same segmental derivation reach those same cells the sensory cortex makes assumptions on the basis of past experience and attributes the source of the pain to that same area of skin. This accounts for the dermatomal reference of pain but the theory can be extended to include the referral of other symptoms.

Knowledge of the nerve supply of soft-tissue structures, coupled with factors affecting dermatomal reference and the general rules of referred pain, is a useful aid to diagnosis. It will help to direct the clinician to the true source of the patient's pain and so facilitate the application of effective treatment.

Several workers have tried to establish patterns of referred pain by examining the dermatomes. However, the dermatomes appear to vary according to the different methods for defining them. These mainly derive from embryonic development, observation of herpetic eruptions, areas of vasodilatation resulting from nerve root stimulation and the areas of tactile sensation remaining after rhizotomies of caudal roots. These dermatomes are referred to as embryonic, herpetic, vasodilatation and tactile respectively.

Sir Henry Head (1900) laid the foundations for the mapping of dermatomes by analysing herpetic eruptions. Herpes zoster is an inflammatory lesion of the spinal ganglia which produces an eruption on the skin in the corresponding segmental cutaneous area. By defining the dermatomes in this way, little overlap was found and there was only slight variation between subjects studied.

The skin is supplied by both ventral and dorsal nerve roots. Foerster (1933) examined the areas of skin supplied by the dorsal roots, which carry the afferent sensory fibres and efferent fibres producing vasodilatation. He described two methods of isolating the area of skin supplied by the dorsal nerve roots using the terms *anatomical* and *physiological*. Foerster described the anatomical method used by Herringham and Bolk which involved the isolation of fibres arising from a single nerve root by dissection through the plexus and the peripheral nerves into the skin. It was impossible to follow the finest ramifications by this method but it largely demonstrated that there was little or no overlap of dermatomes classified in this way.

Within the physiological method of differentiation, Foerster describes how Sherrington divided the nerve roots above and below a single nerve root to map the area supplied by the intervening intact root in the monkey. There was such overlap of different dermatomes identified by this method that division of a single root produced no loss of sensibility. Foerster himself used the same technique in humans and found the same pattern of overlap in the tactile dermatomes.

Stricker and Bayliss, as described by Foerster, used faradic stimulation of the distal part of a divided posterior root to produce vasodilatation. This produced a clearly defined area similar to the dermatomes defined in the isolation method, but slightly smaller in size.

Despite the experimental findings, the extent of individual dermatomes, especially in the limbs, is largely based on clinical evidence. This leads to an often wide variation between the opinions of different disciplines (Williams *et al.*, 1989). The dermatomes given in this book are drawn mainly from the clinical experience of Cyriax and are different from those given in *Gray's Anatomy* (Williams *et al.*, 1989), for example. In the authors' experience, they provide a sound basic guide for clinical practice and are presented as follows.

Nerve root dermatomes (Conesa and Argote, 1976; Cyriax, 1982; Cyriax and Cyriax, 1983) (Fig. 1.1)

C1:   top of head (Note that since there is no disc to provide nerve root compression at this level, this is a comparatively rare area for pain referral. Also C1 dorsal root fibres are sparse and often absent in humans; Poletti, 1991)
(Fig. 1.1a)

C2:   side and back of the head
upper half of the ear, cheek and upper lip
nape of the neck
(similarly, a rare area for referral, as with C1 since there is no disc at this level)
(Fig. 1.1b)

C3:   entire neck
lower mandible, chin, lower half of the ear
(Fig. 1.1c)

C4:   epaulette area of the shoulder
(Fig. 1.1d)

C5:   anterolateral aspect of the arm and forearm as far as the base of the thumb
(Fig. 1.1e)

C6:   anterolateral aspect of the arm and forearm
thenar eminence
thumb and index finger
(Fig. 1.1f)

C7:   posterior aspect of the arm and forearm
index, middle and ring fingers
(Fig. 1.1g)

C8:   medial aspect of the forearm
medial half of the hand
middle, ring and little fingers
(Fig. 1.1h)

T1:   medial aspect of the forearm
upper boundary uncertain
(Fig. 1.1i)

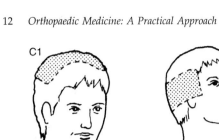

(a)

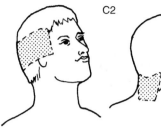

(b)

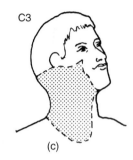

(c)

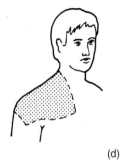

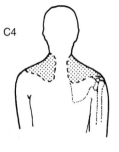

(d)

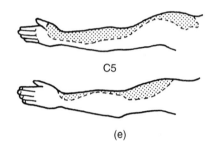

(e)

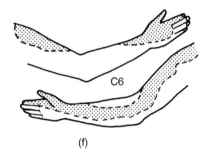

(f)

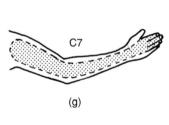

(g)

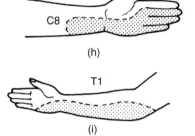

(h)

(i)

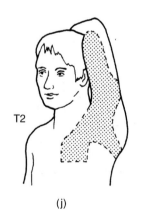

(j)

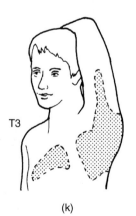

(k)

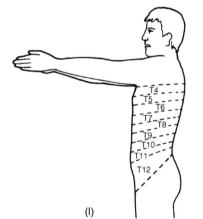

(l)

Fig. 1.1 Dermatomes.

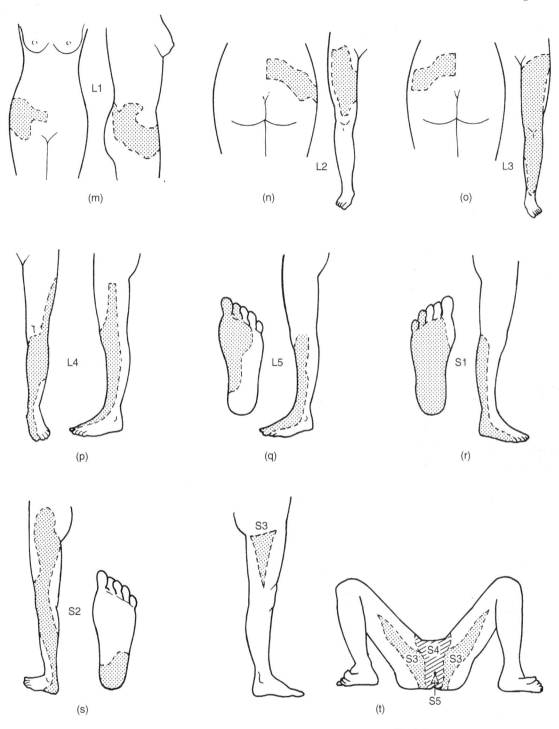

Fig. 1.1

T2:   Y-shaped
        medial condyle of humerus to axilla
        branch to sternum and branch to scapula
        (Fig. 1.1j)

T3:   area at front of chest
        patch in axilla
        (Fig. 1.1k)

T4,5,6: circling trunk above, at and below the nipple area
        (Fig. 1.1l)

T7,8:   circling trunk at lower costal margin
        (Fig. 1.1l)

T9–11: circling the trunk, reaching the level of the umbilicus
        (Fig. 1.1l)

T12:   margins uncertain, extends into groin
        covers greater trochanter and the iliac crest
        (Fig. 1.1l)

L1:   lower abdomen and groin
        lumber region between levels L2 and L4
        upper, outer aspect of the buttock
        (Fig. 1.1m)

L2:   two separate areas:
        lower lumbar region and upper buttock
        whole of the front of the thigh
        (Fig. 1.1n)

L3:   two separate areas:
        upper buttock
        medial aspect and front of the thigh and leg as far as the
        medial malleolus
        (Fig. 1.1o)

L4:   lateral aspect of the thigh
        front of the leg crossing to the medial aspect of the foot
        big toe only
        (Fig. 1.1p)

L5:   lateral aspect of the leg
        dorsum of the whole foot
        first, second and third toes
        inner half of the sole of the foot
        (Fig. 1.1q)

S1:   sole of the foot
        lateral two toes
        lower half of the posterior aspect of the leg
        (Fig. 1.1r)

S2:   posterior aspect of the whole thigh and leg
        plantar aspect of the heel
        (Fig. 1.1s)

S3: circular area around the anus
medial aspect of the thigh
(Fig. 1.1t)

S4: saddle area
anus, perineum, genitals
medial upper thigh
(Fig. 1.1t)

S5: coccygeal area
(Fig. 1.1t)

In general the muscle groups lie under the dermatome which shares the same nerve supply. However, the dermatome and myotome may not overlie each other and there are some apparent discrepancies to this rule. This can cause confusion in the consideration of referred pain, in that lesions in the relevant muscle may appear to refer pain to an unrelated site. The most commonly encountered discrepancies are as follows:

- Scapular muscles are supplied by C4–7, but underlie thoracic dermatomes.
- Latissimus dorsi is supplied by C6–8, but underlies thoracic and lumbar dermatomes.
- Pectoralis major is supplied by C5–T1 but underlies thoracic dermatomes.
- The heart, a thoracic structure, is supplied by C8–T4 and may refer pain into the arm, axilla and chest.
- The diaphragm is supplied by C3–5 and diaphragmatic irritation may lead to pain being felt in the epaulette region of the shoulder.
- The gluteal muscles are supplied by L5, S1–2 but have the dermatomes of L1–3 and S2 overlying them. As a result, pathology in the lumbar spine may wrongly be attributed to a muscle lesion.

Cyriax (1982) and Cyriax and Cyriax (1983) identified several factors that influence the referral of pain:

- The strength of the stimulus.
- Position in the dermatome.
- Depth of the structure.
- Type or nature of the structure.

Strength of the stimulus

The more acutely inflamed or irritable the lesion, i.e. the greater the stimulus, the further into the dermatome will the symptoms be referred (Inman and Saunders, 1944). For example, an acutely inflamed subdeltoid bursitis will refer its pain to the wrist, the distal extent of the C5 dermatome, and a disc protrusion compressing and causing inflammation of the L4 nerve root may refer pain and associated symptoms to the big toe, at the distal end of the L4 dermatome.

Position in the dermatome

Pain and tenderness tend to refer distally. Therefore a structure placed more proximally in the dermatome will be capable of referring its symptoms over a greater distance to the end of the dermatome.

The length or distance of dermatomal referral is particularly obvious in the limbs, where the dermatomes tend to be long. However, if the dermatome is short, even with an acutely inflamed or irritable lesion, the reference will halt at the end of its dermatome, or most distal dermatome in the event of more than one nerve supply.

Structures within the hand and forefoot are already at the distal end of their relevant dermatome. Referral of symptoms is therefore less and such lesions are easier to localize (Inman and Saunders, 1944).

Depth of the structure

Cyriax (1982) proposed that lesions in the more deeply placed structures tended to give greater reference of pain, which was also the finding of Kellgren (1939), and Inman and Saunders (1944). The deeper structures therefore give rise to greater misunderstanding in terms of clinical diagnosis.

Joint, ligament and bursa lesions tend to conform to this assumption but a notable exception is provided by lesions within bone. Pain and tenderness arising from fractures and tumours tend to be well-localized, even though bone itself is the most deeply placed tissue in musculoskeletal terms.

Segmental pain arising from lesions in the deeply sited viscera can also be misleading.

Nature of the tissue

The factor of depth of the structure should perhaps be considered alongside that of the nature of the tissue, since studies to observe the effect of lesions in tissues of different nature and site on patterns of referred pain are hard to dissociate.

Kellgren (1938, 1939) observed patterns of referred pain induced by the injection of 6% hypertonic saline into deeply placed structures including muscle, tendon sheaths, fascia, periosteum and interspinous ligaments. On injection of muscle, diffuse referred pain was produced, which appeared to follow a segmental pattern and was associated with deep tenderness rather than hyperaesthetic skin. It was also observed that pain arising from the limb muscles tended to refer to the region of the joints moved by these muscles, where it could easily be confused as arising from the joint itself.

Tendon sheath and fascia gave sharply localized pain. Stimuli did not produce pain from articular cartilage or compact bone but when applied to cancellous bone a deep diffuse pain was produced, which would appear to contradict the clinical finding mentioned in the previous section. Stimulation of the interspinous ligaments gave rise to segmentally referred pain which, as in muscle, was associated with tenderness in the deeply placed structures.

Inman and Saunders (1944) noted a variability of sensitivity to the different structures beneath the skin, creating a 'league table' of those tissues with the highest sensitivity to the least, as follows: bone, ligaments, fibrous capsules of joints, tendons, fascia and muscle. These findings were supported in part by Kuslich *et al.* (1991), who investigated tissues in the lumbar spine as potential sources of low back pain, using progressive local anaesthetic during operative exploration of the spine. Their emphasis too was that muscles, fascia and the periosteum and compact layer of bone (they did not test cancellous bone) were relatively insensitive.

It had been particularly noted by Inman and Saunders (1944) that capsules and ligaments were most sensitive close to their bony attachments, and therefore most likely to be pain-producing on trauma to these commonly injured sites.

Controversy has existed for many years as to whether the disc or the zygapophyseal joint is the primary source of back pain, especially where associated with pain in the limb. Aprill *et al.* (1989) studied the reference of pain from the cervical zygapophyseal joints to establish whether each joint had a specific area of reference of pain in segmental distribution. They found reasonably distinct and consistent segmental patterns of pain referral associated with joints between each of the levels of C2–7, but there was no referral of pain into the arm from any of the tested levels. The paper acknowledged that the study had not set out to distinguish the pain arising from zygapophyseal joints from other potential sources.

Two pain syndromes of somatic and radicular origin have been described (Bogduk, 1994). In *somatic pain syndromes*, it was proposed that the source of the pain could be in any structure in the spine that receives a nerve supply, i.e. muscles, ligaments, zygapophyseal joints, intervertebral discs, dura mater and dural nerve root sleeve. Somatic pain was not associated with neurological abnormalities and did not involve nerve root compression. The quality of somatic pain was described as dull, diffuse and difficult to localize.

The source of pain in *radicular pain syndromes* was proposed to be compression, but how compression causes pain remains unresolved (see Chapter 13). Experimental compression of dorsal root ganglia or previously damaged nerve root has been shown to cause pain. The clinical experiments of Smyth and Wright show this neuralgic pain to be produced in a particular form, i.e. lancinating and shooting in quality and referred in relatively narrow bands (Bogduk and Twomey, 1991). However, a lesion cannot selectively compress nociceptive axons, therefore for compression to be the source of radicular pain, other neurological abnormalities should be present, e.g. paraesthesia, numbness, muscle weakness and loss of reflexes (Bogduk and Twomey, 1991).

Kellgren (1939), in charting the distribution of pain, demonstrated that injection of the interspinous ligaments of L2–S2 produced pain in the leg. However, Kuslich *et al.* (1991) found that sciatica could only be produced by stretching or direct pressure on an already inflamed nerve root.

In the same study, the zygapophyseal joint capsule was found to be tender in some instances but the pain was never referred to the leg. The zygapophyseal joint's main significance in the production of low back pain was its ability to compress or irritate other local sensitive tissues, particularly with osteophyte formation, including the annulus fibrosus. The annulus fibrosus was demonstrated to be the tissue of origin in most cases of low back pain without pain or symptom referral into the limb. It should be noted that the sacroiliac joint was not included in either study to be able to establish its ability to produce leg pain.

Bogduk (1994) proposed that somatic and radicular pain syndromes can coexist. For example, the annulus fibrosus of the disc may be a source of somatic low back pain, but may also cause secondary compression by a posterolateral displacement causing compression of the nerve root leading to radicular pain.

Other common features of segmentally referred pain were also noted, which Cyriax claimed to be 'rules' of referred pain (Cyriax, 1982; Cyriax and Cyriax, 1983). As with all pronounced rules, exceptions may be noted but, none the less they act as a general guideline in assessing pain behaviour and locating the causative lesion.

A notable exception to the rules of referred pain is provided by the dura mater which, as a centrally placed structure, produces so-called *'extrasegmental reference'* on compression or irritation.

Extrasegmental reference of pain

Throughout his writing Cyriax refers to the phenomenon of *extrasegmental* reference of pain (Cyriax, 1982; Cyriax and Cyriax, 1983). He uses the term to explain the observation that symptoms arising from the dura mater do not obey the rules of referred pain, in terms of referring segmentally, but rather that a pattern of reference is produced which is 'outside' or 'extra' to that of segmental. With another interpretation, the terminology falls short of being ideal since it implies that the pain is not experienced within the segment in which the causative lesion is housed. This is not so and *multisegmental* would perhaps be a more correct term. For consistency amongst orthopaedic medicine texts, the term extrasegmental will be retained here.

The ventral aspect of the dura mater is innervated by the sinuvertebral nerve which sends branches to segments above and below its level of origin (Bogduk and Twomey, 1991). This could account for the extrasegmental reference of pain arising from central compression of the dura mater.

Extrasegmentally referred pain is felt diffusely across several segments usually as a dull background ache, often associated with tenderness or trigger spots (Fig. 1.2). Other unilateral symptoms might be superimposed upon it, as in posterolateral disc protrusions involving pressure on both the dura and the dural nerve root sleeve.

Rules of referred pain

- It does not cross the midline when referred from a unilateral structure.
- It refers distally.
- It refers segmentally.
- It occupies part or all of its dermatome.

The authors suggest that extrasegmentally referred pain may arise from lesions in any structure innervated by the sinuvertebral nerve, including the outer annulus fibrosus, but no evidence can be offered for this hypothesis at the time of writing.

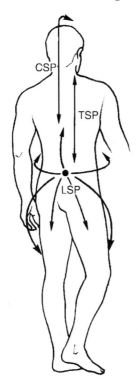

Fig. 1.2 Extrasegmental pain. CSP = cervical spine pain; TSP = thoracic spine pain; LSP = lumbar spine pain.

Mention of the effect of compression of the dura mater leads into the general observation that lesions associated with compression of neural tissue produce varying patterns and nature of symptoms, according to the tissue involved. These will be listed as follows, beginning with the dura mater itself:

Dura mater
- Produces extrasegmental reference of pain and tenderness (Fig. 1.2).

Spinal cord
- Produces no pain but extrasegmental reference of paraesthesia, i.e. in both feet, or all extremities if associated with cervical lesions.
- May produce upper motor neuron lesion with spastic muscle weakness.
- May produce a spastic gait.
- May produce an extensor plantar response.

Dural nerve root sleeve
- Pain produced on compression of the tissue, i.e. the pressure or compression phenomenon (Cyriax, 1982).
- Produces segmental reference of pain in all or part of the dermatome.
- Difficult to ascribe an aspect to the pain, e.g. anterior or lateral.
- Difficult to define an edge to the pain.

Nerve root
- Neurological signs and symptoms produced on compression:
  - Segmental reference of paraesthesia felt at the distal end of the dermatome.
  - Lower motor neuron lesion with flaccid muscle weakness.
  - Absent or reduced reflexes.
- May become pain-sensitive.

Nerve trunk
- Symptoms produced on release of pressure, i.e. the 'release phenomenon' (Cyriax, 1982), e.g. after sitting on a hard gate, placing pressure on the sciatic nerve trunk for a period of time, a shower of 'painful pins and needles' will be experienced in the leg until the nerve recovers.
- Produces sensation of deep painful paraesthesia in the cutaneous distribution of the nerve trunk.
- Some aspect, no edge to the symptoms.
- The longer the compression, the greater the length of time before the onset of pins and needles, e.g. the thoracic outlet syndrome produces diffuse pins and needles in all of the five digits of one or both hands, after going to bed at night, several hours after the compression has been released from the brachial plexus.

Peripheral nerve
- Compression produces paraesthesia and numbness.
- There is a clear edge and aspect to the symptoms, e.g. carpal tunnel syndrome producing paraesthesia and/or numbness in the cutaneous distribution of the lateral three and a half digits on the palmar aspect of the hand, or meralgia paraesthetica involving compression of the lateral cutaneous nerve of the thigh which is associated with a clearly demarcated area of paraesthesia and/or numbness in the anterolateral aspect of the thigh.

Psychogenic pain

Whenever pain itself is the central focus for information towards clinical diagnosis, consideration needs to be given to both its sensory and affective aspects. The discussion within this section, so far, on the characteristics of referred pain has been based on the sensory component of pain, addressing the mechanism and factors of referred pain, particularly relating to its dermatomal distribution.

Consideration has been given to the concept of *central* pain, arising from changes within the central nervous system (Butler, 1995; Mendelson, 1995). However, notwithstanding the contribution of central pain to the chronic state, attention needs to be given to the affective aspects of pain, as an emotional experience rather than as a pure sensation (Butler, 1995). The so-called psychogenic factors can have varying effects on the patient's perception of pain as well as distorting the account given to the clinician.

In addressing this issue in orthopaedic medicine, the term *psychogenic pain* has traditionally been used. The term has survived the controversy on whether or not it exists and, according to the literature review of Mendelson (1995), the work of Engel, Walters and Merskey has led to a general acceptance that pain can be amplified or evoked by psychological factors. Several studies provide evidence that certain personality traits and experiences of individuals have predisposed them to the persisting cycle of chronic pain.

Identification of a significant psychological influence will allow for modification in the treatment approach adopted and certainly may provide a contraindication for some of the techniques used in orthopaedic medicine, most notably the manipulative treatments used for spinal pain.

Cyriax (1982) presented characteristics which, if recognized in patients, give an indication that affective influences are a predominant feature of the complaint and should be taken into account in arriving at a diagnosis, as well as in subsequent treatment selection or appropriate referral.

He suggested that any or all of the following features might be present:

- No recognizable pattern of symptoms or signs in the subjective or objective examination.
- Poor cooperation in both sections of the examination.
- Overenthusiastic assistance from the patient, often accompanied by an element of 'triumph' if the clinical diagnosis remains obscure.
- Patients may seek the answer expected of them.
- Mutually contradictory signs through an incomplete knowledge of the condition.

Juddering is a response occasionally noted on resisted testing but there is no evidence for any neurological condition which allows muscles to work in spasms of effort to produce such a juddering pattern. This is not the cogwheel resistance to movement encountered in Parkinsonism. Severe pain usually produces an 'all-or-nothing' effort where resistance is lost completely as a result of pain, e.g. in resisted wrist extension as a test for tennis elbow where the wrist 'breaks' due to the sharp pain elicited.

Active movements are cited later in this chapter as a useful means of establishing the patient's willingness to perform the movement. This can relate to the psychogenic influence as well as allowing consideration of any unwillingness caused by actual pain, or fear of producing it.

Waddell (1992) listed similar indicators towards the recognition of psychogenic pain. However, he emphasized the need for careful assessment, warning that a 'galaxy of signs does not exclude a remediable condition'. On orthopaedic medicine courses, students are cautioned against the misinterpretation of unusual signs and symptoms by the statement: 'beware of the bizarre but consistent patient', whose behaviour could be indicative of underlying serious pathology.

Several effective approaches have been devised in the treatment of chronic pain, often based on the concept of increasing activity and fitness levels and promoting the maxim that 'hurt does not equate to harm'. Skilled counselling may also be required. This book has set out to acknowledge the possible influence of psychogenic pain but does not intend to expand further on its management.

Onset and duration

The mode of onset of the lesion can provide indicators which lead to a clinical diagnosis and can also contribute to the treatment selection and overall prognosis of the condition. Was the onset sudden or gradual? Meniscal tears and muscle belly lesions come on suddenly whereas overuse tendon and bursa problems and nuclear disc lesions have a gradual onset. Fractures usually have a sudden onset associated with trauma but systemic conditions or serious pathology such as tumours have an insidious onset. None of these latter conditions is suitable for treatment within the specialism of orthopaedic medicine.

In the lumbar spine the mode of onset leads towards a particular hypothesis with regard to pathology, which then provides a guideline for treatment selection. For example, a gradual onset may signify a slow-oozing, nuclear type of protrusion which may respond more effectively to treatment with traction, whilst a sudden onset may indicate a cartilaginous or annular protrusion requiring manipulative treatment, in the absence of any contraindications.

The duration of the symptoms is important as an indicator of the acute or chronic stage in healing which in itself gives guidance for the treatment approach to be adopted, as well as indicating the likely effectiveness and progress of treatment applied. For example, the acutely sprained ligament will require a gentle approach to treatment aiming to reduce swelling, promote healing and to prevent adverse scar tissue formation. In contrast, the chronic ligamentous lesion will require a more aggressive approach to treatment aiming to restore function by breaking down any adverse adhesion formation with stretching and manipulative techniques as appropriate. A lumbar disc lesion of gradual onset and thus of the nuclear type is less likely to respond to traction if it has been present for 3 months rather than for 1 month.

Symptoms and behaviour

The way the pain behaves will assist diagnosis. Mechanical joint lesions are usually better for rest and worse on activity. Also, changing posture can alter the pain. Ligamentous lesions like movement and are usually worse after a period of resting.

Serious pathology may present with unrelenting pain and night pain is likely to be a feature. Generally speaking, benign musculoskeletal lesions do not present with constant, unremitting pain, and there is usually some position of rest which eases pain, or some periods when the pain is easier or even absent.

There will be special questions at each joint which are relevant to the patient's symptoms. For example, how do stairs affect knee pain? How does a cough or sneeze affect back pain? Does the patient with neck pain experience any dizziness? Pertinent questions asked at each joint region will aid diagnosis and, importantly, will also rule out any contraindications to treatment.

The clinician will also wish to investigate if there have been any previous episodes of similar complaints. Spinal pain may be a progression of the same condition and a lumbar disc lesion may characteristically present as increasing episodes of worsening pain.

Past medical history

Asking about the existence of serious illness, operations or accidents gives insight into the patient's past medical record. Past trauma or serious illness may be relevant to current diagnosis, e.g. old fracture of the tibia leading to degenerative changes in the ankle joint, or mastectomy for carcinoma followed by the formation of bony secondaries in the spine.

Other joint involvement

This particularly gives clues to the patient's pain being associated with systemic joint disease. It will alert the examiner to the presence of inflammatory arthritis such as rheumatoid arthritis and ankylosing spondylitis or degenerative osteoarthrosis, all of which have a distinctive pattern of onset and joints affected. Inflammatory joint disease provides a contraindication to manipulative treatment.

Medications

These give a clue to past or underlying disease, e.g. chemotherapy drugs following breast cancer or long-term steroids for inflammatory joint disease. Anticoagulants are in themselves a contraindication for manipulation since manipulation may cause disruption of capillaries and the prolonged bleeding time induced by anticoagulant therapy may lead to haematoma formation. Steroids and chemotherapeutic drugs are not so much a contraindication in themselves but consideration needs to be given to the underlying pathology which necessitates their prescription.

The quantity and regularity of the dose of analgesic and anti-inflammatory drugs provide an indication of the level of pain being experienced by the patient and can be used to monitor the progress of treatment in terms of any change in their requirement.

Inspection

Having completed the history, the patient is inspected, suitably undressed and in a good light, paying particular attention to any *bony deformity, colour changes, muscle wasting* or *swelling*.

Inspection

- Bony deformity
- Colour changes
- Muscle wasting
- Swelling

Bony deformity

This may include spinal asymmetry, leg length discrepancy, excessive valgus or varus deformity at joints, bony lumps or exostoses. Obvious distortion of bony or joint contours following trauma could indicate fracture or dislocation.

Colour changes

Redness may indicate the presence of acute inflammation of the joint being examined as one of the four cardinal signs of inflammation – redness, heat, swelling and pain. There may be signs of bruising following trauma or pallor or reddening associated with circulatory or sympathetic involvement. The presence of scars and rashes may also be indicative of relevant pathology.

Muscle wasting

Any obvious muscle wasting is noted which may have origin in a neurological condition, usually from nerve root compression at the relevant spinal level, as a result of reflex muscle inhibition associated with joint effusion (de Andrade *et al.*, 1965), or as a consequence of disuse.

Swelling

Swelling is indicative of the presence of inflammation resulting from trauma or overuse, as in tenosynovitis and bursitis or arthritis. Other swellings may include ganglia, lipomata and soft-tissue nodules.

Palpation

At this stage of the objective examination, peripheral joints are palpated for signs of inflammatory activity in the form of *heat*, *swelling* and *synovial thickening*. The area is not palpated for tenderness at this stage and this must wait until the end of the examination when the structure at fault has been identified through the rest of the examination procedure.

Palpate a peripheral joint

- Heat
- Swelling
- Synovial thickening

Heat

The joint is palpated for heat using the back of the hand and comparing the same aspect on each side. The same hand is used throughout since the dominant hand may be a few degrees warmer than the non-dominant. Any bandaging or support that the patient has been wearing which could have warmed the area should be taken into account.

Swelling

Swelling is often apparent on inspection alone but may be palpated for, particularly to detect minor swelling, in the knee, for example.

Synovial thickening

Synovial thickening has a 'boggy' feel to it and indicates the presence and level of inflammation in a joint. It is particularly evident in rheumatoid arthritis at the wrist, ankle and knee.

State at rest

The state at rest must be established before any examination requiring joint movement or muscle activity takes place, in order to provide a baseline against which to note the effect of any such movements. Comparison can then be made with subsequent movements which may make the symptoms better or worse.

An open question, such as 'How do you feel as you are standing/sitting there?' usually elicits the status quo and avoids the leading use of the word *pain*.

Based on the observation that normal tissue functions painlessly whereas abnormal tissue does not, Cyriax devised a method of applying appropriate stress to the structures surrounding each joint in order to test their function. Passive movements were employed to test the so-called inert structures such as joint capsules and ligaments, whereas resisted tests were used to test the contractile structures incorporating muscle, tendon and attachments to bone. This then was the method of applying selective tension to tissues

(Cyriax, 1982; Cyriax and Cyriax, 1983) and the movements he propounded will now be described.

Examination by selective tension

Active movements

Active movements
• **Range**
• **Pain**
• **Power**
• **Willingness**

Active movements give an idea of the *range* of movement available in the joint, the *pain* experienced by the patient and the *power* in the muscle groups. They are not carried out routinely at all joints, since they are non-selective and employ both inert and contractile tissues.

They are useful in establishing the *willingness* of the patient to perform the movements as an indicator of the level of pain being experienced within each range. In this role they can act as a guide to the range of movement available before applying passive stresses to the joint.

Active movements can also be used to eliminate neighbouring joints as a potential source of pain. For example, as part of the shoulder examination, six active neck movements are performed. If the patient's pain is not elicited then the cervical spine is eliminated from the enquiry at that initial stage.

They are also most important in illustrating how willing the patient is to move, with respect to the patient's pain tolerance and particularly noting any unusual or bizarre responses. The appropriateness of the patient's response can be significant in the subsequent selection of treatment techniques. This is helpful when assessing the so-called emotional joints, which are prone to psychogenic influence and include all spinal areas, the shoulders and, to a lesser extent, the hips.

A particular sign known as the painful arc is demonstrated by the active movements. By definition a painful arc is an arc of pain with painfree movement on either side. It implies that a structure is being pinched or compressed at that point of the movement and is a useful finding towards diagnosis. For example, a painful arc may be found on active abduction at the shoulder if a lesion lies in the subdeltoid bursa, supraspinatus, infraspinatus or subscapularis teno-osseous attachments, where it may be pinched as it passes under the corocoacromial arch before passing beyond and beneath it, out of harm's way. The painful arc is not usually found in isolation and positive findings on other tests will further incriminate the causative structure.

Passive movements

Passive movements
• **Pain**
• **Range**
• **End-feel**

Passive movements test the *inert structures* which include the joint capsule, joint menisci, ligaments, fascia, bursae, dura mater and the dural nerve root sleeve. Relaxed muscle and tendon can act as inert structures when they are stretched by their opposite passive movement. Passive movements principally give information on *pain, range and end-feel*.

The observation of pain and range of movement will be familiar to all clinicians working with soft-tissue lesions. However, the notion of end-feel may be a new concept which is particularly valuable in the assessment of the soft tissues and is inherent in the orthopaedic medicine approach.

End-feel is the specific sensation imparted through the examiner's hands at the extreme of passive movement (Cyriax, 1982; Cyriax and Cyriax, 1983).

Normal end-feel

Normal end-feel is divided into three categories – hard, soft and elastic. Normal bone-to-bone approximation, as in extension of the elbow, gives a characteristic *hard end-feel* to passive movement. A *soft end-feel* is characteristic of a stop to the movement brought about by approximation of tissue, as in passive knee or elbow flexion. An *elastic end-feel* is felt when the tissues are placed on a passive stretch and is the elastic resistance produced in the inert tissues at the end of range in normal joints. Examples are provided in stretching the end of range of lateral rotation at the shoulder or hip.

Normal end-feel
● Hard
● Soft
● Elastic

There may be a range of end-feels within the 'elastic' group, but all are indicative of normal tissue tension, such as the 'leathery' end-feel of passive pronation and supination of the forearm, or the even tighter 'rubbery' end-feel of plantarflexion and wrist flexion where the resistance to the movement is in part provided by the tendons spanning the joint.

Pain is also a component at the end of range of normal movements, acting as a protection in preventing continuation of movement to the point of producing tissue damage.

Abnormal end-feel

The sensation imparted in the abnormal end-feel falls into four categories – hard, springy, spasm and empty.

The cause of the *abnormal 'hard' end-feel* is different from that of the hard bone-to-bone end-feel and it is a particular feature of the movements limited in arthritis.

Abnormal end-feel
● Hard
● Springy
● Spasm
● Empty

In early arthritis, joint movement is initially limited by pain and involuntary muscle spasm halts the movement. This involuntary muscle spasm provides a brake to the movement and feels 'hard' to the examiner. Certainly the end-feel feels harder than expected, but in the early stages some elasticity is preserved. Early arthritis of the hip, for example, may produce a 'hard' end-feel on either passive flexion or medial rotation but it should be emphasized that this is not caused by bony degenerative change blocking the joint movement. This difference is important as it aids the clinician in the selection of treatment techniques.

In more advanced arthritis, the 'hard' end-feel is also due to capsular contracture. The capsular resistance together with the involuntary muscle spasm may still allow some give at the end of range, but it will not feel as elastic as the earlier stage. In late arthritis, bony changes may occur, leading to a genuine hard end-feel and crepitus associated with advanced arthritis, as well as that arising from involuntary muscle spasm and capsular contracture.

An abnormal *springy end-feel* is associated with mechanical joint displacement, usually a loose body. The sensation imparted to the examiner is one of not quite getting to the end of range, with the joint springing or bouncing back. It is similar to the sensation of trying to close a door with a small piece of rubber caught in the hinge which causes the door to spring back.

The abnormal end-feel associated with *involuntary muscle spasm* is different from that produced by *voluntary muscle spasm*. Voluntary muscle spasm comes in abruptly to halt the movement and indicates acute pain or serious pathology. If the pain is very severe it may also be associated with an empty end-feel.

An *empty end-feel* occurs where the examiner does not have the opportunity to appreciate the true end-feel because the patient calls a halt to the movement prematurely and urgently because of pain, often raising a hand to prevent further movement. The sensation imparted to the examiner is empty, as described, in that the complaint of serious pain comes on before any spasm or tissue resistance.

The empty end-feel is associated with serious pathology such as fracture, neoplasm or septic arthritis. A further cause may be the presence of acute subdeltoid bursitis where the empty end-feel is instantly apparent on passive abduction of the shoulder.

The assessment of end-feel together with the restriction of movement at each joint produces a particular pattern which is either capsular or non-capsular.

The capsular pattern

The capsular pattern is a limitation of movement in a specific pattern which is peculiar to each joint and indicates the presence of an arthritis.

The pattern varies from joint to joint and is characterized by limitation of movement in a fixed proportion. It is the same whatever the cause of the arthritis (Cyriax, 1982; Cyriax and Cyriax, 1983) and the history will suggest the form of arthritis, be it degenerative, inflammatory or traumatic (Table 1.1).

Capsular pattern

- Indicates arthritis
- Varies from joint to joint
- Is limitation of movement in a fixed proportion

Table 1.1 Capsular pattern

Joint	*Capsular pattern*
The movements which become limited in the capsular pattern take on a characteristically 'hard' end-feel	
Shoulder joint	Most limitation of lateral rotation Followed by abduction Least limitation of medial rotation
Elbow joint	More limitation of flexion than extension
Radioulnar joints	Pain at end of range of both rotations
Wrist joint	Equal limitation of flexion and extension Eventual fixation in the mid-position
Trapezio-first metacarpal joint	Most limitation of extension
Metacarpophalangeal joints	Limitation of radial deviation and extension Joints fix in flexion and drift into ulnar deviation
Interphalangeal joints	Equal limitation of flexion and extension
Cervical spine	*Demonstrated by the cervical spine as a whole:* Equal limitation of side flexions Equal limitation of rotations Some limitation of extension Usually full flexion
Thoracic spine	*Demonstrated by the thoracic spine as a whole:* Equal limitation of rotations Equal limitation of side flexions Some limitation of extension Usually full flexion
Hip joint	Most limitation of medial rotation Limitation of flexion and abduction Limitation of extension
Knee joint	More limitation of flexion than extension
Ankle joint	More limitation of plantarflexion than dorsiflexion
Subtalar joint	Increasing limitation of supination Eventual fixation in pronation
Midtarsal joint	Limitation of adduction Limitation of supination Forefoot fixes in abduction and pronation
First metatarsophalangeal joint	Gross limitation of extension Some limitation of flexion
Other metatarsophalangeal joints	*May vary:* More limitation of flexion than extension or joints fix in extension Interphalangeal joints fix in flexion
Lumbar spine	*Demonstrated by the lumbar spine as a whole* Limitation of extension Equal limitation of side flexions Usually full flexion

Characteristically, the movements restricted in the capsular pattern take on the 'hard' end-feel of arthritis, different from the expected normal elastic capsular resistance.

The reason for the development of the capsular pattern could be the presence of joint effusion, causing the joint to assume the position of ease and/or protective muscle spasm (Eyring and Murray, 1964).

An effusion is often present in an arthritis and the acuteness of the condition determines the quantity of the effusion. Joints with symptomatic effusions are held in the position of ease mentioned above and movements out of this position produce pain.

Eyring and Murray (1964) noted a possible relationship between intra-articular pressure and pain. Experiments were conducted to determine the position of minimum pressure in various joints and it was observed that symptomatic joints with effusion spontaneously assume a position of minimum pressure, which coincides with that of minimum pain.

The involuntary muscle spasm, in protecting the painful, inflamed joint, prevents the use of the painful range of movement and if the range of movement is underused it will become limited. In arthritis, the individual joints resent some movements more than others, hence the capsule contracts disproportionately, making some movements more limited than others and giving rise to the characteristic pattern of limitation. For example, the position of minimum pressure for the elbow was found to be between 30° and 70° of flexion. The pressure was not influenced by either pronation or supination. The capsular pattern of the elbow joint is proportionally more limitation of flexion than extension but without involvement of pronation or supination, which conforms to the experimental findings.

Non-capsular pattern

The non-capsular pattern of a joint is, quite simply, anything other than the capsular pattern. That is, it is a limitation of movement that does not conform to the capsular pattern.

An intra-articular displacement produces the non-capsular pattern which may be evident at the spinal joints with a displacement of discal material, in a loose body at the elbow joint or a meniscal tear at the knee leading to limitation of one movement rather than both.

A ligamentous lesion will give pain and possible limitation of the movement which stretches the structure. However, sprains of ligaments which form part of the capsule itself, such as the anterior talofibular ligament of the ankle and the medial collateral ligament of the knee, cause a secondary capsulitis.

Since a contractile unit can be stretched by passive movement, the unit may respond as an inert structure when relaxed, producing pain when it is stretched by the passive movement in opposition to its functional movement. For example, the subscapularis muscle and tendon, which produces medial rotation at the shoulder, will be stretched by passive lateral rotation. This is also particularly evident in acute tenosynovitis when the involved tendon is pulled through its inflamed synovial sheath. In de Quervain's tenosynovitis

---

Non-capsular pattern

- **Intra-articular displacement**
- **Ligamentous lesion**
- **Extra-articular lesion**

at the thumb, for example, pain will be produced on passive adduction and flexion of the thumb, as the tendons of abductor pollicis longus and extensor pollicis brevis are pulled through their shared inflamed sheath, as well as on the appropriate resisted tests.

An extra-articular lesion also produces a non-capsular pattern, e.g. bursitis.

Resisted tests

Resisted tests assess the *contractile unit* comprising the muscle, musculotendinous junction, tendon and the teno-osseous attachment to bone for *pain* and *power*. The tendon is not strictly a contractile structure but is tested as part of the functional contractile unit. When assessing the resisted tests it is important to look for reproduction of the patient's presenting pain and there are specific points to bear in mind which ensure that, as far as possible, only the contractile unit is being tested rather than the inert structures. It is accepted that, although joint movement may not be seen to occur, isometric muscle contraction will cause compression and joint shearing and, in the spinal joints, a rise in intradiscal pressure (Lamb, 1994).

The joint should be placed in the mid-position with the inert structures relaxed so that no stress falls upon them. The muscle group is tested isometrically, as strongly as possible, so encouraging maximal voluntary contraction, but without allowing movement to occur at the joint. This also ensures that minor lesions will be detected. Patient and examiner's body positioning should be such that all muscles not being tested are eliminated from the testing procedure.

Resisted tests may produce any of several findings, each of which has a different implication. The test may be:

- Strong and painless – normal.
- Strong and painful – contractile lesion.
- Weak and painless – neurological weakness.
- Weak and painful – partial rupture, fracture, bone tumour.
- Painful on repetition – claudication or provocation of overuse injury.
- All resisted tests about the joint painful or juddering – serious pathology, psychogenesis.

In addition to the active, passive and resisted tests, a brief neurological examination is included as part of the routine examination for a spinal joint, testing for root signs.

Having completed the subjective and objective examination sequence the causative structure, if not its pathology will, in almost all cases, have been identified (Cyriax, 1982; Cyriax and Cyriax, 1983).

Palpation

At this stage palpation of the structure determined to be at fault may be made to identify the site of the lesion to which appropriate treatment can be applied.

Resisted tests

- Pain
- Power

If the diagnosis is still unclear, further tests may be added either mechanically, for example using techniques of neural tension tests, combined, repeated or accessory movements, or with the use of blood tests, X-rays, electromyograph (EMG) or scanning techniques.

References

Aprill, C., Dwyer, A., Bogduk, N. (1989) Cervical apophyseal joint pain patterns II: a clinical evaluation. *Spine* **15**: 458–461.

Beckman, H.B., Frankel, R.M. (1984) The effect of physician behaviour on the collection of data. *Annals of Internal Medicine,* **101**: 692–696.

Blau, J.N. (1989) Time to let the patient speak. *British Medical Journal* **298**: 39.

Bogduk, N. (1994) Innervation, pain patterns and mechanisms of pain production. In: *Clinics in Physical Therapy, Physical Therapy of the Low Back,* 2nd edn. (Twomey, L.T., ed.). Churchill Livingstone. pp. 93–109.

Bogduk, N., Twomey, L.T. (1991) *Clinical Anatomy of the Lumbar Spine,* 2nd edn. Churchill Livingstone.

Butler, D. (1995) Moving in on pain. In: *Moving in on Pain* (Shacklock, M. ed.). Butterworth-Heinemann, pp. 8–12.

Conesa, S.H., Argote, M.L. (1976) *A Visual Aid to the Examination of Nerve Roots.* Baillière Tindall.

Cyriax, J. (1982) *Textbook of Orthopaedic Medicine,* Vol. 1, 8th edn. Baillière Tindall.

Cyriax, J.H., Cyriax, P.J. (1983) *Illustrated Manual of Orthopaedic Medicine.* Butterworths.

de Andrade, J.R., Grant, C., Dixon, A. St J. (1965) Joint distension and reflex muscle inhibition in the knee. *Journal of Bone and Joint Surgery* **47-A**: 313–322.

Eyring, E.J., Murray, W.R. (1964) The effect of joint position on the pressure of intra-articular effusion. *Journal of Bone and Joint Surgery* **46-A**: 1235–1241.

Foerster, O. (1933) The dermatomes in man. *Brain* **56**: 1–39.

Head, H. (1900) The pathology of herpes zoster and its bearing on sensory localization. *Brain* **16**: 353–523.

Hunter, D., Bomford, R.R. (1963) *Hutchison's Clinical Methods,* 14th edn. Baillière Tindall & Cassell.

Inman, V.T., Saunders, J.B. de C.M. (1944) Referred pain from skeletal structures. *Journal of Nervous and Mental Disease* **99**: 660–667.

Kellgren, J.H. (1938) Observations on referred pain from muscle. *Clinical Science* **3**: 175–190.

Kellgren, J.H. (1939) On the distribution of pain arising from deep somatic structures with charts of segmental pain areas. *Clinical Science* **4**: 35–46.

Kuslich, S.D., Ulstrom, C.L., Michael, C.J. (1991) The tissue origin of low back pain and sciatica. *Orthopaedic Clinics of North America* **22**: 181–187.

Lamb, D.W. (1994) A review of manual therapy for spinal pain. In: *Grieve's Modern Manual Therapy,* 2nd edn. Churchill Livingstone.

McMahon, S.B., Dmitrieva, N., Koltzenburg, M. (1995) Visceral pain. *British Journal of Anaesthesia* **75**: 132–144.

Mendelson, G. (1995) Psychological and psychiatric aspects of pain. In: *Moving in on Pain* (Shacklock, M. ed.). Butterworth-Heinemann, pp. 66–89.

Poletti, C.E. (1991) C2 and C3 pain dermatomes in man. *Cephalalgia* **11**: 155–159.

Waddell, G. (1992) Understanding the patient with back pain. In: *The Lumbar Spine and Back Pain,* 4th edn (Jayson, M. ed.). Churchill Livingstone, pp. 469–485.

Wilkinson, C. (1989) Time to let the patient speak (letter). *British Medical Journal* **298**: 389.

Williams, P.L., Warwick, R., Dyson, M., Bannister, L.H. (1989) *Gray's Anatomy,* 37th edn. Churchill Livingstone.

2 Soft tissues of the musculoskeletal system

Summary

Orthopaedic medicine is concerned with the examination, diagnosis and treatment of soft-tissue lesions. In order to understand the relevant mechanisms of injury and repair and the rationale for treatment of soft-tissue lesions, the soft tissues themselves need to be defined and examined. The principal soft tissues of orthopaedic medicine encompass the connective tissues, muscle tissue and nervous tissue.

Within this chapter, the histology and biomechanics of the soft tissues relevant to orthopaedic medicine will be studied to provide background knowledge for clinical practice.

Connective tissue

The connective tissues form a large class of tissues responsible for providing tensile strength, substance, elasticity and density to the body, as well as facilitating nourishment and defence. Connective

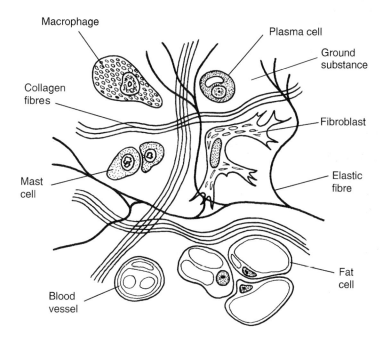

Macrophage

Plasma cell

Ground substance

Collagen fibres

Fibroblast

Mast cell

Elastic fibre

Fat cell

Blood vessel

Fig. 2.1 Irregular connective tissue, cellular and fibre content. Adapted from Cormack (1987) with permission.

tissue has a major role in the repair mechanisms of the body following trauma and a mechanical role to provide connection and leverage for movement, as well as preventing friction, pressure and shock between mobile structures. Connective tissue is the main focus of treatment procedures in orthopaedic medicine.

Connective tissue consists primarily of cells embedded in a matrix of extracellular fibres and amorphous ground substance (Fig. 2.1).

Not all types of connective tissue cell are found in each tissue, and the cell content can alter, with some cells being resident in the tissue and others brought to specific areas at times of need. Generally, the cells make up approximately 20% of the tissue volume and mainly consist of fibroblasts, macrophages and mast cells.

Connective tissue cells

Fibroblasts

Fibroblasts (Latin: *fibra* = fibre; *blastos* = germ), usually the most abundant of the connective tissue cells, are responsible for producing the contents of the matrix, namely fibres and amorphous ground substance. They are found lying close to the bundles of fibres they produce and are closely related to chondroblasts and osteoblasts, the cells responsible for producing cartilage and bone matrix. The less active mature fibroblasts are known as fibrocytes.

Since fibroblasts produce the contents of the matrix, they play a key role in the repair process after injury. Stearns (1940b) observed that, once fibre formation was initiated, the fibroblast was able to produce an extensive network of fibrils in a remarkably short time.

Myofibroblasts are specialized cells which contain contractile filaments producing similar properties to smooth-muscle cells. They assist wound closure after injury.

Macrophages (histiocytes)

Macrophages may be resident in the connective tissues or circulating as monocytes, which migrate to an area of injury and modulate into tissue macrophages (Fowler, 1989). They are large cells that have two important roles. The first is phagocytosis and the second is to act as director cells, in which role they have a considerable influence on scar formation (Hardy, 1989).

As a phagocyte, the macrophage acts as a housekeeper to the wound, ingesting cellular debris and subjecting it to lysosomal hydrolysis, thus debriding the wound in preparation for the fibroblasts to begin the repair process. Matter such as bacteria and cellular debris is engulfed by the phagocyte on contact.

As a director cell, the macrophage chemically activates the number of fibroblasts required for the repair process. Corticosteroids can inhibit the function of the macrophage in the early inflammatory stage, resulting in a delay in fibre production (Dingman and Arbor, 1973; Leibovich and Ross, 1974; Fowler, 1989). This should be taken

Clinical tip
Treatment techniques that agitate tissue fluid increase the chance contact of the macrophage with debris and can be applied during the early stages of inflammation to promote phagocytosis (Evans, 1980), e.g. gentle transverse friction massage and grade A mobilization (see Chapter 4) as well as heat, ice, ultrasound, pulsed electromagnetic energy, etc.

into consideration when exploring treatment options in the early stage.

Mast cells

Mast cells are large, round cells containing secretory granules that manufacture a number of active ingredients including heparin, histamine and possibly serotonin. The contents of the mast cell granules are released in response to mechanical or chemical trauma and they therefore play a role in the early stages of inflammation. Heparin temporarily prevents coagulation of the excess tissue fluid and blood components in the injured area (Wilkerson, 1985) whilst histamine causes a brief vasodilatation in the neighbouring non-injured area (Hardy, 1989). Serotonins are internal nociceptive substances released during platelet aggregation in response to tissue damage. They cause contraction of blood vessels and activate pain signals (Kapit *et al.*, 1987).

Connective tissue matrix

The matrix accounts for about 80% of the total tissue volume, with approximately 30% of its substance being solids and the remaining 70% being water. It consists of fibres and amorphous ground substance, the extracellular substances responsible for supporting and nourishing the cells. The amorphous ground substance also determines the connective tissue's compliance, mobility and integrity.

The fibrous portion of connective tissue is responsible for determining the tissue's biomechanical properties. Two major groups of fibres exist – collagen fibres and elastic fibres.

Collagen fibres

Collagen is a protein in the form of fibre and is the body's 'glue' (Greek: *kolla* = glue). It provides great tensile strength and movement and forms the major fibrous component of connective tissue structures, i.e. tendons, ligaments, fascia, sheaths, bursae, bone and cartilage.

Individual collagen fibres are normally mobile within the amorphous ground substance, producing discrete shear and gliding movement as well as dealing with compression and tension. Collagen is also the main constituent of scar tissue, in which it demonstrates its great versatility by attempting to mimic the structure it replaces.

Collagen fibres are large in diameter and appear to be white in colour. They do not branch or anastomose. They are flexible but inelastic individually.

The arrangement and weave of individual collagen fibres and collagen fibre bundles give the connective tissue structure elastic qualities. For example, nylon thread is inelastic, but when woven to produce nylon stockings, the weave gives the material elasticity

(Peacock, 1966). Collagen fibre bundles elongate under tension to their physiological length and recoil when tension is released.

The bundles of fibres are laid down parallel to the lines of main mechanical stress, often in a wavy, sinusoidal or undulating configuration. This gives the tissue an element of crimp when not under tension. Crimp provides a buffer so that longitudinal elongation can occur without damage, as well as acting as a shock absorber along the length of the tissue, to control tension (Amiel *et al.*, 1990).

Collagen fibre structures are strong under tensile loading but weak under compressive forces, when they have a tendency to buckle. The orientation of the collagen fibrous structure determines the properties that that structure will have. Crimp patterns are different in ligaments and tendons and even between different ligaments and different tendons, depending on function. For example, tendons have great tensile strength for transmitting loads and resisting pull, whilst the arrangement in articular cartilage provides a cushioning force for weight-bearing.

Production and structure of collagen fibres and collagen cross-linking

Procollagen, the first step in collagen fibre formation, is produced intracellularly by the fibroblast. Amino acids are assembled to form

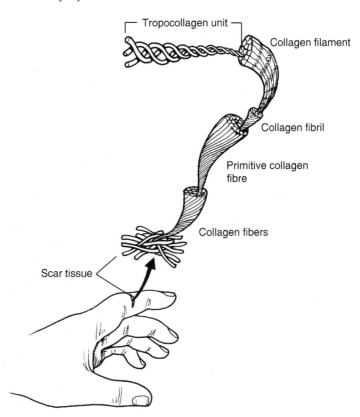

Fig. 2.2   Intramolecular cross-links. From Hardy (1989) with permission.

polypeptide chains, which are attracted and held together by weak intramolecular hydrogen bonds known as cross-links (Fig. 2.2). Three polypeptide chains bond to form a procollagen molecule in the form of a triple helix, which is exocytosed by the fibroblast into the extracellular space.

Once outside the cell the chains are known as tropocollagen molecules and several tropocollagen molecules become bonded by intermolecular cross-links to form a filament or microfibil (Fig. 2.3).

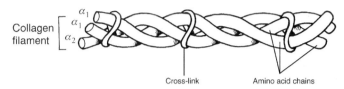

Collagen filament $\begin{bmatrix} \alpha_1 \\ \alpha_1 \\ \alpha_2 \end{bmatrix}$

Cross-link   Amino acid chains

Fig. 2.3 Collagen aggregation. From Hardy (1989) with permission.

With the maturation into tropocollagen, stronger covalent bonds occur at specific nodal intercept points, making the structure more stable (Nimni, 1980; Donatelli and Owens-Burkhart, 1981; Hardy, 1989).

Cross-links exist at every level of organization of the collagen structure (Fig. 2.4). Intermolecular cross-linking in particular gives

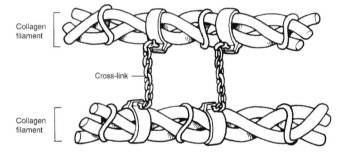

Collagen filament

Cross-link

Collagen filament

Fig. 2.4 Intermolecular cross-links. From Hardy (1989) with permission.

collagen its great tensile strength as it matures. The greater the intermolecular cross-linking the stronger the collagen fibrils, with bone being considered to be the most highly cross-linked tissue (Hardy, 1989).

Immature collagen tissue possesses reducible cross-links and as collagen matures these reducible links stabilize to form stronger non-reducible cross-links. Excessive cross-link formation can be prevented in immature scar tissue by mobilization, whilst established cross-links in scar tissue must be mobilized before longitudinal orientation of the fibres can be encouraged.

Many microfibrils make up a collagen fibril and many collagen fibrils make up a collagen fibre. Collagen fibres continue to aggregate together into larger and larger bundles and the production, aggregation and orientation of collagen are strongly influenced by mechanical tension and stress. Bundles of collagen are arranged in a specific pattern to accommodate to the function of each individual connective tissue structure (Chamberlain, 1982).

It has been shown that when fibroblasts grown in tissue culture are subjected to regional tension, the cells exposed to the tensile

> *Clinical tip*
> Transverse friction massage and mobilization techniques used in orthopaedic medicine aim to affect the reducible and mature scar tissue cross-linking.

forces multiply more rapidly and orient themselves in parallel lines in the direction of the tension (Le Gros Clark, 1965).

Stearns (1940a, 1940b) identified that internal and external mechanical factors influence fibre orientation. Cell movement and occasional cytoplasmic retraction produced early local orientation of fibres, whilst a period of secondary orientation of fibres into heavy parallel layers was probably the result of external mechanical factors. This secondary orientation of fibres appeared to take place during the remodelling phase of wound healing and is the way in which soft-tissue structures develop in response to intermittent stress and mechanical tension.

Collagen takes on many forms and functions. In tendons it is tough and inelastic, in cartilage it is resilient, whilst in bone it is hard. This difference in structure is related to the diameter, orientation and concentration of the fibres. Collagen fibres have been classified into groups (Nimni, 1980). The most common form is type I collagen consisting of large diameter fibres, found abundantly in structures subjected to tensile forces. Type II collagen consists of a mixture of large and narrow diameter fibres and is abundant in structures subjected to pressure or compressive forces. Reticulin is considered to be a delicate supporting network of fragile type III collagen fibres; it may be present in the earliest stages of soft-tissue repair.

Elastic fibres

Elastic fibres, consisting of the protein elastin, are yellow in colour and much thinner and less wavy than collagen fibres. Elastic fibres run singly, never in bundles, and freely branch and anastomose.

Elastic fibres provide the tissue with extensibility so that it can be extended in all directions but, if tension is constantly exerted in one direction, the elastic fibres may be laid down in sheets known as lamellae, e.g. ligamentum flavum (the 'yellow ligament'). Elastic fibres make up some of the connective tissue fibres of ligaments, joint capsules, fascia and connective tissue sheaths.

Amorphous ground substance of connective tissue

The amorphous ground substance (Greek: *amorphous* = without form) with its fibrous content comprises the connective tissue matrix. As well as maintaining the mobility and integrity of the tissue structure at a macrostructural level, it is responsible for nourishing the living cells by facilitating the diffusion of gases, nutrients and waste products between the cells and capillaries.

It contains carbohydrate bound to protein (Williams *et al.*, 1989). The carbohydrate is in the form of polysaccharides, hexuronic acid and amino sugars, alternately linked to form long-chain molecules called glycosaminoglycans (GAGs). The main GAGs in connective tissue matrix are hyaluronic acid, chondroitin-4-sulphate, chondroitin-6-sulphate and dermatan sulphate (Donatelli and Owens-Burkhart, 1981).

When GAGs are covalently bonded to proteins, the molecules are called proteoglycans (Cormack, 1987). These proteoglycan molecules have the property of attracting and retaining water (Bogduk and Twomey, 1991) and this strong water-binding property of the amorphous ground substance allows it to exist as either a viscous semisolution, known as a sol, or a semisolid substance, or gel. Sols act as a filling material between cells and fibres and are found in ligaments and tendons. Gels act as a resilient surface for weight-bearing, as may be found in bone and cartilage.

The concentration of GAGs present in tissues is related to their function and gives connective tissue structures viscous properties. More water is associated with a higher GAG concentration and rabbit ligamentous tissue has a significantly greater water content than that in rabbit tendinous tissue (Amiel *et al.*, 1982). This increase in GAG and water content alters the viscoelastic properties and may provide the ligament with an additional shock-absorbing feature that is unnecessary in most tendons.

The amorphous ground substance forms a lubricant, filler and spacing buffer system between collagen fibres, fibrils, microfibrils and the intercellular spaces (Akeson *et al.*, 1980). It reduces friction and maintains distance between fibres as well as facilitating the discrete shear and gliding movement of individual collagen fibres and fibrils. It is the lubrication and spacing at the fibre–fibre interface that are crucial to the gliding function at nodal intercept points where the fibres cross in the tissue matrices (Amiel *et al.*, 1982).

If the tissues are allowed to adopt a stationary attitude, anomalous cross-links form at the nodal intercept points. This is most important to normal connective tissue mobility where a balance must be maintained in the cross-link formation relative to the tissue's tensile strength and mobility. Excessive cross-linking adheres fibres closer and closer together and, where not desirable, will alter tissue function and cause pain.

The elasticity of connective tissue fibres together with the viscosity of the amorphous ground substance gives connective tissue structures viscoelastic properties that ensure that normal connective tissues are mobile.

The biomechanical properties of connective tissue depend on the number and orientation of collagen fibres and the proportion of amorphous ground substance present. Each connective tissue structure is specifically designed for function but the tissues can be simply grouped into irregular and regular connective tissue.

> *Clinical tip*
> The aim in orthopaedic medicine is to maintain normal connective tissue mobility through the phases of acute inflammation, repair and remodelling, and to regain mobility in the chronic inflammatory situation. This mobility is essential to function and the bias of orthopaedic medicine treatment techniques is towards preserving the mobility of connective tissue structures.

Irregular connective tissue

Irregular connective tissue consists of a mixture of collagen and elastic fibres interwoven to form a loose meshwork that can withstand stress in any direction. Its main function is to support and protect regular connective tissue structures.

The following examples of irregular connective tissue are commonly encountered in orthopaedic medicine.

The *dura mater* is the outermost of three irregular connective tissue sleeves which enclose the brain and the spinal cord. It is extended to form the dural nerve root sleeve that invests the nerve roots within the intervertebral foramen. At or just beyond the intervertebral foramen the dural nerve root sleeve fuses with the epineurium of the nerve root. The dura mater and dural nerve root sleeve extensions are formed of sheets of collagen and elastic fibres providing a tough, but loose fibrous tube. The dura mater is separated from the bony margins of the vertebral canal by the epidural space that contains fat, loose connective tissue and a venous plexus. These structures are mobile in a non-pathological state and can accommodate normal movement (Netter, 1987; Williams *et al.*, 1989; Palastanga *et al.*, 1994). Adhesions may develop in the dura mater and dural nerve root sleeve, compromising this mobility and giving rise to clinical symptoms.

An *aponeurosis* is a sheet of fibrous tissue that increases the tendinous attachment to bone (Greek: *neuron* = nerve or tendon). It distributes the tendon forces, increasing the tendon's mechanical advantage, and needs to retain mobility in its attachment to perform its function.

The *epimysium* is a layer of irregular connective tissue surrounding the whole muscle; the *perimysium* surrounds the fascicles within the muscle and the *endomysium* surrounds each individual muscle fibre. In a similar arrangement, a fibrous sheath, the *epineurium*, surrounds each nerve, the *perineurium* surrounds each fascicle and each individual nerve fibre is invested in a delicate sheath of vascular loose connective tissue, the *endoneurium*. Since connective tissue mobility is important to the function of muscle, its arrangement in nerve structure implies that it is also important to the function of nervous tissue.

The *paratenon* is an irregular connective tissue fibroelastic sheath, adherent to the outer surface of all tendons. It is composed of relatively large amounts of proteoglycans to provide a gliding surface around the tendon, allowing it to move freely amongst other tissues with a minimum of drag (Merrilees and Flint, 1980). The paratenon becomes a true double-layered *synovial sheath* surrounding all tendons subjected to frictional and compressive forces, i.e. under retinacula and at deflections around bones. This synovial sheath is protective but also facilitates the gliding function of tendons that might be impaired by compression or friction. The tendon synovial sheath is an irregular connective tissue envelope lined with synovial cells. It consists of an inner visceral layer which is the paratenon adherent to the tendon, and an outer parietal layer which attaches to the surrounding tissues.

Like the synovial tendon sheaths, *bursal sacs* also prevent friction and pressure and facilitate movement between adjacent connective tissue structures. Bursae can be subcutaneous, e.g. the olecranon bursa, subtendinous, e.g. psoas bursa, sub- or intermuscular, e.g. gluteal bursa or adventitious (i.e. developing in response to trauma or pressure), e.g. subcutaneous Achilles bursa.

Fascia lies in sheets to facilitate movement between the various tissue planes. *Deep fascia* has a more regular formation as it forms a tight sleeve to retain structures, adds to the contours of the limbs and is extended to form the intermuscular septa. It provides a compressive force which facilitates venous return and may act as a mechanical barrier preventing the spread of infection.

Fascia may develop *retinacula* which hold tendons in place, preventing a bowstring effect on movement, e.g. the retinacula at the ankle. It may produce thickenings forming protective layers such as the *palmar and plantar aponeuroses*, or it may form envelopes to enclose and protect major neurovascular bundles, e.g. the femoral sheath in the femoral triangle.

Regular connective tissue

In contrast to irregular connective tissue, this group of tissues has a highly organized structure with fibres running in the same linear direction, in a precise arrangement that is related to function. The main collagen fibre bundles will be aligned parallel to the line of major mechanical stress, which functionally suits such structures as tendons and ligaments that are mainly subjected to unidirectional stress (Donatelli and Owens-Burkhart, 1981).

The following examples of regular connective tissue are commonly encountered in orthopaedic medicine.

Tendons

Muscles and tendons are distinct tissues, although they functionally act as one structure, the contractile unit. The tendon cells are derived from the embryonic mesenchyme, the tissue occupying the areas between the embryonic layers (Williams *et al.*, 1989), classifying tendon as a connective tissue. Muscle cells are derived from mesoderm, the intermediate embryonic layer, such that muscle itself belongs to a separate tissue group.

The tendon is an inert structure which does not contract, but as part of the contractile unit it is directly involved in muscle action. Therefore the tendon is assessed by resisted testing via the muscle belly. Active movement does not produce transverse movement within the tendon but its fibrous structure can be moved passively by transverse friction massage, to prevent or to mobilize adhesions.

Tendons are exposed to strong, unidirectional forces and to function they require great tensile strength and inelastic properties. They are able to withstand much greater tensile forces than ligaments and are composed of closely packed parallel bundles of collagen microfibrils, fibrils and fibres, bound together by irregular connective tissue sheaths into larger bundles (Fig. 2.5). Tendons do not usually contain any elastic fibres since their muscle belly acts as an energy damper such that elastic fibres are not required (Akeson, 1990).

The fibres are large-diameter type I collagen, well-suited to accept tensile forces. The proteoglycan molecules are packed in between the fibres and because the tendon is so compact, there is little room for the tendon cells or an adequate blood supply. The tendon's blood vessels lie in the epitenon (adherent to the surface of the

---

Clinical tip
Tissue injury involves the surrounding and supporting irregular connective tissue as well as the regular connective tissue structure itself. It is therefore important to recognize the extensive nature of irregular connective tissue and its close relationship with the regular connective tissue structures encountered in orthopaedic medicine.

Functions of tendons:

- **To attach a muscle to bone.**
- **To transmit the force of muscle contraction to the bone to produce functional movement.**
- **To set the muscle belly in the optimum position for functional movement and to affect the direction of muscle pull.**
- **To be able to glide within the surrounding tissues, accepting stress and tensile forces with minimal drag.**

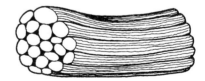

Fig. 2.5 Structure of a tendon. Adapted from Williams *et al.* (1989).

tendon) and the endotenon (a division between collagen fibre bundles) (Gelberman *et al.*, 1983).

All tendons are surrounded by a fibroelastic paratenon to facilitate their gliding properties and stress is borne by the whole tendon. Tendinitis, i.e. inflammation of a tendon, most commonly occurs at the teno-osseous site.

Tenosynovitis occurs in ensheathed tendons and involves the synovium rather than the tendon itself. Inflammation of the synovium can produce adhesions between the two layers of the sheath which may produce a palpable crepitus (Cyriax, 1982). Adhesion formation interferes with the normal function of the tendon sheath, which is to allow controlled movement of the sheath around the tendon and to facilitate nutrition by forcing synovial fluid into the tendon (Barlow and Willoughby, 1992).

Tenovaginitis is a term used to describe thickening of the synovial sheath (Cyriax, 1982) and is associated with chronic tenosynovitis, e.g. de Quervain's stenosing tenosynovitis of the sheath containing the abductor pollicis longus and extensor pollicis brevis tendons.

As with all other connective tissues structures, tendons remodel in response to mechanical demand and they are sensitive and responsive to changes in physical load, a property which may be demonstrated by a difference in structure within one tendon unit. Merrilees and Flint (1980) looked at the macrostructural features of different regions of the flexor digitorum profundus tendon in the rat. This tendon, in common with most tendons, is subjected to longitudinal stress throughout its length, but it also possesses a sesamoid-like area as it passes under the calcaneum and talus. In this area the tendon is subjected to compressive forces, as well as to the normal longitudinal stress.

In the zone subjected to tension, the collagen fibres were arranged in longitudinal bundles, but in the zone subjected to pressure the sesamoid-like area took on a form similar to that of fibrocartilage, i.e. a loose weave of collagen fibres and chondrocyte-like cells arranged in columns perpendicular to the main fibre axis. The proteoglycan content was also different, containing dermatan sulphate as the main GAG in the tensile zone and chondroitin sulphate as the main GAG in the pressure zone.

This illustrates the ability of connective tissue structures to adapt to different functions and to changes in physical loads in a normal situation. In abnormal situations, such as a period of immobility when physical demand is reduced, adaptations in collagen turnover occur. When physical demand is increased, collagen production increases. This turnover (synthesis and lysis) of collagen is a continuing process allowing the remodelling and adaptation of structures to suit demand.

Ligaments and joint capsules

The joint capsule and its supporting ligaments are similar in function, both allowing and restraining movement at the joints. Ligaments can be considered to be a reinforcement of the joint capsule in an

---

Clinical tip

In order to maintain or restore the gliding properties of the tendon within its synovial sheath, transverse friction massage is applied with the tendon on the stretch. This position allows the therapist to roll the sheath over a firm tendon base, imitating the function of the tendon sheath.

Functions of ligaments and joint capsules:

- **Flexibility, requiring elastic properties, to allow normal movement to occur at a joint.**
- **Resilience, requiring tensile strength, to be tough and unyielding to excessive movement at a joint.**

area of special stress. As inert tissue structures they are assessed by passive movements which should be applied at the extremes of range to test function.

The ligaments, together with the fibrous capsule, guide and stabilize the tracking articular surfaces. When excessive stresses are applied to a joint, proprioceptive impulses recruit a muscle response so that the passive stabilizing effect of the ligament is reinforced by dynamic muscle stabilization (Akeson *et al.*, 1987).

To meet its functional requirements the structure of a ligament will be different from that of a tendon. The main ligamentous fibres are 70–80% collagen laid down in bundles, which assume a wavy configuration providing an element of elongation and recoil to facilitate movement (Fig. 2.6). Interwoven with these main fibre bundles are 3–5% elastic fibres, to enhance extensibility and elasticity (Akeson *et al.*, 1987). When ligaments are put under longitudinal tensile stress the parallel wavy bundles of collagen straighten out to prevent excessive movement and to provide tensile strength.

Although the joint capsule is similar in function to ligaments, its structure is slightly different. The capsule consists of sheets of collagen fibres which form a fibrous cuff joining opposing bony surfaces. The fibrous structure is predominantly collagen but, rather than a parallel array of fibres, its pattern is more a criss-cross weave, with the fibres becoming more parallel as the capsule is loaded (Fig. 2.7) (Amiel *et al.*, 1990; Woo *et al.*, 1990). The ability of the fibres to change and straighten depends on them being mobile and able to slide independently of one another. Capsular contractures in the form of disorganized collagen will prevent independent fibre gliding at the nodal intercept points, considerably reducing function and causing pain.

The joint capsule has two layers – an outer fibrous capsule and an internal synovial membrane. The outer fibrous capsule is strong and flexible but relatively inelastic. It is supported functionally by its ligaments which may be intrinsic, forming an integral part of the joint capsule, e.g. coronary and medial collateral ligaments of the knee, or accessory, being either intracapsular, e.g. the cruciate ligaments, or extracapsular, e.g. lateral collateral ligaments of the knee. The fibrous capsule is perforated by vessels and nerves and contains afferent sensory nerve endings, including mechano-receptors and nociceptors.

The synovial membrane is mainly a loose connective tissue membrane with a degree of elasticity to prevent its folds and villi becoming nipped during movement. It covers all surfaces within the joint except the articular surfaces themselves and menisci. Adipose fat pads may exist in the joint, acting as shock absorbers, and distinct fringes of synovium may be present, e.g. the plicae of the knee joint. These folds, fringes and villi allow the joints to accommodate to movement.

The synovium is a highly cellular membrane containing synoviocytes, i.e. the synovium-producing cells, and collagen fibres. It has a rich nerve, blood and lymphatic supply. A capillary network is situated on the inner surface of the synovium to produce synovial fluid. Synovial fluid is pale yellow and viscous. It lubricates the

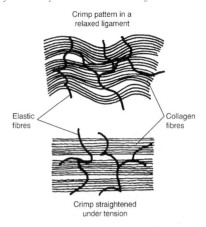

Fig. 2.6 Structure of a ligament. Adapted from Nordin and Frankel (1989).

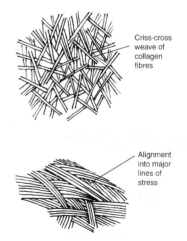

Fig. 2.7 Structure of the joint capsule.

Clinical tip
Trauma can cause a haemarthrosis and the difference between this and a trauma-induced synovial effusion is indicated clinically by the immediate onset of swelling as a result of bleeding into the joint, as opposed to the more slowly developing synovial effusion, sometimes over several hours.

ligamentous structures of the joint and nourishes cartilage and menisci through a mechanism of transsynovial flow aided by movement (Akeson *et al.*, 1987).

In an arthritis or inflammation of a joint, the inflammation causes pain and involuntary muscle spasm which prevents full range of movement. The relative immobility causes changes to occur in the connective tissue which lead to capsular contracture, further loss of function and pain.

Cartilage

Cartilage is a weight-bearing connective tissue displaying a combination of rigidity, which is resistant to compression, resilience and some elasticity. It is relatively avascular and relies on tissue fluid for nourishment. There are three main types of cartilage:

- Elastic cartilage.
- Fibrocartilage.
- Hyaline cartilage.

Elastic cartilage consists of a matrix of yellow elastic fibres and is very resilient. It is found in the external ear, the epiglottis and the larynx.

Fibrocartilage has a large proportion of type I collagen fibres in its matrix, providing it with great tensile strength. Examples are the annulus fibrosus of the intervertebral discs, the menisci of the knee joint, the acetabular and glenoid labra, the articular disc of the acromioclavicular and wrist joints, the lining of the grooves which house tendons, and as a transitional cartilage at the teno-osseous junction of the tendons (Cormack, 1987; Williams *et al.*, 1989; Palastanga *et al.*, 1994). The annulus fibrosus in particular has a unique geometrical pattern of collagen fibres.

Hyaline cartilage is articular cartilage. Its relatively solid gel-like matrix provides a weight-bearing surface which is elastic and resistant to compression. It moulds to the shape of the bones, presenting a smooth articular surface for movement.

Hyaline articular cartilage is composed of scantily deposited chondroblasts and chondrocytes which produce the gel matrix consisting of type II collagen fibres and amorphous ground substance. The matrix contains distinctive large supermolecular proteoglycan aggregates which resemble bottle brushes (Fig. 2.8). These provide a network for trapping and retaining water which significantly contributes to the resilience of cartilage (Cormack, 1987). The collagen fibres themselves are relatively weak under compression, therefore the water-enhanced matrix compensates for this by providing a resilient weight-bearing surface.

Three separate structural zones exist in hyaline cartilage which contribute to its biomechanical functions (Nordin and Frankel, 1989). A superficial zone is approximately 10–20% of the total thickness of the cartilage. It consists of fine, tangential, densely packed fibres

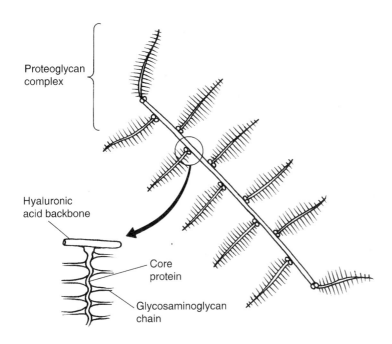

Proteoglycan complex

Hyaluronic acid backbone

Core protein

Glycosaminoglycan chain

Fig. 2.8 Proteoglycan complex of hyaline cartilage. Adapted from Netter (1987).

lying in a plane parallel to the articular surface (Fig. 2.9). A middle, vertical zone is approximately 40–60% of the total thickness with the cells arranged in vertical columns, perpendicular to the surface, with scattered collagen fibres. The deep zone is approximately 30% of the total thickness and forms a transition between the articular cartilage and the underlying calcified cartilage layer. The fibres are arranged in radial bundles.

The zonal arrangement of cartilage provides a 'well-sprung mattress' arrangement to cope with compression forces. The variation in collagen fibre orientation in each zone enables the articular cartilage to vary its material property with direction of the load.

> *Clinical tip*
> Articular cartilage requires movement for nutrition and to maintain fluid levels within its matrix in order to withstand compressive forces. Prolonged loading reduces fluid levels in the matrix through the action of tissue creep, which may lead to degenerative changes. It is essential therefore to maintain mobilization of inflamed or degenerate joints.

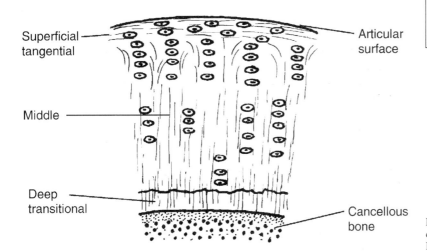

Superficial tangential

Middle

Deep transitional

Articular surface

Cancellous bone

Fig. 2.9 Zonal arrangement of articular cartilage. Adapted from Nordin and Frankel (1989).

The fluid content of articular cartilage is responsible for its nutrition as well as its mechanical properties, allowing diffusion of nutrients and products between the cells and the synovial fluid. When cartilage is loaded, the fluid in the 'sponge' moves, which is important for the mechanical properties of the cartilage as well as for joint lubrication. Intermittent loading creates a pumping effect but prolonged loading will eventually press fluid out of the cartilage without allowing new fluid to be taken up, leading to degeneration.

Muscle

Muscle tissue is a separate tissue group responsible for contraction and functional movement. It consists of cells known as muscle fibres due to their long, narrow shape.

Muscle has a large connective tissue component which supplies its nutrients for its metabolism and facilitates contraction by providing a continuous connective tissue harness (Fig. 2.10). This continuous harness consists of the epimysium, perimysium and endomysium. Each end of the harness is continuous with strong connective tissue structures which anchor it to its attachments.

Skeletal muscle is of obvious concern in orthopaedic medicine and following trauma it is capable of some regenerating properties. However, large muscle belly lesions, due to major trauma, will be filled with a mixture of disorganized scar tissue and new muscle fibres.

> *Clinical tip*
> Connective tissue mobility is important to the normal muscle function. Although skeletal muscles have some regenerating properties, healing of large muscle belly lesions is largely through the formation of scar tissue. Disorganized scar tissue alters function and acts as a physical barrier to regenerating muscle fibres.

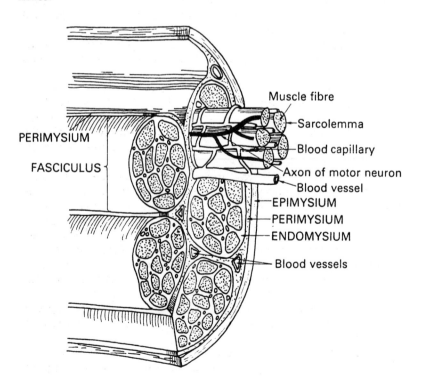

Fig. 2.10 Connective tissue component of skeletal muscle. From Palastanga *et al.* (1994) with permission.

Nervous tissue

Nervous tissue is designed for the conduction of nerve impulses and initiation of function. The central nervous system is largely devoid of connective tissue being made up of specialized tissue held together by neuroglia. Three connective tissue meninges (pia mater, arachnoid mater and dura mater) and the cerebrospinal fluid protect the system inside its bony framework.

The peripheral nervous system is not as delicate, with connective tissue constituting part of the nerves, providing strength and resilience. The epineurium is an outer connective tissue sheath enclosing large nerves. The perineurium surrounds each fascicle or bundle of nerve fibres and the endoneurium invests each individual nerve fibre.

> *Clinical tip*
> Connective tissue mobility is essential to the normal function of the central and peripheral nervous systems. Compression of any part of the system or reduction in connective tissue mobility will compromise function.

Behaviour of connective tissues to mechanical stress

Excessive mechanical stress is responsible for connective tissue injury and manual techniques utilize mechanical stresses to mobilize, permanently elongate or rupture scar tissue, where the adhesions formed are preventing full painless function. Understanding the mechanical response of connective tissue structures to stress is helpful in interpreting mechanisms of injury and rationalizing treatment programmes. However, it should be appreciated that most experimental evidence has been derived from animal and cadaveric specimens in the laboratory setting, and the physical principles have been adapted in order to explain the mechanical properties demonstrated.

The *stress, or load*, is the mechanical force applied to the tissue. The strain is the resultant deformation produced by the applied stress.

The *stress–strain curve* is a way of illustrating the reaction of connective tissue structures to loading (Fig. 2.11). Experimentally, a tensile stress is applied to collagen until it ruptures. The applied stress or elongating force is plotted on the *y* axis and the strain, the extent to which collagen elongates, measured as a percentage of its original length, is plotted along the *x* axis.

Collagen at rest is crimped and, as stress is applied, the fibres straighten and the crimp pattern is lost (Akeson *et al.*, 1987; Bogduk and Twomey, 1991). The straightening out of the fibres is represented by the first part of the curve, known as the *toe region*. Crimp straightens easily and there is little or no resistance to the applied stress. At the end of the toe region some of the elongation may be due to sliding and shear of the collagen fibres in the interfibrillar gel (Nordin and Frankel, 1989). The more regularly oriented the collagen fibres, the shorter the toe region, e.g. a ligament displays a shorter toe region than the more loosely woven joint capsule, but a longer toe region than the more regularly arranged tendon (Threlkeld, 1992).

The second part of the curve is known as the *linear region*. The straightened fibres realign in the linear direction of the applied

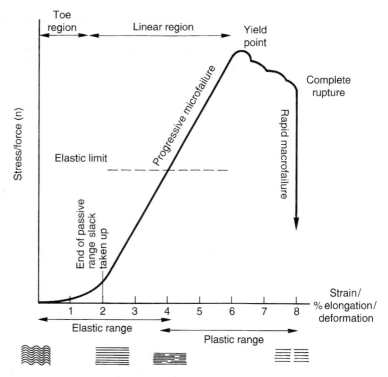

Fig. 2.11 Stress–strain curve. Adapted from Bogduk and Twomey, 1987; Nordin and Frankel, 1989; Keir, 1991; Kisner and Colby in Norris (1993) with permission.

stress and the structure becomes longer and thinner. Water and proteoglycans are displaced and the chemical cross-links between fibres and fibrils are strained, producing a resistance or stiffness in the tissue, so that a progressively greater stress is required to produce equivalent amounts of elongation.

Collagen exhibits *elastic properties* and, if the deforming stress is removed, the structure will return to its original resting length. In the early part of the linear region a point is reached at which slack is taken up in connective tissue and this represents the end of passive range.

In the second half of the linear region, stress causes some of the strained cross-links to break and microfailure begins to occur in a few overstretched fibres. *Microfailure* is said to occur somewhere after 4% of elongation has been achieved (Bogduk and Twomey, 1991), at which point the collagen is said to have reached its *elastic limit*. A traumatic stress applied at this stage produces minor pain and swelling, but no clinical laxity.

Once the elastic limit of collagen has been exceeded, collagen exhibits *plastic properties* and progressive microfailure produces permanent elongation once the deforming stress is removed. A traumatic stress applied within the plastic range produces more pain and swelling, together with some clinical laxity.

A further increase in stress causes major collagen fibre failure and the *yield point* is reached, represented by the peak of the stress–strain curve, where a large number of cross-links are irreversibly broken. The stress–strain curve drops rapidly, indicating *macrofailure* or complete rupture, where the structure is unable to sustain further stress even though it may remain physically intact. Threlkeld (1992), reporting Noyes *et al.*, stated that the estimated macrofailure of connective tissue occurs at approximately 8% of elongation. A traumatic stress that produces complete rupture causes severe pain initially which is followed by less pain and gross clinical laxity.

The stress applied to tissues can be divided into several categories (Bogduk and Twomey, 1991; Norris, 1993):

- *Tensile stress* – a pulling or elongating force applied longitudinally parallel to the long axis of the structure.
- *Compressive stress* – a pushing or squashing force applied perpendicular to the long axis of the structure.
- *Shear stress* – a sliding force applied across the long axis of the structure.
- *Torsional stress* – a twisting force or torque applied in opposite directions about an axis of rotation.

The type of stress applied and the speed of application influence the outcome of the different mobilization techniques. The mechanical behaviour of connective tissue is influenced by other mechanisms which will be applied to the graded mobilizing techniques used in orthopaedic medicine in Chapter 4.

The stiffness of a structure is its resistance to deformation under the applied stress. A stiff structure displays reduced elastic properties and a shorter toe phase. Scar tissue, which forms within a connective tissue structure, is not as elastic as the surrounding normal tissue. Therefore, slack will be taken up sooner and mobilization techniques can be applied to the adherent scar tissue to produce elongation or rupture. Tough scar tissue requires considerable force or stress to deform it and it does not easily resume its original shape. Once the failure point of scar tissue is reached it ruptures relatively quickly (Norris, 1993).

Connective tissue structures have viscoelastic properties which cause them to behave differently under different loading rates. If the structure is loaded quickly it behaves more stiffly than the same tissue loaded at a slower rate (Threlkeld, 1992). This behaviour of the tissue is utilized in tissue mobilization techniques. Adhesions may be ruptured by a quickly applied shear stress, or stretched by a slow sustained tensile stress. Increasing the temperature of a structure allows lower sustained loads to achieve greater elongation (Warren *et al.*, 1971).

Creep is a property of viscoelastic structures which occurs when a prolonged stress is applied in the linear phase. Further deformation occurs through a gradual rearrangement of the collagen fibres, proteoglycan gel and water and/or through straining and perhaps breaking some of the collagen fibre cross-links (Bogduk and Twomey, 1991). When the stress is released, resumption of the original length of the structure occurs at a slower rate than its deformation and this mechanical behaviour is known as hysteresis. The original length may not be achieved and the difference between the two lengths is known as set.

Repeated or cyclical loading may achieve an increment of elongation with each loading cycle. This may lead to eventual failure of the structure through accumulated fatigue. A larger load requires fewer repetitions to produce failure, but a minimum load, the endurance limit, must be applied to achieve this effect (Norris, 1993).

Mobilization to maintain tissue function should remain within the elastic range, whilst mobilization aimed at elongating or rupturing established adhesions occurs at the end of the linear region and within the plastic range of the tissue.

The principles of creep and cyclical loading are applied to facilitate permanent lengthening of the tissues.

References

Akeson, W. (1990) The response of ligaments to stress modulation and overview of the ligament healing response. In: *Knee Ligaments: Structure, Function, Injury and Repair* (Daniel, D. *et al.*, eds). Raven Press, pp. 315–327.

Akeson, W., Amiel, D., Woo, S. L.-Y. (1980) Immobility effects on synovial joints, the pathomechanics of joint contracture. *Biorheology* **17**: 95–110.

Akeson, W., Amiel, D., Abel, M.F. *et al.* (1987) Effects of immobilisation on joints. *Clinical Orthopaedics and Related Research* **219**: 28–37.

Amiel, D., Woo, S.L.-Y., Harwood, L., Akeson, W.H. (1982) The effect of immobilisation on collagen turnover in connective tissue: a biochemical–biomechanical correlation. *Acta Orthopaedica Scandinavica* **53**: 325–332.

Amiel, D., Billings, E., Akeson, W. (1990) Ligament structure, chemistry and physiology. In: *Knee Ligaments: Structure, Function, Injury and Repair* (Daniel, D. *et al.*, eds). Raven Press, pp. 77–90.

Barlow, Y., Willoughby, J. (1992) Pathophysiology of soft tissue repair. *British Medical Bulletin* **48**: 698–711.

Bogduk, N., Twomey, L.T. (1991) *Clinical Anatomy of the Lumbar Spine.* Churchill Livingstone.

Chamberlain, G.J. (1982) Cyriax's friction massage: a review. *Journal of Orthopaedic and Sports Physical Therapy* **4**: 16–22.

Cormack, D.H. (1987) *Ham's Histology*, 9th edn. J.B. Lippincott.

Cyriax, J. (1982) *Textbook of Orthopaedic Medicine*, vol. 1, 8th edn. Baillière Tindall.

Dingman, R.O., Arbor, A. (1973) Factors of clinical significance affecting wound healing. *Laryngoscope* **83**: 1540–1554.

Donatelli, R., Owens-Burkhart, H. (1981) Effects of immobilisation on the extensibility of periarticular connective tissue. *Journal of Orthopaedic and Sports Physical Therapy* **3**: 67–72.

Evans, P. (1980) The healing process at cellular level: a review. *Physiotherapy* **66**: 256–259.

Fowler, J.D. (1989) Wound healing: an overview. *Seminars in Veterinary Medicine and Surgery* **4**: 256–262.

Gelberman, R.H., Vande Berg, J.S., Lundberg, G.N., Akeson, W.H. (1983) Flexor tendon healing and restoration of the gliding surface. *Journal of Bone and Joint Surgery* **65(A)**: 70–83.

Hardy, M.A. (1989) The biology of scar formation. *Physical Therapy* **69**: 1014–1023.

Kapit, W., Macey, R., Meisami, E. (1987) *The Physiology Coloring Book.* Harper Collins.

Keir, K.A.I. (1991) Introduction to manipulation. *British Journal of Sports Medicine* **25**: 221–225.

Le Gros Clark, W.E. (1965) *The Tissues of the Body*, 5th edn. Oxford University Press.

Leibovich, S.J., Ross, R. (1974) The role of the macrophage in wound repair. *American Journal of Pathology* **78**: 71–91.

Merrilees, M.J., Flint, M.H. (1980) Ultrastructural study of tension and pressure zones in a rabbit flexor tendon. *American Journal of Anatomy* **157**: 87–106.

Netter, F.H. (1987) Musculoskeletal system, part 1. *The Ciba Collection of Medical Illustrations*, vol. 8. Ciba-Giegy.

Nimni, M.E. (1980) The molecular organisation of collagen and its role in determining the biophysical properties of the connective tissues. *Biorheology* **17**: 51–82.

Nordin, M., Frankel, V.H. (1989) *Basic Biomechanics of the Musculoskeletal System*, 2nd edn. Lea & Febiger.

Norris, C.M. (1993) *Sports Injuries: Diagnosis and Management for Physiotherapists*. Butterworth-Heinemann.

Palastanga, N., Field, D., Soames, R. (1994) *Anatomy and Human Movement*, 2nd edn. Butterworth-Heinemann.

Peacock, E.E. (1966) Some biochemical and biophysical aspects of joint stiffness. *Annals of Surgery* **164**: 1–12.

Stearns, M.L. (1940a) Studies on the development of connective tissue in transparent chambers in the rabbit's ear, I. *American Journal of Anatomy* **66**: 133–176.

Stearns, M.L. (1940b) Studies on the development of connective tissue in transparent chambers in the rabbit's ear, II. *American Journal of Anatomy* **67**: 55–97.

Threlkeld, A.J. (1992) The effects of manual therapy on connective tissue. *Physical Therapy* **72**: 893–902.

Warren, C.G., Lehmann, J.F., Koblanski, J.N. (1971) Elongation of the rat tail tendon: effect of load and temperature. *Physical Medicine and Rehabilitation* **52**: 465–474.

Wilkerson, G.B. (1985) Inflammation in connective tissue: etiology and management. *Athletic Training* 298–301.

Williams, P.L., Warwick, R., Dyson, M., Bannister, L.H. (1989) *Gray's Anatomy*, 37th edn. Churchill Livingstone.

Woo, S.L.-Y., Wang, C.W., Newton, P.O., Lyon, R.M. (1990) The response of ligaments to stress deprivation and stress enhancement. In: *Knee Ligaments: Structure, Function, Injury and Repair*. (Daniel, D. *et al.*, eds). Raven Press, pp. 337–349.

3 Connective tissue inflammation, repair and remodelling

Summary

An injury causes disruption of connective tissue unity. The body's response to this is one of inflammation, repair and remodelling ultimately to restore anatomical structure and normal function to the damaged tissue.

This chapter examines the different phases of healing and explores the process of scar tissue formation and its implication in restoring or preventing painfree function. General principles of treatment are applied to each phase, aiming to facilitate healing, and the factors which promote or impede healing are considered.

The different phases of connective tissue healing are not separate and each is overlapped by the other, with one response signalling another until the wound is bridged by scar tissue. The inflammatory phase prepares the area for healing, the repair phase rebuilds the structure and the remodelling phase provides the final form of the tissue (Hardy, 1989).

The degree of inflammation in response to injury depends on the degree of trauma. A minor injury causes a minimal response whereas a major injury will produce a significant inflammatory response which will pass through acute, subacute and chronic phases. A repetitive injury develops gradually through overuse, causing microtrauma and chronic self-perpetuating inflammation which may last for months, or even years, particularly if the aggravating activity or trauma is continued.

Lesions encountered in orthopaedic medicine include acute and chronic muscle belly lesions, ligamentous lesions, tendinitis, tenosynovitis, arthritis, bursitis and mechanical joint displacements.

Acute inflammation is significant and the patient can usually recall the precise time and mode of onset. Following injury the inflammatory response is rapid with noticeable pain and swelling, which can last for hours or days. With chronic inflammation associated with overuse injury, the patient cannot usually recollect the onset and the reaction is low-grade with less noticeable pain and swelling. Chronic inflammation may occur as a progression from acute inflammation or as a result of overuse, and can last for weeks, months or even years.

The most marked feature of chronic inflammation is the mild inflammatory process which continues simultaneously with repair (Peery and Miller, 1971). Fibrous scar tissue is produced which interferes with function and can rupture, even with minor trauma, leading into the perpetual cycle of recurrent injury and eventual tissue failure.

The inflammatory phase

The initial inflammatory reaction involves vascular and cellular changes. Injury is rapidly followed by transient vasoconstriction, lasting for 5–10 min, and is succeeded by vasodilatation which may result in haemorrhage. If the lesion is still bleeding at the time of treatment this will necessitate careful management.

In the early stage of inflammation the blood vessel walls become more permeable and plasma and leukocytes leak into the surrounding tissues as inflammatory exudate or oedema. Swelling may take a few hours to develop and the amount of swelling is determined by the type of tissue involved in the injury. For example, muscle bellies may produce considerable swelling and bleeding but the structure of tendons prevents the collection of fluid and they do not easily swell. Similarly, ligaments themselves do not usually show dramatic swelling but intrinsic joint ligaments, e.g. the medial collateral ligament of the knee, may provoke a traumatic arthritis of the joint causing considerable pain and swelling. Swelling may also be restricted physically by fascial bands and intermuscular septa.

The vascular response is directly due to damage of blood vessel walls and indirectly due to the influence of chemical mediators. These chemical mediators include heparin and histamine, released by the mast cells, bradykinin originating from plasma and plasma proteins, serotonin from platelets and prostaglandins, which are hormone-like compounds, produced by all cells in the body.

Heparin temporarily prevents coagulation of the excess tissue fluid and blood in the area. Bradykinins have multiple effects. They are potent mediators of the inflammatory response, can directly cause pain and vasodilatation, can activate the production of substance P and can enhance prostaglandin release. Substance P promotes vasodilatation, increases vascular permeability and stimulates phagocytosis and mast cell degranulation, with the subsequent release of histamine and serotonin. Prostaglandins may provoke or inhibit the inflammatory response.

Histamine and serotonin produce a short-lived vascular effect whereas both bradykinins and prostaglandins promote more long-term vasodilatation. The overall vascular activity is responsible for the gross signs of inflammation: heat (*calor*), redness (*rubor*), swelling (*tumor*), pain and tenderness (*dolor*) and disturbed function (*functio laesa*) (Peery and Miller, 1971).

Inflammation causes pain and tenderness. Mechanical pain is due to mechanical stress, tissue damage, muscle spasm and the accumulated oedema causing excess pressure on surrounding tissues. Chemical pain arises through chemosensitive nerve receptors which are sensitive to histamine, serotonin, bradykinins and prostaglandins which are released into the tissues during this inflammatory phase. However, most nociceptors (pain receptors) are sensitive to more than one type of stimulus. The inflammatory substances may cause extreme stimulation of nerve fibres without necessarily causing them damage.

The nociceptors become progressively more sensitive the longer the pain stimulus is maintained and proinflammatory prostaglandins are believed to sensitize nociceptors leading to a state of hyperalgesia, an increased response to a painful stimulus (Wilkerson, 1985; International Association for the Study of Pain (IASP) definition, 1986; Kloth and Miller, 1990).

If the tissue is still haemorrhaging, attempts must be made to stop this as blood is a strong irritant and will cause chemical and mechanical pain, as well as prolonging the inflammatory process (Dingman and Arbor, 1973; Evans, 1980). This is particularly true of a haemarthrosis which, if present, must be aspirated immediately.

In the first few hours of the early inflammatory phase fibronectin, a structural glycoprotein which acts as a tissue 'glue', appears in the wound, deposited along strands of fibrin in the clot (Williams *et al.*, 1989). This fibrin–fibronectin meshwork is associated with immature fibroblasts, which are thought to deposit type III collagen fibres to provide a scaffold for platelet adhesion and anchorage for further invading fibroblasts (Nimni, 1980; Lehto *et al.*, 1985).

In minor injury, the inflammatory process is short and the scar tissue produced is minimal. The red blood cells break down into cellular debris and haemoglobin pigment, and the platelets release thrombin, an enzyme which changes fibrinogen into fibrin. The fibrin forms a meshwork of fibres which trap the blood clot and an early scar is formed.

If the injury is major, the next stage of the inflammatory phase is phagocytic. Circulating monocytes modulate into macrophages (Fowler, 1989) and join the resident macrophage population to clear the debris from the site of injury through phagocytic action (Leibovich and Ross, 1974). The macrophages increase in great numbers during the first 3 or 4 days (Dingman and Arbor, 1973). They engulf any matter with which they come into contact, clearing the wound environment and preparing it for subsequent repair. As well as performing a phagocytic role, the macrophage acts as a director cell, directing the repair process by chemically influencing the number of fibroblastic repair cells activated in the area.

A stage of neovascularization is also reached, with capillaries starting to develop after about 12 h and continuing to develop for a further 2 or 3 days (Daly, 1990). The new vessels supply oxygen and nourishment to the injured tissues, but are delicate and easily disrupted. Relative immobilization is necessary at this stage and heat is contraindicated as it will cause increased bleeding from the fragile vessels (Hardy, 1989).

Inflammation is a normal response to either trauma or infection and to have no inflammatory response would mean that healing would not occur. Too little inflammation will delay healing and too much inflammation will lead to excessive scarring. The so-called RICE principle of employing relative rest, ice, compression and elevation in the first 2–3 days can help to control heat, swelling and pain and to reduce, but not abolish, inflammation.

The control of swelling is important towards regaining function since the greater the amount of inflammatory exudate, the more fibrin will be found in the area which becomes organized into scar tissue (Evans, 1980). Although pain inhibits normal movement, it should be encouraged at an early stage to promote healing and to avert adverse scar tissue formation.

Pain itself can be further reduced by analgesic drugs. Non-steroidal anti-inflammatory drugs (NSAIDs) modify the inflammatory response, reduce chemical pain and reduce temperature by inhibiting the production of prostaglandins. There are exponents of the so-called NICE principle, adding in the prescription of non-steroidal drugs to the usual first-line after-care of injury. However, a counter view is that these should not be prescribed for the first 2 or 3 days after injury since they will tend to delay healing (Boruta *et al.*, 1990). It may be more appropriate to allow the body's natural inflammatory response to proceed, with analgesics such as paracetamol and/or physical measures such as mobilization, massage and electrotherapy as appropriate methods of pain control.

Corticosteroids should not be used in the acute inflammatory phase as they inhibit macrophage activity which delays debridement of the wound and scar tissue production by delaying the onset and proliferation of the fibroblasts (Leibovich and Ross, 1974; Hardy, 1989). Each stage of the inflammatory phase is essential to the repair process and suppression in the early stages will delay healing.

Gentle friction massage and controlled mobilization should be initiated early to stimulate the healing process in the presence of movement. Mobilization should begin very gently, to start moving the injured connective tissue towards regaining painless function, but without stressing the healing breach. Overstressing the healing tissue would disrupt the early fragile scar and set up a secondary inflammatory response, leading to excess scar tissue formation. Mobilization also has an effect on the mechanoreceptors which helps to reduce pain.

The inflammatory process is a prerequisite to repair with the macrophage directly stimulating the repair process to begin.

> *Clinical tip*
> Gentle friction massage together with gentle mobilization will agitate tissue fluid and increase the chance contact of the macrophage with cellular debris, so promoting healing (Evans, 1980). Physical or electrical modalities that also achieve this effect, e.g. ice, ultrasound, etc., will be an appropriate adjunct to the treatments of orthopaedic medicine.

Repair phase

The repair process is simultaneous with the inflammatory phase and overlaps the remodelling phase.

Some tissues are capable of direct regeneration, e.g. the synovial lining of the joints, bone and skeletal muscle. All other connective tissues are incapable of regeneration, and repair of these structures involves a reconstruction process of the damaged tissue by collagen fibre or scar tissue formation. Scar tissue does not have exactly the same properties or tensile strength of the tissue it is rebuilding, but its structure comes to resemble that tissue closely to ensure that normal function is regained (Douglas *et al.*, 1969; Hardy, 1989).

Once the wound has been prepared by phagocytosis, the macrophage becomes the director of repair and signals an appropriate number of fibroblasts to the area. As the inflammatory phase subsides the fibroblast becomes the dominant cell in the repair phase and synthesizes the connective tissue matrix, comprising the amorphous ground substance and collagen. Fibroblasts may appear in the wound during the first 24 h after injury, but maximum numbers are not achieved until 5–10 days (Bryant, 1977; Chamberlain, 1982; Fowler, 1989). They do not decrease in number until 3 weeks after the injury (Chamberlain, 1982).

Fibroblasts secrete the amorphous ground substance which provides the cross-linking mechanism for the collagen fibres it also synthesizes. This arrangement 'glues' the wound together, with cross-links forming at appropriate nodal intersect points. Once the fibroblasts are stimulated to produce collagen there is rapid closure of the healing breach. Collagen fibres proper are laid down approximately 5–10 days after injury and the repair process continues as they arrange themselves into larger units or bundles (Stearns, 1940b; Chamberlain, 1982).

The rate of repair is directly related to the size of the wound (Stearns, 1940a, 1940b). A small wound with approximated edges will heal quickly with a minimal inflammatory response and collagen fibres will be laid down early to bind the edges together, providing that the edges remain in apposition. Consider a clean, stitched skin wound, when the stitches are usually safely removed after 7 days and the wound has sufficient tensile strength to withstand movement.

Large, unapproximated wounds are deep as well as wide and healing initially requires the formation of granulation tissue. It may be several days after injury before the fibroblasts initiate fibre formation and several weeks before there is sufficient collagen to provide enough tensile strength for the wound to withstand normal movement.

During the early part of the repair process, a stage of wound contraction occurs assisted by the contractile action of myofibroblasts (Gabbiani *et al.*, 1971; Daly, 1990). Linear wounds contract rapidly whilst circular or rectangular wounds contract relatively slowly (Grillo *et al.*, 1958; Fowler, 1989; Hardy, 1989; Williams *et al.*, 1989; Daly, 1990). Wound contracture, as distinct from contraction, results from fibrosis or adhesion formation and this will be discussed later in this chapter.

Initial collagen fibre formation is random. The number of collagen fibres and the tensile strength of the wound increase substantially during the first 3 weeks after injury, to become approximately 15–20% of the normal strength of the tissue (Hardy, 1989; Daly, 1990). However, the tensile strength does not depend on the number of fibres, since after this time the number of collagen fibres stabilizes but the tensile strength of the wound continues to increase. Tensile strength is related to a balance between the synthesis and lysis of collagen, the development of collagen cross-links and the orientation of collagen fibres into the existing weave. This process of maturation is known as the remodelling phase (van der Meulen, 1982; Williams *et al.*, 1989).

Remodelling phase

The remodelling phase sees the new collagen or scar tissue attempt to take on the physical characteristics of the tissue it is replacing. It begins in earnest approximately 21 days after injury and continues for 6 months or more, or possibly for several years. Remodelling is responsible for the final structural orientation and arrangement of the fibres as well as its tensile strength.

Initial, immature scar tissue is weak and the fibres are oriented in all directions through several planes. Remodelling allows these randomly arranged fibres to become rearranged in both a linear and a lateral orientation. The orientation of collagen fibres occurs in two ways, through induction and through tension.

Normal tissue adjacent to the wound induces structure in the replacement scar tissue. Thus dense tissue induces dense, highly cross-linked scar tissue whilst pliable tissue induces loose, coiled, less cross-linked scar tissue (Hardy, 1989). The final physical weave of the collagen so formed is responsible for the functional behaviour of the wound within the connective tissue it is replacing.

Internal and external stresses apply tension to the wound during the remodelling phase, e.g. muscle tension, joint movement, passive gliding of fascial planes, connective tissue loading and unloading, temperature changes and mobilization (Hardy, 1989). It is recognized that both mobilization and immobilization can strongly influence the structural orientation of collagen fibres (Stearns, 1940a, 1940b; Akeson *et al.*, 1987).

During the maturation phase of scar formation, immature scar tissue is converted to mature scar tissue and the cross-linking system changes from weak hydrogen bonding to strong covalent bonding (Price, 1990). Whilst the scar tissue is relatively immature the weak electrostatic bonding forms reducible cross-links which allow scar tissue to be mobilized with a gentle, steady stress. During this stage friction massage and mobilization within the limits of pain are appropriate to maintain the mobility of immature scar tissue and to promote alignment of fibres.

Remodelling involves the reorganization of scar whilst it matures with fibres being absorbed, replaced and reoriented. When stresses arising from mobilization are applied to collagen fibres, the resultant piezoelectric effect, generating small voltages called streaming potentials, is believed to be responsible for the production, maintenance, alignment and absorption of collagen fibrils (Williams *et al.*, 1989; Price, 1990).

Cross-linking is responsible for the tensile strength of new, desirable scar tissue, but if the cross-linking becomes excessive it will be responsible for the toughness and lack of resilience of unwanted fibrous adhesions (Kloth and Miller, 1990). Immobilization causes loss of the ground substance (Akeson *et al.*,

> *Clinical tip*
> The application of appropriate stress by performing painfree movements ensures that collagen fibre orientation occurs throughout the tissue and matches its function.

1967; Akeson, 1990), which reduces the interfibrillar distance and causes friction between the collagen subunits, facilitating the formation of excessive cross-links.

Collagen fibre formation and orientation conform to lines of stress within connective tissue, and are similar in this respect to osseous alignment (Le Gros Clark, 1965; Williams *et al.*, 1989; Price 1990).

Ligaments must have strong scar tissue fibres within their parallel wavy weave to be capable of resisting excessive joint stresses as well as being able to relax and fold when the tension is removed. The scar tissue formed between the ligament and bone must be randomly oriented and loose to allow movement of the joint (Hardy, 1989).

Scar tissue formed within a muscle belly needs to be flexible to allow the muscle fibres to broaden as the muscle contracts and extensible enough to allow the muscle to lengthen when stretched. Scar tissue within tendons must be oriented in a parallel weave along the lines of mechanical stress to ensure maximum tensile strength of the tendon, whilst also maintaining the gliding properties of the tendons.

Collagen synthesis and remodelling continue in the 6 months following injury with the tissue returning to its normal state of activity 6–12 months after injury under normal conditions (Daly, 1990). However, the increase in tensile strength in fascia and other dense connective tissues is thought to take much longer (Dingman and Arbor, 1973). Fully repaired skin wounds eventually achieve only approximately 70% of their original strength (Douglas *et al.*, 1969; Bryant, 1977; Daly, 1990).

As the scar matures, it becomes dense, tough and less resilient than immature scar tissue. The developing stable cross-links become more prolific and the stronger covalent bonds which form do not yield as readily to applied stresses (Price, 1990).

An increasing depth of transverse friction massage provides pressure and gentle lateral stretch to the maturing scar. Deeper friction massage and more vigorous mobilization are required to mobilize mature scar tissue.

> **Clinical tip**
> To avoid adverse scar tissue formation, gentle friction massage and a progressively increasing range of mobilization should be continued until a full, painfree range of movement is restored. This aims to prevent excessive cross-links occurring between individual fibres and encourage fibre alignment.

Adhesion formation and contracture

The process of collagen synthesis and lysis and orientation of fibres, i.e. remodelling, ensures the final form of scar tissue. A balance is needed between collagen synthesis and lysis for an appropriate turnover of collagen and sufficient stresses should be applied to the tissue to stimulate fibre orientation but without disrupting the healing breach.

Increasing the size of the healing breach would set up secondary inflammatory changes, leading to excessive scar tissue formation and eventual contracture, adhesions and fibrosis. Excessive scar tissue, adhesions or contracture within any soft-tissue structure will impede function and cause pain. Pain itself, as a characteristic of inflammation, acts as an inhibitor to normal function and if a state of chronic inflammation is maintained the function of the tissue will continue to deteriorate. This self-perpetuating inflammation presents an ongoing chronic functional problem which may be difficult to treat.

An abnormal excessive production of scar tissue may result in hypertrophic or keloid scars (Daly, 1990; Price, 1990). Hypertrophic scars develop when excessive collagen is deposited within the original wound site whilst keloid scarring involves excessive collagen deposits in the tissues surrounding the scar. In the connective tissue structures important in orthopaedic medicine this excessive production of scar tissue may be seen as adhesion formation and contracture either within the healing structure or within the surrounding tissues.

In the treatment of hypertrophic scarring, prolonged pressure has been used to restore the balance between collagen synthesis and lysis (Hardy, 1989). In a chronically inflamed wound where excessive scar tissue has been produced, the technique of deep transverse friction massage applies pressure to the area of scar tissue as well as providing a lateral stress to the scar to mobilize adhesions.

The use of intralesional corticosteroid is said to produce keloid regression through its multiple steroid effects which include inhibition of fibroblast migration, decreased collagen synthesis and increased collagenase activity (Carrico *et al.*, 1984). This effect may be transferred to the use of intralesional steroid for chronic inflammation in chronic connective tissue lesions such as tendinitis, bursitis and some chronic ligament strains.

> *Clinical tip*
> In chronic lesions, deep friction massage and vigorous mobilization are applied to mobilize the existing scar tissue. Alternatively, an intralesional injection of corticosteroid may be given.

Factors which may affect wound healing

Chronic trauma can cause excessive movement or tension on devitalized tissues promoting unwanted scarring. This is the mechanism of chronic overuse syndromes in which repetitive trauma disrupts tissue unity, causing microtrauma and setting up secondary inflammatory changes.

Haematoma formation retards the healing process by acting as an irritant, producing a mechanical blockage which separates the torn edges and provides a medium for infection (Dingman and Arbor, 1973).

Infection of the injured tissue presents a serious complication which delays the healing process.

Age, according to Mulder (1990), can delay cell migration and proliferation, wound contracture and collagen remodelling, and decrease the tensile strength of the wound, so increasing the chance of wound dehiscence or splitting. Experimental wounds in young rats showed better mechanical properties in terms of greater strength, elastic stiffness and energy absorption, than those in older rats. The fibre organization was more complex and better organized in the young rats and healing was observed to be faster (Holm-Pedersen and Viidik, 1971).

Changes in the gel–fibre ratio occurring with age are consistent with the changes occurring with immobilization. Contractures tend to occur more frequently, after less trauma and after shorter periods of time in the relatively immobile joints of the elderly. Chemical changes in the gel–fibre ratio have been noted in such tissues as the skin and the nucleus pulposus of older individuals (Akeson *et al.*, 1968).

The following medications, therapies and conditions may also affect wound healing.

Whilst anti-inflammatory medication may not be the most appropriate treatment for acute inflammation, its use in chronic lesions is most appropriate for suppressing inflammation and relieving pain. NSAIDs, either taken orally or topically applied, may be used in conjunction with physical measures (RICE). NSAIDs do not cause a significant change in collagen synthesis; they inhibit production of histamine, serotonin and prostaglandins (Wilkerson, 1985). Aspirin, in addition to its anti-inflammatory function, inhibits platelet aggregation and may help to prolong bleeding (Rang *et al.*, 1995).

The oral intake of corticosteroids inhibits collagen synthesis, reduces tensile strength and delays wound healing (Dingman and Arbor, 1973; Ahonen *et al.*, 1980; Mulder, 1990). Corticosteroids administered in the acute inflammatory phase interfere with macrophage migration but if delivered after the macrophage invasion, i.e. after 3 days, their effect on wound healing is much less severe (Fowler, 1989).

Anticoagulants, e.g. heparin and warfarin, prolong the bleeding and delay wound healing.

The effect of chemotherapy depends on the drugs used and their dosage, but fibroblast proliferation may be affected and therefore collagen synthesis (Carrico *et al.*, 1984).

Radiotherapy radiation can damage fibroblasts, cause vascular damage and decrease collagen production, but it depends on the dose, frequency and location of the irradiated area in relation to the injury site (Mulder, 1990).

Acquired immunodeficiency syndrome (AIDS) patients are in a state of immunosuppression and this will delay the healing process.

Diabetes appears to affect the inflammatory stage rather than collagen synthesis, implying that insulin is important in the early phase of healing (Carrico *et al.*, 1984).

Other factors which could affect healing include vitamin A and C deficiency, protein deprivation, systemic vascular disorders and systemic connective tissue disorders.

The summary below lists the principles of treatment to be applied in the different phases of healing:

Clinical tip

In considering various factors which can promote or delay or lead to poor repair, assessment of connective tissue lesions should take into account the following factors:

- Time of onset and the time lapse since injury.
- Extent of the lesion.
- Stage reached in the inflammation, repair, remodelling phases.
- Anatomical structures involved directly and indirectly in the lesion.
- Medical conditions which may affect wound healing, e.g. circulatory disorders, clotting disorders, diabetes.
- Age.
- Medications which might affect management and healing, e.g. anticoagulants, analgesics, anti-inflammatory drugs.

Summary

Early acute inflammatory phase
- Relative rest.
- RICE.
- Gentle transverse friction massage.
- Gentle mobilization within the painfree range.

Repair
- Gradual increase of functional movement (when there is enough tensile strength in the wound to withstand this).
- Gradual increase in the depth of transverse friction massage.
- Gradual increase in the range of mobilization.

Remodelling
- A return to normal stress to generate the piezoelectric effect, encouraging fibre alignment.
- Deeper transverse friction massage to prevent excessive cross-links.

References

Ahonen, J., Jiborn, H., Zederfeldt, B. (1980) Hormone influence on wound healing. In: *Wound Healing and Wound Infection: Theory and Surgical Practice* (Hunt, T.K., ed.). Appleton Century Croft, pp. 95–105.

Akeson, W. (1990) The response of ligaments to stress modulation and overview of the ligament healing response. In: *Knee Ligaments: Structure, Function, Injury and Repair* (Daniel, D. *et al.*, eds). Raven Press, pp. 315–327.

Akeson, W., Amiel, D., La Violette, D. (1967) The connective tissue response to immobility: a study of chondroitin-4 and 6-sulfate and dermatan sulfate changes in periarticular connective tissue of control and immobilised knees of dogs. *Clinical Orthopaedics* **51**: 183–197.

Akeson, W., Amiel, D., LaViolette, D., Secrist, D. (1968) The connective tissue response to immobility: an accelerated ageing response? *Experimental Gerontology* **3**: 289–301.

Akeson, W., Amiel, D., Abel, M.F. *et al.* (1987) Effects of immobilisation on joints. *Clinical Orthopaedics and Related Research* **219**: 28–37.

Boruta, P.M., Bishop, J.O., Braly, W.G., Tullos, H.S. (1990) Acute lateral ankle ligament injuries: a literature review. *Foot and Ankle* **11**: 107–113.

Bryant, W.M. (1977) Wound healing. *Clinical Symposia* **29**: 2–28.

Carrico, T.J., Mehrhof, A.I., Cohen, I.K. (1984) Biology of wound healing. *Surgical Clinics of North America* **64**: 721–731.

Chamberlain, G.J. (1982) Cyriax's friction massage: a review. *Journal of Orthopaedic and Sports Physical Therapy* **4**: 16–22.

Daly, T.J. (1990) The repair phase of wound healing – re-epithelialization and contraction. In: *Wound Healing: Alternatives in Management* (Kloth, L.C., McCullock, J.M., Feedar, J.A., eds). F. A. Davis, pp. 14–29.

Dingman, R.O., Arbor, A. (1973) Factors of clinical significance affecting wound healing. *Laryngoscope* **83**: 1540–1554.

Douglas, D.M., Forrester, J.C., Ogilvie, R.R. (1969) Physical characteristics of collagen in the later stages of wound healing. *British Journal of Surgery* **56**: 219–222.

Evans, P. (1980) The healing process at cellular level: a review. *Physiotherapy* **66**: 256–259.

Fowler, J.D. (1989) Wound healing: an overview. *Seminars in Veterinary Medicine and Surgery* **4**: 256–262.

Gabbiani, G., Ryan, G.B., Majno, G. (1971) Presence of modified fibroblasts in granulation tissue and their possible role in wound contraction. *Experientia* **27**: 549–550.

Grillo, H.C., Watts, G.T., Gross, J. (1958) Studies in wound healing: I. contraction and the wound contents. *Annals of Surgery* **148**: 145–152.

Hardy, M.A. (1989) The biology of scar formation. *Physical Therapy* **69**: 1014–1023.

Holm-Pedersen, P., Viidik, A. (1971) Tensile properties and morphology of healing wounds in young and old rats. *Scandinavian Journal of Plastic Reconstructive Surgery* **6**: 24–35.

Kloth, L.C., Miller, K.H. (1990) The inflammatory response to wounding. In: *Wound Healing: Alternatives in Management* (Kloth, L.C., McCullock, J.M., Feedar, J. eds). F. A. Davis, pp. 3–13.

Le Gros Clark, W.E. (1965) *The Tissues of the Body*, 5th edn. Oxford University Press.

Lehto, M., Duance, V.C., Restall, D. (1985) Collagen and fibronectin in a healing skeletal muscle injury. *Journal of Bone and Joint Surgery* **67-B**: 820–827.

Leibovich, S.J., Ross, R. (1974) The role of the macrophage in wound repair. *American Journal of Pathology* **78**: 71–91.

Mulder, G.D. (1990) Factors complicating wound repair. In: *Wound Healing: Alternatives in Management* (Kloth, L.C., McCullock, J.M., Feedar, J. eds). F.A. Davis, pp. 43–51.

Nimni, M.E. (1980) The molecular organisation of collagen and its role in determining the biophysical properties of the connective tissues. *Biorheology* **17**: 51–82.

Peery, T.M., Miller, F.N. (1971) *Pathology: A Dynamic Introduction to Medicine and Surgery*, 2nd edn. Little & Brown.

Price, H. (1990) Connective tissue in wound healing. In: *Wound Healing: Alternatives in Management* (Kloth, L.C., McCullock, J.M., Feedar, J. eds). F.A. Davis, pp. 31–41.

Rang, H.P., Dale, M.M., Ritter, J.M. (1995) *Pharmacology*, 3rd edn. Churchill Livingstone.

Stearns, M.L. (1940a) Studies on the development of connective tissue in transparent chambers in the rabbit's ear, I. *American Journal of Anatomy* **66**: 133–176.

Stearns, M.L. (1940b) Studies on the development of connective tissue in transparent chambers in the rabbit's ear, II. *American Journal of Anatomy* **67**: 55–97.

van der Meulen, J.H.C. (1982) Present state of knowledge on processes of healing in collagen structures. *International Journal of Sports Medicine* **3**: 4–8.

Wilkerson, G.B. (1985) Inflammation in connective tissue: etiology and management. *Athletic Training* 298–301.

Williams, P.L., Warwick, R., Dyson, M., Bannister, L.H. (1989) *Gray's Anatomy*, 37th edn. Churchill Livingstone.

4 Orthopaedic medicine treatment techniques

Summary

Over the years the emphasis of treatment for musculoskeletal lesions has moved from one of total immobilization to one of early mobilization. The benefits of early mobilization have become clear and, whilst a short period of immobilization may still be necessary, the overall aim of orthopaedic medicine treatment techniques is to restore full painless fuction to the connective tissues.

The selection of techniques depends on several factors that include the stage the lesion has reached in the healing cycle and the overall irritability. An accurate clinical diagnosis allows the effective application of the selected treatment techniques and the development of a carefully rationalized treatment programme.

The treatment techniques used in orthopaedic medicine fall into two broad categories of mobilization and injection and within this chapter the techniques will be considered in turn, on the basis of the theory presented in the preceding chapters, with notes on their application.

The treatment techniques used in orthopaedic medicine may be categorized as follows:

Mobilization
- Transverse friction massage.
- Grade A mobilization.
- Grade B mobilization.
- Grade C mobilization (manipulation).
- Traction.

Injection
- Local anaesthetic.
- Corticosteroid.
- Sclerosant therapy.

Mobilization

Connective tissue structures are more responsive to a decrease in mechanical demand than they are to progressive increases (Tipton *et al.*, 1986). Therefore, depriving the healing soft tissues of motion and stress can lead to a number of structural changes within the articular and periarticular connective tissues that may be difficult to reverse. These changes may include all or some of the following:

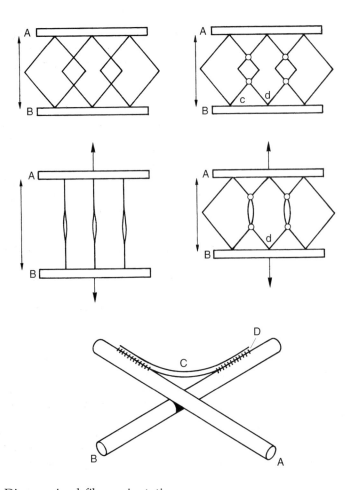

Fig. 4.1 Adhesion formation at the fibre–fibre interface. Adapted from Akeson *et al.* (1980) with permission.

- Disorganized fibre orientation.
- Adhesion formation at the fibre–fibre interface (Fig. 4.1).
- Adhesion formation between ligaments, tendons and their surrounding connective tissue.
- Reduced tensile strength of ligaments, tendons and muscles.
- Loss of the gliding capacity of connective tissue, especially tendons.
- Weakening of ligament and tendon insertion points.
- Inhibition of muscle fibre regeneration by scar tissue.
- Proliferation of fibrofatty tissue into the joint space and adherence to cartilage surfaces.
- Decrease in the volume of synovial fluid with adhesion formation between synovial folds.
- Cartilage erosion and osteophyte formation.

(Burke-Evans *et al.*, 1960; Enneking and Horowitz, 1972; Akeson *et al.*, 1973, 1980, 1986; Videman, 1986; Hardy, 1989; Järvinen and Lehto, 1993.)

It is noticeable that this list of connective tissue changes, associated with immobilization, is similar to the changes seen with the degenerative ageing process.

The length of connective tissue structures tends to adapt to the shortest distance between origin and insertion, which produces the consequences of immobilization that can lead to pain and long-term loss of function (Videman, 1986).

Several authors have discussed the effects of stress and motion deprivation on healing connective tissues in animal experiments (Akeson *et al.*, 1967, 1973, 1986; Woo *et al.*, 1975, 1990; Arem and Madden, 1976; Woo, 1982; Akeson, 1990). During a 9-week period of immobilization, dysfunction was not simply due to connective tissue atrophy, as there was no statistical difference in the quantity of collagen fibres, but due to other more consequential changes within the connective tissue matrix. Loitz *et al.* (1988) noticed similar changes within a 3-week period of immobilization.

The changes noted were:

- Development of anomalous cross-linking of existing and new collagen fibres (Fig. 4.2).
- Alteration of the dynamics of collagen turnover (synthesis/lysis).
- Random deposition of new collagen fibres within the existing collagen weave.

In explanation of the changes a difference was noted in the quantity and quality of the amorphous ground substance, consistent in all connective tissue structures, which amounted to a reduced concentration of water and glycosaminoglycans (GAGs). As a result, the critical distance and separating effects between adjacent collagen fibres were reduced and the interfibrillar lubrication was lost. Friction developed at the fibre–fibre interface leading to the development of anomalous cross-links which altered the gliding function of the collagen fibres. This formation of cross-links was observed to be time-dependent and occurred when fibres remained stationary for a period of time, i.e. assumed a stationary attitude.

The incorporation of new, disorganized collagen fibres into the existing collagen weave physically restrains mobility. Overall this has an effect of altering the plasticity and pliability of the connective tissue structures. It is important to note that adhesion formation is a normal part of the repair process and it cannot be prevented entirely. However it is possible to prevent excessive or unwanted adhesions, or to mobilize them if they develop unwittingly. Treatment aims to maintain or regain the anatomy and biomechanical function of collagen fibres, enabling them to deal with tension, compression, shear and glide.

Collagen turnover (synthesis/lysis) is a normal process that is influenced by stress and motion. When deprived of these physical forces through immobilization, the balance of collagen turnover is lost and a greater ratio of immature collagen fibres is present with a potential for the formation of increased anomalous, reducible cross-links. Pliable young scar tissue is ripe for early mobilization techniques that will reduce the formation of anomalous cross-links.

Stress and motion deprivation is also responsible for the random, disorganized deposition of new collagen fibres within the existing weave, that results in an overall reduction in tensile strength.

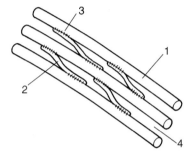

Fig. 4.2 The anomalous cross-link formation within existing collagen fibres. 1 = Existing fibre; 2 = newly synthesized fibril; 3 = cross-links created as the fibril becomes incorporated into the fibre; 4 = fibres normally move freely past one another (ligament, tendon, muscle) or separate (muscle belly). Adapted from Akeson *et al.* (1980) with permission.

Collagen tissue is elastic mainly by virtue of the weave of its collagen subunits, and it will become relatively inelastic if that weave is altered (Peacock, 1966). The careful, controlled application of normal stress and motion will stimulate new collagen to be laid down in parallel with the existing weave and the collagen tissue will maintain its elasticity and tensile strength. Wolff's law, relating to laying down of trabeculae in cancellous bone along the lines of stress, could be broadened to encompass the response of the musculoskeletal system to stress as a whole (Akeson, 1990).

Immobilization affects the gliding function of tendons and ligaments by virtue of the restricting adhesions failing to elongate to permit painfree function (Weiner and Peacock, 1971). In orthopaedic medicine the principles of mobilization can be applied to healing tendons in both tendinitis and tenosynovitis. The application of treatment techniques to rupture adhesions to permit normal gliding function may be necessary in lesions of tennis elbow and some chronic ligamentous strains.

In muscle lesions, collagen or scar tissue formation provides a necessary framework for muscle fibre regeneration. However, excessive scar tissue forms a physical barrier and hinders the progress of the regenerating muscle fibres. The connective tissue component of muscles is subject to the usual deleterious changes of immobilization. An adequate period of relative rest (1–5 days depending on the injury) is required to allow the muscle to regenerate sufficiently to combat the mechanical forces of mobilization (Lehto *et al.*, 1985; Järvinen and Lehto, 1993). The early application of graded mobilization will maintain muscle function and stimulate structural orientation without the excessive formation of scar tissue.

Articular changes during periods of immobilization depend on the restriction of the movement, the length of the immobilization period and the amount of contact, pressure and friction between the joint surfaces. The amount of synovial fluid is reduced, which renders the articular cartilage more vulnerable to injury by friction and pressure. Longer periods of immobilization (45–60 days) show cartilage erosion, subchondral cyst and osteophyte formation, consistent with the changes observed clinically in joints affected by osteoarthrosis and age-related changes. Studies involving the immobilization of rat knee joints showed that if immobilization did not exceed 30 days, the changes due to immobilization were somewhat reversible. The longer the joints were immobilized, the longer it took to remobilize them, irrespective of the method used (Burke-Evans *et al.*, 1960). Degenerative changes occurring during immobilization can be partly inhibited by traction and continuous passive motion (Videman, 1986).

The beneficial effects of intermittent and continuous passive motion have been well-documented (Loitz *et al.*, 1988; Takai *et al.*, 1991). The original concept of continuous passive motion was developed by Salter in 1970 (Salter, 1989) to reduce the harmful effects of immobilization. He moved joints continuously through a predetermined range of movement. This application of cyclical tensile loading facilitates the orientation of collagen fibres providing tensile strength and a stronger functional and structural repair of connective tissue, including articular cartilage.

In summary, the aim of mobilization treatment techniques applied in orthopaedic medicine is to prevent or to reverse the connective tissue changes associated with a period of immobilization. It is important to recognize that stress deprivation causes rapid structural changes and recovery is much slower, which must be taken into account when preparing treatment programmes.

Careful consideration should be given to the application of other treatment modalities either simultaneously or consecutively with the application of appropriate mobilization. Abusive use of movement can produce mechanical forces sufficient to stretch or disrupt the healing breach, producing excessive scar tissue formation. Additional soft-tissue trauma leads to secondary inflammation and the vicious circle of chronic inflammation (Noyes, 1977). The correct amount of movement applied at the appropriate time is the key.

Mobilization should be used at optimum levels, with appropriate grade, range, force, direction, speed and duration to achieve the specific treatment aims (Arem and Madden, 1976). Hunter (1994), however, correctly points out that, although soft-tissue mobilization techniques are known to be clinically effective, no research has been conducted to establish the grade of mobilization required for each stage of the healing process. Orthopaedic medicine mobilization techniques (transverse friction massage and specific mobilization techniques) are graded on the basis of patient feedback and observation against the underpinning knowledge of the different phases of healing and the experience of the clinician.

Transverse friction massage

Transverse friction massage is a specific type of connective tissue massage applied precisely to the soft-tissue structure of tendons, muscles and ligaments, for a specific purpose. It is applied prior to and in conjunction with mobilization techniques to gain its effects.

Massage is the manipulation of the soft tissues of the body with the hands using varying degrees of force (Carreck, 1994). You will note that the term deep friction massage has been deliberately avoided to prevent the abuse of this technique. Unfortunately, deep friction massage has been taught to many therapists as just that, and it has not been adapted or graded to suit the lesion to gain specific purpose. Consequently, the technique has developed a reputation for being very painful for the patient and tiring for the therapist (Ingham, 1981; Woodman and Pare, 1982; Cyriax and Cyriax, 1983; de Bruijn, 1984) often being abandoned for these reasons. It is an underrated modality at our fingertips (pun intended) and, applied correctly, it is an extremely useful technique.

Transverse friction massage can be graded in depth for acute and chronic lesions. If correctly applied, it achieves a numbing or analgesic effect and does not have to be a painful experience for the patient. In this text, the terms *gentle transverse friction massage* and *deep transverse friction massage* will be used to give an indication of the grade required for specific treatments.

A review of the literature provides very little scientific evidence on the effectiveness of friction massage. The few studies that have been undertaken show little support for the modality (Stratford *et al.*, 1989; Schwellnus *et al.*, 1992; Vasseljen, 1992; Pellecchia *et al.*, 1994), but these studies were not ideally conducted and left many questions unanswered, with the result that more research is urgently needed.

Some studies have looked at the physiological effects of massage and the numerous studies on the use of mobilization have already been discussed. It may be hypothesized that since transverse friction massage is a massage technique that aims to produce therapeutic movement, some of the proven effects of massage and mobilization must apply. However, this must be recognized for what it is – hypothesis, not scientific proof.

To produce therapeutic movement

Transverse friction massage aims to achieve a transverse sweeping movement of the collagenous structure of the connective tissues. This, together with graded mobilization, discourages the stationary attitude of fibres that promotes anomalous cross-link formation. The therapeutic movement facilitates the shear and gliding properties of collagen, allowing subsequent longitudinally applied stresses to stimulate fibre orientation to enhance tensile strength. In this way adhesion formation is prevented in acute situations and mobilized in chronic situations.

Gentle transverse friction massage applied in the early inflammatory phase causes an agitation of tissue fluid that may increase the rate of phagocytosis by chance contact (Evans, 1980). It is a useful treatment to apply in the first day or two following injury, before scar tissue formation has truly begun, providing it is graded appropriately to avoid increased bleeding or disruption of the healing breach.

In the chronic inflammatory phase, deep transverse friction massage produces therapeutic movement that softens and mobilizes adhesions. This prepares the structure for other graded mobilizations that aim to apply longitudinal stress or selectively rupture the unwanted adhesions.

To produce a traumatic hyperaemia in chronic lesions

Deep, as distinct from gentle, transverse friction massage produces a controlled traumatic hyperaemia and is used exclusively for chronically inflamed lesions.

An erythema develops in the skin and it is assumed that the same reaction is occurring in the deeper tissues where the effect is required (Winter, 1968). The area of redness that develops under the finger may be slightly raised and warm, indicating vasodilatation and increased blood flow to the area, facilitating the removal of chemical irritants responsible for producing the pain. Massage, which

---

Aims of transverse friction massage

- **To produce therapeutic movement.**
- **To produce a traumatic hyperaemia in chronic lesions.**
- **To induce pain relief.**
- **To improve function.**

increases blood flow in this way, may also produce a decrease in pain by transportation of endogenous opiates.

The increased inflammatory response is desirable in chronic lesions, but not in acute lesions where the response is already excessive. Gentle transverse friction massage applied to acute lesions is performed with reduced depth and time, to avoid producing a traumatic hyperaemia.

To induce pain relief

Pain relief following the application of transverse friction massage has been clinically observed and a number of hypotheses are proposed to substantiate this.

The gate control theory proposed by Melzack and Wall in 1965 is a theory of pain modulation that affects the passage of sensory information at spinal cord level, especially nociceptive impulses. Within the spinal cord there are mechanisms which 'open the gate' to impulses provoked by noxious stimuli, and mechanisms which 'close the gate', thus reducing the awareness of noxious stimuli. Pressure stimulates low-threshold mechanoreceptors in the skin that reduce the excitability of the nociceptor terminals by presynaptic inhibition, effectively 'closing the gate' on the pain. The greater the mechanoreceptor stimulation, the greater the level of pain suppression (Bowsher, 1988; Wells, 1988). Quite simply, rubbing a painful spot reduces pain, enabling the transverse friction massage to be graded in depth, specific to individual lesions, and thus to produce its beneficial effects.

A reduction in pain is experienced as a numbing effect by the patient and is so obvious that the patient will often acknowledge this by saying you have 'gone off the spot'. However, with faith in diagnosis and accurate knowledge of anatomy, this should be the signal to grade the friction more deeply to apply beneficial treatment appropriate to the lesion. Following treatment the comparable signs can be reassessed and a reduction in pain and increase in strength is usually noted.

The reduction in pain achieved seems to have fairly long-lasting effects, possibly longer than expected. Transverse friction massage, like rubbing or scratching the skin, is considered to be a form of noxious counterirritation that leads to a desired analgesic effect (de Bruijn, 1984). Inhibition, which produces lasting pain relief is believed to be through diffuse noxious inhibitory controls (de Bruijn, 1984; Melzack and Wall, 1988), a descending pain suppression mechanism that releases endogenous opiates. Endogenous opiates are inhibitory neurotransmitters which diminish the intensity of the pain transmitted to higher centres (Goats, 1994).

de Bruijn (1984) treated 13 patients with deep transverse friction massage to various soft-tissue lesions. The time required to produce analgesia during the application of deep transverse friction massage was noted to be 0.4–5.1 min (mean 2.1 min) whilst the post-massage analgesic effect lasted 0.3 min–48 h (mean 26 h).

Carreck (1994) evaluated the effect of a 15-min general lower-limb massage (*effleurage* and *pétrissage*) on pain perception threshold in 20 healthy volunteers and showed that the massage significantly increased the pain perception threshold for experimentally induced pain. Conversely, Kelly (1997), using deep transverse friction massage, reported no significant change in the pain pressure threshold, although there was an improvement in function that will be discussed below.

Massage in its various forms is considered to be a placebo, having a therapeutic effect on the psychological aspects of pain. Transverse friction massage as a form of massage may also have this effect.

To improve function

The therapeutic movement achieved and the pain relief induced by transverse friction massage produces an immediate clinical improvement in function of the structure treated. This can be demonstrated by reassessment immediately after treatment and provides an optimum situation for the application of other graded mobilizing techniques.

Kelly (1997) studied a group of 46 normal volunteers to investigate the effects of deep transverse friction massage to the gastrocnemius muscle. The treatment group received 5 min deep transverse friction massage, deep enough to achieve movement of the muscle fibres but not deep enough to cause discomfort. The control group were placed in the treatment position, for 5 min. The results of this study showed improved function with an increase in force of muscle contraction and an increased range of dorsiflexion.

> *Clinical tip*
> The exact grade of transverse friction massage is determined by the irritability of the lesion and through feedback from the patient, but to be effective, it must be deep enough to reach the target tissue.

Principles of application of transverse friction massage

Transverse friction massage should be applied to the exact site of the lesion. This relies on clinical diagnosis and palpation of the lesion, based on anatomical knowledge and the structural organization of the tissue. Tenderness is not necessarily an accurate localizing sign, therefore palpation must reproduce the patient's pain and be different in comparison with the other limb.

Transverse friction massage is always applied transversely across the longitudinal fibre orientation of the structure (Fig. 4.3). This aims to prevent or mobilize adhesion formation between individual fibres and between fibres and the surrounding connective tissues. Application of the technique in this manner deters a stationary attitude of fibres and prevents or mobilizes anomalous cross-links. This transverse sweep, together with longitudinal stress applied in accompanying graded mobilization techniques, stimulates fibre orientation within the collagen weave and increases tensile strength.

Transverse friction massage must be applied with sufficient sweep or amplitude to separate the individual connective tissue fibres of the affected structure. The therapist must be positioned to ensure that this sweep is maintained through the application of body weight.

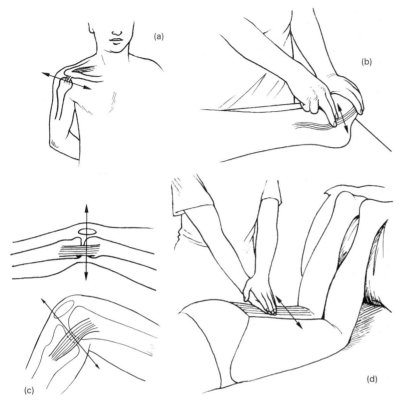

Fig. 4.3 Transverse friction massage of: (a) a tendon (supraspinatus); (b) a tendon in sheath (peronei); (c) a ligament (medial collateral) in flexion and extension; (d) muscle belly (hamstring).

Transverse friction massage must be applied with effective depth to reach and benefit the target tissue. Knowledge of anatomy is again paramount. The depth is maintained by applying the technique slowly and deliberately. The grading of friction massage is intended as a clinical guide, the depth of technique being dependent upon the irritability of the lesion and feedback from the patient. The depth of the initial sweeps should always be gentle to gain some numbing effect before proceeding with the effective massage. Application in this way will dispel the myth that transverse friction massage is a painful treatment.

The patient is positioned, taking into account the situation in which the structure is most accessible and the degree of stretch or relaxation appropriate.

- Tendons in a sheath are placed on the stretch to allow the transverse friction massage to roll the sheath around the firm base of the tendon, facilitating functional movement between the tendon and its sheath.
- Tendons are placed into a position of accessibility, with the lesion commonly lying at the teno-osseous junction. Consideration is given to anatomy.
- Muscle bellies are always placed in a shortened, relaxed position to facilitate broadening of the muscle fibres, imitating function.
- Ligaments are put under a small degree of tension to tighten the overlying soft tissues, allowing the target tissue to be reached.

The therapist should adopt a position that utilizes body weight to an optimum, ensuring sufficient sweep and depth. Sitting is possible, but the most effective position to apply body weight is with the patient situated on a plane lower than the therapist. Consideration should be given to the variety of ways the hands can be used to avoid fatigue and overuse (Fig. 4.4). The therapist's finger and the patient's skin should move simultaneously to avoid raising a blister. The most efficient way of achieving this is to apply the

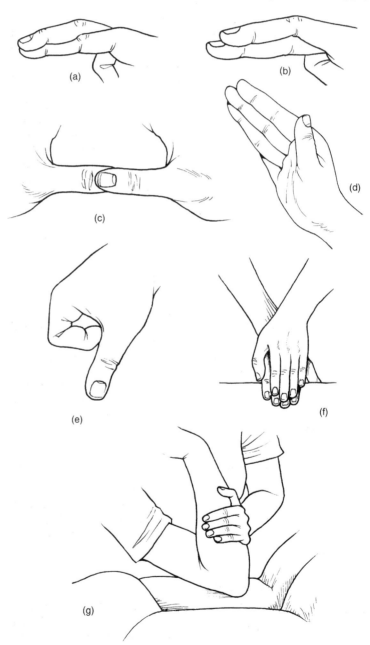

Fig. 4.4 Hand positions for transverse friction massage. (a) Index finger reinforced by middle finger; (b) middle finger reinforced by index finger; (c) thumbs; (d) ring finger; (e) pinch grip; (f) hands; (g) hand guiding the flat of the elbow.

technique in two directions. Pressure is first directed down on to the structure and maintained whilst the transverse sweep is applied.

As a general guideline, deep transverse friction massage is applied to chronic lesions for 10 min after the numbing effect has been achieved. Due to the traumatic hyperaemia induced, treatment is repeated at a minimum interval of 48 h. Gentle transverse friction massage is applied to acute lesions for six effective sweeps once some numbing is achieved and the target tissue reached. Treatment can be on a daily basis, if practically possible, to promote pain relief and therapeutic movement. Only empirical evidence supports the above suggested times, although students on courses often report better results with increased time of application. From the practical aspect, the duration of application fits in with appointment times and allows for both reassessment and the application of other modalities of treatment judged to be appropriate.

Transverse friction massage makes other graded mobilization techniques possible, therefore it is applied first. Acute lesions are followed by painfree mobilization, whilst chronic lesions may require manipulation to rupture unwanted adherent scar tissue.

Absolute contraindications to transverse friction massage are few. It is never applied to active conditions, active infection or rheumatoid arthritis. Care is required if there is fragile skin or the patient is currently involved in anticoagulant therapy.

Grade A, B and C mobilizations are specific mobilization techniques applied to achieve a particular purpose.

Grade A mobilization

Grade A mobilization is a passive, active or active/assisted mobilization performed within the patient's painfree range of movement. At the spinal joints Grade A technique indicates mid-range, painfree mobilization.

It is usually applied to acutely inflamed or painful lesions and it may be made possible by the previous application of transverse friction massage. A degree of mechanical stress is applied to stimulate orientation of collagen fibres.

To promote tissue fluid agitation

Grade A mobilization, either active or passive, produces a gentle soft-tissue movement agitating tissue fluid in the acute inflammatory phase and facilitating phagocytic action (Evans, 1980). The movements are of small amplitude, slow, painfree, without force and repeated often.

To prevent a stationary attitude of fibres

Grade A mobilization will promote movement within connective tissue structures to prevent a stationary attitude of fibres. In the acute phase of inflammation, the movement should occur without

Aims of Grade A mobilization

- To promote tissue fluid agitation.
- To prevent a stationary attitude of fibres.
- To apply longitudinal stress.
- To promote normal function.
- To reduce a loose body.

stress or disruption of the healing breach. The patient is instructed to exercise up to the point of discomfort, but not into or through pain, and must understand the importance of this controlled, precise movement. In this way a critical amount of movement is applied to encourage function but not to delay healing.

The function of a muscle belly is maintained by performing active inner-range, isometric, painfree contractions aiming to broaden muscle fibres. The function of a ligament is promoted by performing active isotonic painfree movement, maintaining the ligament's ability to glide over the underlying bone. In overuse lesions, e.g. tenosynovitis or tendinitis, the patient maintains normal function by performing movement within the painfree range, and avoiding the painful movements.

To apply a longitudinal stress to connective tissue structures

Grade A mobilization can impart sufficient longitudinal stress to promote orientation of collagen fibres within the existing parallel collagen weave. From 3 to 5 days after injury there should be sufficient tensile strength in the wound for the patient to 'nudge' pain so providing minimal longitudinal stress, without disrupting the healing breach. These movements are of short duration, with sufficient amplitude to apply a minimum of stress. They are repeated often, but are not forceful. This is appropriate for the repair phase of connective tissue injuries, and as progress is made an increasing range of movement is encouraged. In this way the developing scar tissue is stressed, not stretched, aiming to restore full range.

To promote normal function

Grade A mobilization is applied early in the inflammatory phase to ensure function is rapidly regained. Healing within the presence of movement promotes a return to function. The range of movement is gradually increased, applying sufficient stress to the wound to promote orientation of fibres. Daily treatment is ideal to restore full range of painfree movement. Controlled mobilization of acute lesions should prevent the need for stretching tissue.

In chronic injuries, once rendered painfree by transverse friction massage or corticosteroid injection, normal movement will promote remodelling and alignment of fibres and restoration of function. However, until signs and symptoms subside, overuse activity must be avoided in lesions aggravated by repetitive movements.

To reduce a loose body or bony subluxation in a peripheral joint

To reduce a peripheral joint loose body or a bony subluxation (e.g. capitate), a Grade A mobilization is performed under strong traction, giving the fragment space to move, which is the principal component of this technique.

Grade B mobilization

A Grade B mobilization is a mobilization performed at the end of available range. It is a specific sustained stretching technique that aims to cause permanent elongation of connective tissue. At the spinal joints a Grade B technique indicates a mobilization performed to the end of range.

To stretch capsular adhesions

In the early stages of an arthritis, pain causes the joint to be held in a position of ease, restricting movement of some parts of the joint capsule. This promotes a disordered deposition of collagen fibres and the normal flexibility of the joint capsule is impeded by anomalous cross-link formation. The changes in the capsule contribute to contracture and the capsular adhesions severely restrict the range of movement, causing pain and altered function. The aim of treatment by Grade B mobilization is to lengthen the capsular contracture permanently to restore normal movement.

Adhesions that develop within the capsules of the synovial joint tend to be tough and unyielding. The shoulder and hip joints commonly demonstrate this gross loss of function and respond well to Grade B mobilization, providing the joints are in a non-irritable state. However, the technique could be applied to any non-irritable capsulitis in which pain and loss of movement are clinical features. Characteristically the joint is limited in the capsular pattern with the restricted movements demonstrating a 'hard' end-feel (see Chapter 1). Grade B mobilization is aimed at restoring the movements limited in the capsular pattern.

Grade B mobilization is applied at the end of available range, appreciating the end-feel and the patient's pain response. To be successful, the end-feel should still have some elastic quality, but the sensation of muscle spasm may also be apparent as the technique is applied within a painful range. The technique is a slow, sustained and repeated stretch, performed at the end of available range for the duration of the patient's pain tolerance. As soon as the end-range position is released, an immediate relief of pain should be felt. If pain lingers at this stage, the joint may be too irritable and the technique may not be appropriate. Successful treatment is dependent upon patient compliance as the management of the condition is long-term.

To stretch tough, relatively unyielding capsular adhesions a number of factors need consideration relating to the behaviour of connective tissue under mechanical stress (see Chapter 2).

Sufficient force must be applied to break collagen cross-links, producing microfailure and thus producing permanent elongation of the capsular adhesions. The force must be strong enough to take the capsular adhesions at least into the latter part of the linear phase and possibly beyond the elastic limit into the early plastic range. As the technique is applied into a painful range, the patient's pain tolerance will determine the amount of force possible for each sustained stretch. Microfailure produces a low-grade inflammatory

Aims of Grade B mobilization
• **To stretch capsular adhesions.** • **To reduce pain.** • **To improve function.**

response and some discomfort may be noticeable for a few hours after treatment. It is essential that this is explained to the patient, since mobilization must continue whilst the discomfort persists to maintain the elongation achieved.

A slow, sustained force utilizes the viscous flow phenomenon related to connective tissue structures (Amis, 1985). A slowly applied force is met with less resistance or stiffness (it is easier to move slowly through a viscous medium) and the tough adhesions gradually give under the slow, sustained stretch.

The application of heat relieves pain and lowers the viscosity of collagen tissue, allowing a greater elongation of collagen tissues for less force. Warren *et al.* (1971) considered the effect of temperature and load on elongation of the collagen fibre structure of rat tail tendon. Heat and load were applied at selected temperatures of 39, 41, 43 and 45°C. The greatest elongation with least microdamage was achieved with lower loads at the higher therapeutic temperatures. The mechanism of a combined application of temperature and load affected the viscous flow properties of collagen.

Raising local temperature to between 40 and 45°C (40°C is the temperature of a very hot bath) achieves this useful therapeutic effect. Ultrasound can be applied to produce this thermal effect and it has a preference for heating collagen tissue (Low and Reed, 1994). To achieve its best effects, heat should be applied concurrently with the Grade B mobilization; however, for practical purposes it is usually applied before.

Viscoelastic structures display the properties of creep, hysteresis and set. A prolonged Grade B stretch applied into the linear region produces deformation through creep. The collagen fibres line up in the direction of the applied stress, water and proteoglycans are displaced and the cross-links strain and may break. When the force is released, recovery occurs at a slower rate, i.e. hysteresis occurs and some increased length may remain.

The technique is repeated often in each treatment session. If each cycle of loading is applied before the tissue has recovered its original length, an increment of lengthening is achieved each time.

To reduce pain

In arthritis the inflammatory changes involve both the synovial lining of the joint and the fibrous capsule. The capsule develops small lesions that undergo scar tissue formation, producing adhesions or capsular thickenings. The adhesions are affected by joint movement that, through abnormal tension, stimulates the free nerve endings lying in the capsule, producing mechanical pain. The nerve endings also respond to the chemical products of inflammation – histamine, kinins and prostaglandins. Impulses are transported in the non-myelinated C fibres and a 'slow', aching, throbbing pain is produced which is poorly defined, i.e. chemical pain (Norris, 1993). The pain and associated involuntary muscle spasm reduce movement, allowing healing to occur in a shortened position. Over time the patient will develop a restriction of movement in the capsular pattern.

The permanent lengthening achieved by Grade B mobilization reduces the mechanical stress and therefore inflammation, which in turn relieves pain. Normal movement applied to collagen fibres produces alignment and orientation of the fibres within the collagen weave.

> *Clinical tip*
> Grade B mobilization produces some treatment soreness that is acceptable for 2–4 h after treatment. This gives a guide to irritability of the lesion and progression of treatment.

To improve function

The increase in joint range and pain relief achieved by Grade B mobilization improves overall function. However, the gradual onset of loss of movement through capsular contraction can considerably alter movement patterns. Careful assessment of the patient is necessary and a treatment programme planned which considers all components of the dysfunction, including altered biomechanics, muscle imbalance and neural tension.

Grade B mobilization is not used exclusively for capsular contractures. In chronic lesions, adaptive shortening may be part of an overall dysfunction. The shortened tissues can be stretched by applying the principles of Grade B mobilization both by the therapist and as a home treatment regime. Grade B mobilization is applied after the structure has been rendered functionally painfree by deep transverse friction massage.

Grade C mobilization

Grade C mobilization is a manipulative technique and will be referred to as such. It is a passive movement performed at end of range, i.e. once all the slack has been taken up, and is a minimal-amplitude, high-velocity thrust. Most importantly, its principles of application are different in spinal and peripheral lesions.

To reduce a spinal or sacroiliac joint intra-articular displacement

In the spinal or sacroiliac joints, manipulation aims to 'unblock' the joint, reducing intra-articular displacement, relieving compression and restoring full, painless function. Spinal manipulation can produce an immediate and dramatic restoration of range of movement and pain relief. The mechanism by which manipulation achieves this is not well-understood, but may be related to many factors rather than a single mechanism. A major factor towards successful manipulation is in the selection of patients with a small, uncomplicated intra-articular displacement of recent onset.

Pain relief may also occur through stimulation of the mechanoreceptors effecting the pain-gate mechanism or through stimulation of the descending inhibitory controls.

Mechanoreceptors within the joint capsule and spinal ligaments are stimulated by the tension created by spinal manipulation. This inhibits the small-diameter nociceptor afferent input to the ascending pathways at spinal cord level. The relief of pain achieved reduces

Aims of manipulation

- **To reduce a spinal or sacroiliac joint intra-articular displacement.**
- **To rupture unwanted peripheral adhesions.**

the reflex muscle spasm and an increase in the range of movement occurs.

The periaqueductal grey (PAG) area of the brain, as a control centre for endogenous analgesia, is considered to play an important role in the control of pain. Two different forms of analgesia may be produced: an opioid form that seems to be associated with sympathetic inhibition and takes a period of time to develop and a non-opioid form that is associated with sympathetic excitation that has a more rapid onset. Spinal manipulation has an immediate effect, producing pain relief within seconds or minutes due to the non-opioid form, associated with sympathetic excitation that is related to mechanical nociception. Over a period of about 20–45 min the analgesia changes to the opioid form associated with sympathetic inhibition. Spinal manipulation provides an appropriate stimulus to activate the descending pain-inhibitory systems from the PAG to the spinal cord (Wright, 1995).

It must not be forgotten that spinal manipulation can also relieve pain through the placebo effect of skilful handling and care. It is not possible to quantify this effect.

Certain principles need to be considered in order to apply the technique effectively.

A short- or long-lever arm is used and a torque or twisting force is usually applied, taking up the slack in the surrounding connective tissue to induce a passive movement at one or more spinal joints (Hadler *et al.*, 1987). The minimal-amplitude, high-velocity thrust is of great importance since tissues loaded quickly behave more stiffly and have a higher ultimate strength (see Chapter 2). Thus, as the spinal manipulative technique is applied, the force needed to affect the target tissue does not cause damage to the surrounding structures (Threlkeld, 1992), i.e. the weak link in the chain effect.

Manipulative reduction is more likely to succeed if the fragment is given room to move. Therefore an element of traction is usually included. Spinal manipulation, in particular, requires skilful handling that takes time and practice to acquire. The hands must be continuously sensitive to the end-feel of the joints and any abnormal end-feel, e.g. bony resistance or muscle spasm, should alert the manipulator to abandon the procedure.

Successful manipulation requires accurate clinical diagnosis and the choice of the right patient with knowledge of the effects, contraindications and limits of the technique. Thought, care and expert skill are essentials, together with an explanation to the patient of the diagnosis, treatment and possible complications, in order to gain informed consent. Safety is essential and the precautions necessary will be discussed in the appropriate chapters.

Much of the rationale for Cyriax manipulative techniques is based on clinical observation and his hypothesis on spinal disc pathology has received criticism for its lack of sound scientific backing. There is no conclusive evidence that manipulation will alter the size or shape of a bulging annulus or that the herniated nucleus can be relocated (Zusman, 1994), but neither is there conclusive evidence that manipulation will not achieve these effects. Despite manipulative techniques being in use for hundreds of years, the authors recognize that scientific proof is sadly lacking.

Many authors have reviewed clinical manipulation trials (Abenhaim and Bergeron, 1992; LaBan and Taylor, 1992; Barker, 1994; O'Donaghue 1994; Shekelle, 1994), but most of these fall short of the ideal scientific criteria necessary for good-quality research. However, it is generally accepted from the scientific data produced to date that spinal manipulation has shown short-term benefits of improvement in pain, movement and functional ability. The long-term benefits of manipulation remain unknown although, if the aim of manipulation is to expedite recovery, these are of little significance. There is insufficient evidence to support or to refute the use of manipulation for chronic low back pain but manipulation is particularly appropriate for patients with uncomplicated acute back pain with symptoms of short duration (Shekelle, 1994). Until soundly disproved, the authors endorse the benefit of Cyriax manipulation techniques, based on many years of clinical experience.

Manipulation is often associated with an audible 'crack', said to be due to cavitation of the joints. The forces applied increase the joint volume with a corresponding decrease in fluid partial pressure, creating a gas bubble as the intra-articular gases are drawn out of the solution. As the fluid rushes into the area of low-pressure volume, the gas bubble collapses, producing the 'crack' (Herzog *et al.*, 1993).

To rupture unwanted peripheral adhesions

In peripheral lesions, the aim of the technique is to manipulatively rupture unwanted adhesions, producing permanent elongation and restoring full painless function. The short toe-phase of the adhesions ensures that the slack is taken up more rapidly than in the surrounding normal tissue and the minimal-amplitude, high-velocity thrust causes macrofailure, or rupture, of the adhesions whilst the normal tissue remains intact. It is important that the elongation achieved should be maintained by the patient. In orthopaedic medicine manipulative rupture of unwanted adhesions is applied in two situations:

1. *Manipulative rupture of unwanted adhesions between a ligament and bone.* Peripheral manipulation is applied to a chronic ligamentous sprain of two ligaments in the lower limb, the medial collateral ligament at the knee and the lateral collateral ligament at the ankle. Unwanted adhesions have developed between the ligament and the underlying bone that disrupt the normal functional movement of the joint and a non-capsular pattern of pain and limitation will be found on examination.

   The ligament is prepared by deep transverse friction massage to soften and numb the ligament; the manipulation follows immediately. Effective manipulation should achieve instant results and vigorous exercise is required to maintain the lengthening achieved. Rehabilitation must address all components contributing to the dysfunction.

2. *To rupture adherent scar tissue at the teno-osseous junction of the common extensor tendon (tennis elbow).* A special manipulation (Mills' manipulation) is applied at the teno-osseous junction of the common extensor tendon as a treatment for tennis elbow (Chapter 6). The manipulation aims to elongate adhesions interfering with the mobility of the tendon at its insertion and within the adjacent tissues. The tendon is first prepared by deep transverse friction massage, followed by the manipulation. The elongation gained must be maintained through exercise.

Traction

The terms traction and distraction have the same meaning in describing a force applied to produce separation of joint surfaces and widening of the joint space. There is a convention that 'traction' is applied to spinal joints and 'distraction' to peripheral joints, but this is not a hard and fast rule.

This section considers the theory underpinning the traction and distraction techniques used in orthopaedic medicine. Emphasis will be placed on the use of traction as a treatment for back and neck pain. Many other treatment modalities employ distraction in the treatment of peripheral joint lesions and the aims and effects will be described only briefly here.

The general indications for traction and distraction will be mentioned, but these, together with the contraindications for treatment, will be discussed in greater detail in the following chapters.

The aims of traction were originally devised from Cyriax's hypotheses of the effects on the spinal joints. They have been developed subsequently to encompass the peripheral joints, where appropriate, and may be stated as follows.

To relieve pain

Pain relief through the use of traction is gained by relieving pressure. Traction reduces the compression force, muscles relax and the pressure on the joint and pain-sensitive structures is reduced.

Aims of distraction/traction

- **To relieve pain.**
- **To create space.**
- **To produce negative pressure within a joint.**
- **To tighten ligaments around a joint.**
- **To reduce a peripheral loose body.**

To create space

The application of distraction/traction creates a degree of space within the joint, allowing a displaced bulge or fragment, a loose body or a displaced carpal bone room to move.

To produce negative pressure within a joint

Creating space within the joint creates a suction effect that helps to move a displaced intra-articular fragment.

To tighten the ligaments around a joint

Tightening up of the ligaments around the joint produces a centripetal force. A disc displacement will tend to be pushed towards the centre as the traction is applied.

To reduce a peripheral loose body

Distraction is the main element of the manoeuvre, with a Grade A mobilization applied during traction. The aim is to move the displaced fragment to another area of the joint where it does not block joint movement.

Discussion on the aims and effects of traction

To provide some support for the aims, the following paragraphs set out to review the evidence for the effects and effectiveness of traction, particularly as a treatment for back and neck pain.

'Traction is generally considered to be an empirical treatment' stated Colachis and Strohm (1965) and, in spite of several well-organized trials to demonstrate to the contrary, this statement unfortunately continues to be true.

In these days of evidence-based practice, demands have been made for traction, as an expensive, time-consuming modality, to be stopped as a treatment until evidence for its effectiveness has been produced. Mathews and Hickling's presentation of their paper (1975) was criticized for not honestly stating that no evidence had been found and an article in the *British Medical Journal* ('Trial by Traction' *BMJ* Jan. 1976) urgently called for thorough research into traction to avoid further waste of resources.

Swezey (1983) represented the views of the many who use traction when he acknowledged that 'there is a consensus amongst thoughtful clinicians that traction is useful, and until further study argues to the contrary, it deserves a place in our therapeutic armamentarium'.

Traction has been documented as a treatment for back pain at least since the time of Hippocrates (Hume Kendall, 1955). Cyriax himself developed his first traction bed in 1949 and collaborated with his physiotherapists on how it could be used to relieve the symptoms produced by nuclear disc protrusion.

His belief was that pain of gradual onset, usually associated with leg pain, was due to nerve root compression from herniated nuclear material through a tear in the annulus, i.e. a disc protrusion (see Chapter 13).

His hypothesis was that effective traction could produce a suction effect within the disc to draw the nuclear material centrally and away from the nerve root. At the same time a mechanical 'push' would be given to the herniated material by tightening the ligaments spanning the bulge – the posterior longitudinal ligament in particular. In order to achieve these effects traction would need to produce separation of the intervertebral and zygapophyseal joints between the vertebrae accompanied by tensioning of the intervertebral ligaments.

To demonstrate the separation of the vertebrae Cyriax (1982) compared two X-rays of the cervical spine taken before and after the application of 'fairly' strong manual traction for several seconds. He measured an increase of 2.5 mm at each of the joints between the fourth cervical and first thoracic vertebrae. His maximum manual traction had previously been estimated to be 140 kg, in an experiment in 1955, but his use of the term 'fairly' implies something less than that. Similarly, before and after X-rays of the lumbar spine were superimposed upon each other after 50 kg of traction had been applied for 10 min, and a widening of the disc space was observed.

Judovitch (1952) took a series of X-rays as progressive poundages were applied to the cervical spine of seven patients. He observed that with 45 lb (20.5 kg) of static, vertical traction there was separation of the interbody joints of C2–7 and a small widening of the zygapophyseal joints. A similar serial study was performed by Colachis and Strohm (1966), but using 30 lb (14 kg) of intermittent cervical traction at a 24° angle of pull. In all 10 subjects the mean separation of the vertebrae increased proportionally, both anteriorly and posteriorly, to a maximum at 25 min.

On the assumption that increased disc space with traction would be manifest in an increase in height, Worden and Humphrey (1964) applied sustained traction of up to 132 lb (60 kg) to normal fit males. The traction was divided between the head and thorax and pelvis and ankles for 1 h on each of several consecutive days. They demonstrated an average increase in height of 8 mm.

They continued to observe two subjects and noted that they lost their increased height at a rate of 4 mm per hour. In the Colachis and Strohm study, mentioned above, no increase in posterior separation remained at 20 min after the cessation of traction but the residual anterior separation was statistically significant (Colachis and Strohm, 1966).

Mathews (1968) used epidurography, involving the injection of radiopaque contrast medium into the epidural space for subsequent radiological investigation, and applied 120 lb (55 kg) of lumbar traction to three patients, two with suspected disc protrusions and one control. In one patient the bulge of the protrusion began to decrease in depth from 4 min and was further decreased at 20 min, with partial recurrence on release.

Evidence was provided for Cyriax's proposed suction effect on observing a second patient where not only was there a reduction in the depth of the multiple protrusions, but contrast medium appeared to have been drawn into the disc spaces, implying the production of negative pressure within the disc.

The apparent suction effect may be a sequel to the reduction of load on the disc when traction is applied. Nachemson (1980), with the use of a miniature intradiscal pressure transducer, measured the approximate load on the L3 disc in a 70 kg individual, in different postures and exercises. Minimal load of 30 kg was recorded on the disc with the subject in supine lying; this was reduced to 10 kg on the application of 30 kg of traction.

This finding provided foundation for Cyriax's suggestion that the same effect on a disc prolapse could be achieved in a short time with sustained traction as that brought about by weeks or months of bed rest. Bed rest had disadvantages in terms of expense, if prolonged hospitalization was involved, as well as incapacitating the patient. Lumbar traction, on the other hand, would allow the patient to continue with daily activities and commitments.

However, since the ambulant position subjects the disc to compressive forces, certain considerations need to be applied to prevent the loss of the benefits of traction between treatments.

Cyriax (1982) claimed that traction needs to be:

- As strong as possible.
- Applied for as long as was both practicable and tolerable.
- Applied daily, or at least five times a week.
- Applied continuously.

When Cyriax proposed that the physiological and biomechanical effects of static traction were more effective at reducing a nuclear protrusion, the debate of continuous (static) versus intermittent traction had little evidence to support either side.

Wyke, referred to in Cyriax (1982), observed that motor activity in the sacrospinalis muscles increased as the distracting force was increased, until the mechanoreceptors in the tendons were stimulated, producing an inhibitory effect after which the stress was allowed to fall on the spinal joints. Cyriax claimed that electromyographic (EMG) silence in the sacrospinalis was not achieved until 3 min into the application of traction. For this reason he proposed that intermittent traction would not be as suitable to produce nuclear movement, since repeated pulls of shorter duration would continually elicit the stretch reflex, producing muscular contraction and preventing joint distraction.

Cyriax's argument for wanting to avoid muscular contraction is supported by the study of Goldie and Reichmann (1977) to examine the influence of traction on the cervical spine. They observed that the force of muscle contraction in the cervical spine could overcome a traction force in excess of 30 kg (66 lb).

However, Hood and Chrisman (1968) used EMG recordings of lumbar sacrospinalis activity to compare the effect of static and intermittent traction and found no difference. Moreover, Klaber Moffatt *et al.* (1990) investigated the effects of sustained cervical traction on neck musculature using EMG recordings. They applied 6–12 lb (3–5 kg) of traction for 20 min in the recumbent position, but found that relaxation was not induced.

Support for sustained, as opposed to intermittent, traction may lie in the hydrostatic behaviour of the disc (Nachemson, 1980). Sustained traction would be expected to be more effective in producing creep in the tissues gradually to reduce the herniation by the combined effect of both suction from within the disc and the 'push' produced by the tightening of the tissues spanning the joint.

Onel *et al.* (1989) performed computed tomographic investigation of 30 patients diagnosed as having disc prolapse to observe the effect of traction on lumbar disc herniations. Whilst establishing that 45 kg of traction was effective in reducing disc herniations, it was also apparent that intervertebral joint and zygapophyseal joint space was increased, with associated stretching of all anatomical structures of the spine. Grieve (1981) had already acknowledged the much wider range of application of traction, irrespective of the disc. The effect of traction on other tissues would suggest that it should be seen as a useful and adaptable method of mobilization of the motion segment, or segments, as a whole. This being so, intermittent traction would also have a place in mobilizing stiffness in the motion segments, relieving pain through the stimulation of the mechanoreceptors and by increasing circulation, as well as by reducing the compressive effects.

Indications for spinal traction

Cyriax (1982) identified factors from the patient's history, together with certain symptoms and signs, which he believed were characteristic of a nuclear disc protrusion. Treatment with sustained traction was therefore indicated to reduce the protrusion.

He described that with a nuclear protrusion, the pain is usually of gradual onset, with no recollection of the mode or time of onset. There is usually little central pain, but referred pain is usually present in the arm or leg. The pattern of spinal movement is non-capsular and the movements provoke the limb pain.

Cyriax ascribed the pathology to posterolateral movement of the protrusion, compressing the dural nerve root sleeve and producing unilateral pain. Smyth and Wright (1958) had also proposed this mechanism but when, in the light of investigation, opinion moved away from the notion of a 'jelly-like' nucleus, thus refuting the possibility of a nuclear ooze, Cyriax's hypothesis was largely rejected. The empirical findings none the less remained that traction could afford relief with that particular onset and pattern of pain.

Mathews and Hickling (1975) suggested that traction should be applied to a defined syndrome rather than a specific condition. This would appear to be a more satisfactory premise against which clinicians from the myriad of musculoskeletal backgrounds can apply the basic principles, whilst the debate on pathology continues as fresh evidence emerges.

Apart from the application of mechanical traction, in the cervical spine most of the mobilization and manipulation techniques are performed under manual traction. In the rotational techniques in the lumbar spine, a degree of distraction is applied to the joints with the Grade C manipulation.

Indications for traction at peripheral joints

Stiff osteoarthritic joints respond well to distraction, as do joints demonstrating the capsular pattern following adaptive changes in response to traumatic arthritis. The distraction is applied to increase

Clinical tip

When applying the techniques of traction or distraction to the cervical spine or peripheral joints, the following principles should be employed:

- Maximum body weight should be used.
- The application of body weight should be achieved by leaning out with straight arms.
- The distraction/traction should be sustained a moment or two to become established before proceeding with the manoeuvre.

mobility, using longitudinal or lateral distraction techniques, which produce separation of joint surfaces and assist mobilization by stretching the joint capsule and capsular ligaments.

It may be applied manually as a treatment in itself or in conjunction with mobilization and manipulation techniques.

Where signs and symptoms indicate the presence of a loose body in a joint, or a carpal bone needs to be relocated, distraction before Grade A mobilization is applied. The distraction of joint surfaces allows space for movement of the fragment, assisted by the accompanying suction effect, which distraction tends to produce.

Orthopaedic medicine injection techniques

In orthopaedic medicine, injection techniques are often an alternative treatment to transverse friction massage and mobilization techniques. Whereas transverse friction massage and mobilization appear to be most efficacious when used together or with other physiotherapy modalities, injection techniques stand alone. The drugs administered often have effects for some time after the application of treatment and they must be given time to achieve these beneficial effects. In many instances the orthopaedic medicine clinician has a choice of treatment, either injection or transverse friction massage and mobilization, e.g. tendinitis. In some cases an injection is more appropriate, e.g. bursitis, and in others, transverse friction massage may be more appropriate, e.g. musculotendinous lesions. Injections tend to be more cost-effective when compared to manual therapy, e.g. capsulitis. The need for collaboration between the patient, physician and physiotherapist is emphasized to ascertain the best mode of treatment for the patient.

> **Types of injection applied in orthopaedic medicine**
>
> - Local anaesthetic.
> - Corticosteroid.
> - Sclerosant.

Local anaesthetic

The earliest local anaesthetic, cocaine, first used in 1860, was used as a local anaesthetic for surgery. A synthetic substitute, procaine, was developed in 1905 and many other compounds have since been produced.

Local anaesthetics work by penetrating the nerve sheath and axon membrane. In the normal resting state, the membrane of a nerve is polarized. The membrane is permeable to potassium ions and relatively impermeable to sodium ions, and the inside of the nerve fibre is negatively charged in relation to the outside, which is positively charged.

Stimulation of the nerve causes changes in the resting state called depolarization. The permeability of the membrane is altered, opening the channel to sodium ions which then pass freely across the membrane. This inflow of positive ions means that the inside of the fibre becomes relatively positively charged. Excitation of nerve and muscle fibres is brought about by this sequential opening and closing of the sodium and potassium channels in the cell

> **Uses in orthopaedic medicine**
>
> - Used alone for diagnostic purposes.
> - Used together with corticosteroids for diagnostic purposes and therapeutic pain relief for the patient.
> - To treat chronic bursitis.
> - As part of an epidural injection via the sacral hiatus.

membrane, which is interrupted by the use of local anaesthetics that specifically block sodium channels.

A change in cell membrane potential that accompanies these activities is called an action potential. Each region of the nerve fibre, in turn, excites the next and a nerve impulse is propagated along the fibre. Local anaesthetics inhibit the initiation and propagation of the action potential.

Local anaesthetics tend to block conduction more readily in small-diameter, myelinated and unmyelinated nerve fibres. Nociceptive and sympathetic impulses are therefore blocked more readily (Rang *et al.*, 1995).

This pain-relieving effect of local anaesthetic is utilized in orthopaedic medicine for its therapeutic and diagnostic effects. Given together with corticosteroid it allows immediate reassessment of the patient to confirm diagnosis and to ensure that the lesion has been completely infiltrated. It gives the patient initial pain relief and may reduce the effects of post-injection flare from corticosteroid injection.

Two local anaesthetics used in orthopaedic medicine

Procaine	Lignocaine
Moderate rate of onset	Rapid rate of onset
Short duration	Moderate duration
Used mainly as 0.5% solution	Used as 0.5%, 1% or 2% solution
Maximum dose 1 g*	Maximum dose 200 mg*
Acidic	

* These maximum doses apply to local anaesthetic given by infiltration to a fit adult of average weight. It would be unsafe to give such doses intravenously.

Unwanted side-effects of local anaesthetic

It is important to recognize the maximum dose of local anaesthetic in order to avoid the unwanted side-effects (Rang *et al.*, 1995) and patients should always be questioned about sensitivity to previous injections.

Central nervous system effects

Local anaesthetics cause stimulation of the central nervous system in the first instance and this may be displayed as restlessness and tremor, confusion and agitation. Tremor may progress to convulsion and increasing doses lead to respiratory depression.

Cardiovascular effects

Local anaesthetic administration may cause a combination of myocardial depression and vasodilatation producing sudden hypotension which may be life-threatening. Myocardial depression occurs as a result of inhibition of sodium current in cardiac muscle. Vasodilatation is due to the local anaesthetic effect on the smooth muscle of the arterioles and sympathetic inhibition.

Corticosteroid injections

Corticosteroids have a potent anti-inflammatory effect, much more dramatic than the anti-inflammatory effect of non-steroidal anti-inflammatory drugs (NSAIDs), and are therefore used therapeutically to achieve this effect in orthopaedic medicine. They are applied intra-articularly or intralesionally for chronic inflammatory lesions. The intense anti-inflammatory effect is beneficial in some acute lesions (e.g. acute bursitis, rheumatoid arthritis) but is unwanted in other conditions (e.g. acute muscle belly lesion and acute ligamentous lesions) because of its detrimental effects on collagen production.

As well as its anti-inflammatory effect, corticosteroids have other potent effects, including immunosuppression and a delay in the normal physiological process of healing. These effects cannot be separated from the beneficial effects of corticosteroids. Much of the reported unwanted effects of corticosteroids involve systemic, high-dose applications of the drugs for long periods of time.

A locally applied injection of corticosteroid in orthopaedic medicine aims to achieve a rapid and intense local anti-inflammatory effect. The local effect will depend on the dose applied, the relative potency of the corticosteroid and its solubility, which determines the length of time it stays in the tissues. In orthopaedic medicine the aim is to give the smallest dose that will achieve the desired effects. Intra-articular injections are most appropriate if there is an inflammatory component, therefore they are indicated whenever a joint capsule is inflamed, e.g. in rheumatoid arthritis traumatic arthritis and acute episodes of osteoarthrosis. Intralesional injections are applied to chronic tendinitis, tenosynovitis, bursitis and some ligamentous sprains.

The use of corticosteroids would seem to affect all stages of the inflammatory process, the initial acute phase of heat, redness, swelling and pain, as well as the proliferative phases of repair and remodelling.

The effects of corticosteroids may be due to one or more of the following.

- Vasoconstriction of the small blood vessels which reduces fluid exudation and leukocyte infiltration in the acute inflammatory phase.
- Reduction in the permeability of the synovial membrane, with the corticosteroid being taken up selectively by the synovium.
- In arthritis, corticosteroids are most effective in the presence of active inflammation.
- Reduction in the activity of the macrophages, which delays the clearing up operation. This in turn delays the repair phase.
- Inhibition of the macrophage, which also acts as a director cell. Impairing its function of initiating the number of fibroblasts directed to the area will delay the repair process. Corticosteroids administered after the macrophage invasion have much less influence on wound healing (Fowler, 1989).

Uses in orthopaedic medicine

- **Chronic enthesitis, tendinitis and tenosynovitis.**
- **Acute and chronic bursitis.**
- **Inflammatory arthritis and acute episodes of degenerative osteoathrosis.**
- **Epidural, via sacral hiatus.**
- **Nerve entrapment syndromes.**
- **Some ligament sprains.**

At a cellular level corticosteroids reduce the production of the chemical mediators of inflammation – prostaglandins, histamine and kinins. They directly penetrate the cell wall and modify protein synthesis to produce anti-inflammatory mediators called lipocortins which in turn inhibit the production of prostaglandins and leukotrienes (Agambar and Flower, 1990; Grillet and Dequeker, 1990).

During the repair phase the net result of a reduced number of fibroblasts is to reduce the quality and quantity of the matrix, collagen fibres and ground substance (Stephens *et al.*, 1971; Noyes, 1977; Priestley, 1978; Van Story-Lewis and Tenenbaum, 1986). Corticosteroids are thought to reduce the tensile strength of closed wounds, but generally this effect only occurs if the corticosteroid is administered in the first 2–3 days following injury, when it affects the early inflammatory phase and the macrophage function.

There is a difference of opinion in the literature about the effect of corticosteroids on collagen synthesis in the repair and remodelling phases (Sandberg, 1964; Ehrlich and Hunt, 1968; Ehrlich *et al.*, 1972; Kulick *et al.*, 1984). Cohen *et al.* (1977) measured collagen synthesis and found it was suppressed by long-term large doses of a sustained-release form of methylprednisolone. Intermittent doses appeared not to alter collagen synthesis. Human keloid scar formation was softened and reduced by intralesional doses of corticosteroids.

Collagen synthesis is thought to be altered, but not inhibited by, the action of corticosteroids, with a greater degradation of collagen fibres. This leads to the production of new immature scar tissue which is pliable and influenced by movement. This effect can be applied to the use of intralesional corticosteroid administration for chronic soft-tissue lesions such as tendinitis, where the degradation of mature collagen fibres softens the scar and new, immature collagen is laid down to be influenced by normal movement.

This effect of softening collagen tissue and reducing its tensile strength affects the normal collagen tissue as well as the scar tissue collagen. It is important that this should be recognized and the patient instructed to rest from the aggravating factors following administration of corticosteroids. Marks *et al.* (1983) showed that wound healing was significantly delayed by the application of topical steroids.

Corticosteroid injections seem to be most appropriate for chronic lesions where the inflammation is excessive. Their potent anti-inflammatory effect inhibits the normal inflammatory phase required to produce healing in acute soft-tissue lesions involving disruption.

Corticosteroids also produce a potent immunosuppressive effect which is why it is so important to pay attention to aseptic technique.

The relative potency is available for corticosteroids administered systemically, but not for their intra-articular or intralesional use. The box gives the relative potency of corticosteroids, which have been licensed for use where there is an inflammatory component, using hydrocortisone as the standard (Rang *et al.*, 1995).

Steroid	Relative potency
Hydrocortisone	1
Prednisolone	4
Methylprednisolone	5
Triamcinolone	5
Dexamethasone	30

Hydrocortisone acetate is a relatively soluble, weak anti-inflammatory agent which is usually absorbed within 36 h. The synthetic corticosteroids are more potent but generally less soluble than hydrocortisone acetate and their anti-inflammatory effects are more prolonged. Triamcinolone hexacetonide takes 14–21 days to be absorbed from a joint; triamcinolone acetonide takes slightly less time (Cameron, 1995). The duration of action of the corticosteroids is qualified in terms of their biological half-life but this relates to systemic application of the drugs.

Least prolonged	**Hydrocortisone**
(about 36 h) *Relatively soluble*	**Prednisolone acetate**
More prolonged **(about 14–21 days)**	**Methylprednisolone** **Dexamethasone** **Triamcinolone acetonide**
Most prolonged **(weeks–months)** *Most insoluble*	**Triamcinolone hexacetonide**

In this text the corticosteroid referred to is triamcinolone acetonide. The two different concentrations of triamcinolone acetonide, Adcortyl and Kenalog, provide versatility for different applications. Table 4.1 lists the preparations currently used for soft-tissue lesions (other drugs and information are available on current data sheets).

Table 4.1 Drugs used in soft-tissue lesions

Generic name	Trade name	Presentation
Hydrocortisone acetate 25 mg/ml	Hydrocortistab injection	1-ml ampoules
Prednisolone acetate BP 25 mg/ml	Deltastab	1-ml ampoules
Methylprednisolone acetate 40 mg/ml	Depo-Medrone	1-, 2- and 3-ml vials
Triamcinolone acetonide 10 mg/ml	Adcortyl	1-ml ampoules
Triamcinolone acetonide 40 mg/ml	Kenalog	1-ml vials
Triamcinolone hexacetonide 20 mg/ml	Lederspan 20 mg/ml	1- and 5-ml vials
Dexamethasone sodium phosphate 4 mg/ml	Decadron injection	2-ml vials
Dexamethasone sodium phosphate 5 mg/ml	Dexamethasone injection (Organon)	2-ml vials and 1-ml ampoules

Corticosteroid injection technique

The appropriate dose (corticosteroid alone, or mixed with local anaesthetic) will be determined by the size of the joint or lesion to be injected and the previous response to injection, if any.

Triamcinolone acetonide

- Adcortyl 10 mg/ml for large-volume injections.
- Kenalog 40 mg/ml for small-volume injections.

Accurate needle placement is essential. This depends on clinical diagnosis.

Knowledge of anatomy will allow accurate location of the lesion and avoid unnecessary complications. Points worth considering are:

- The tissue in which the lesion lies.
- How deep the lesion lies.
- The extent of the lesion.
- The position of the patient to make the site of the lesion accessible.
- The direction in which the needle should be inserted.
- The length of needle and the size of syringe required.

Needle size

	Imperial size	Metric size	Hub colour
Fine-bore	$25G \times \frac{5}{8}$ in	0.5×16 mm	Orange
	$23G \times 1$ in	0.6×25 mm	Blue
	$23G \times 1\frac{3}{4}$ in	0.6×30 mm	Blue
	$21G \times 1\frac{1}{2}$ in	0.8×40 mm	Green
	$21G \times 2$ in	0.8×50 mm	Green
Large-bore	$19G \times 1\frac{1}{2}$ in	1.1×40 mm	White

Spinal needles

Various sizes from $1\frac{1}{2}$ to $3\frac{1}{2}$ in.
$20G \times 3\frac{1}{2}$ in $(0.9 \times 90$ mm) is a useful size for orthopaedic medicine.

Syringes

Relevant sizes for orthopaedic medicine are: 1-, 2-, 5-, 10-, 20- and 50-ml syringes.

To inject a relatively tough tendon, pressure is required. This can be achieved by using a 1-ml syringe which has a smaller piston, producing a higher pressure for a given force.

An aseptic no-touch technique is essential to avoid introducing infection. Avoid injecting in the presence of infection because the corticosteroid also has an immunosuppressive effect.

- Explain the procedure to the patient.
- Position patient with the lesion accessible and mark the injection site (pen, thumb nail).
- Ensure that the injection site is medicolegally clean using an appropriate antiseptic (e.g. chlorhexidine in spirit).
- Wash and dry hands, preferably using surgical scrub.
- Draw up the appropriate dosage of corticosteroid and local anaesthetic using disposable syringes and needles. Single-dose

containers should be used wherever possible and discarded after use.

- Change the needle, discarding the one used for drawing up the dose.
- Give the injection without touching the needle or the injection site.
- Withdraw the needle and apply the appropriate dressing.
- Issue the patient with instructions to rest from aggravating factors and avoid painful movements for up to 2 weeks.

Two techniques are generally used to deliver the injection. A *bolus technique* is used for joint spaces and bursae, where no resistance is felt on pressing the plunger. A *peppering technique* is used for tendons and ligaments where a series of small droplets is delivered throughout the substance of the structure to cover the extent and depth of the lesion.

Lack of response to corticosteroid injection may require a review of the diagnosis and the technique. It is fairly common to have a relapse or recurrence of symptoms in soft-tissue lesions. This is particularly likely if the patient returns to the overuse activity too soon or the cause of the problem is not properly investigated and remedied.

Unwanted side-effects of corticosteroid therapy

Most of the unpleasant side-effects of corticosteroid therapy relate to large, long-term doses of the drugs taken systemically. It is rare to produce systemic side-effects from a single local corticosteroid injection, but it can happen.

Systemic effects include:

- Hyperglycaemia in a diabetic patient.
- Suppression of endogenous cortisol may be deleterious to patients who develop infection or require surgery within 3 days of corticosteroid injection. The attending doctor should be made aware of this recent treatment.
- Facial flushing in the first 2–3 days and lasting a day or two.
- Menstrual disturbance, including postmenopausal bleeding. Generally, doses in excess of 40 mg may produce an effect on menstruation but occasionally even 20 mg can upset the cycle.

Afterpain

This is caused by a post-injection flare which is usually a localized response of increased pain occurring up to 12 h, and occasionally up to 48 h, after injection when the local anaesthetic effect has worn off. It is something the patient should be warned about to prevent alarm and the appropriate use of analgesics explained. This flare tends to be less common with those corticosteroids with a more prolonged effect, e.g. triamcinolone acetonide. Berger and Yount (1990) reported a case of a patient who developed a general post-injection flare 90 min after injection of 40 mg triamcinolone hexacetonide and rare cases of anaphylactic shock have also been reported in the use of systemic corticosteroids (Larsson, 1989).

Dermatological changes

Inaccurate needle placement and/or leakage of fluid, particularly of long-acting corticosteroids, into subcutaneous tissue have been documented to promote fat necrosis, dermal atrophy, senile purpura, depigmentation and subcutaneous atrophy (Ponec *et al.*, 1977; Marks *et al.*, 1983; Grillet and Dequeker, 1990). These subcutaneous changes may be reversible, although the patient may be left with long-lasting evidence of injection.

Tendon rupture

Corticosteroids have an effect on the fibroblasts and collagen. They are given to reduce chronic inflammation and pain and have a potent effect. The balance of collagen synthesis is altered to produce degradation of fibres and new immature scar tissue is laid down. Appropriate mobilization is required at the right time to encourage alignment of fibres and increased tensile strength.

The corticosteroid will affect the normal tissue as well as the damaged tissue. During its time of action, corticosteroid potentially causes a weakening of collagen fibres, damaged and normal, and this should be recognized as a potential hazard. The patient is instructed to rest from aggravating activities whilst normal, painfree function is encouraged, to provide mechanical stimulus for the new fibres. Since triamcinolone acetonide is absorbed within approximately a 2-week period, it would seem appropriate to advise the patient to rest for up to 2 weeks if practical.

Cases of tendon rupture have been reported following corticosteroid injection. However, chronic inflammation of a tendon and its inherent poor blood supply make it susceptible to rupture in any event and rupture may be a coincidence rather than directly caused by injection (Kleinman and Gross, 1983).

A mailing from the Committee on Safety of Medicines (1995) drew attention to tendon damage associated with quinolone antibiotics, e.g. Ciproxin. Although inflammation and rupture of tendons may be rare, the elderly and those treated concurrently with corticosteroids were considered to be at particular risk of tendon rupture.

Steroid arthropathy

There is a general consensus that repeated corticosteroid injections into weight-bearing joints should be limited to a maximum of two, or perhaps three, per year because of the risk of steroid arthropathy. A Charcot-type arthropathy has been reported in association with corticosteroid injections; however more recent reports have refuted this (Grillet and Dequeker, 1990; Cameron, 1995). It has been considered that the deterioration in the cartilage and joint may be more likely to be due to the underlying inflammatory or degenerative condition rather than the treatment with corticosteroids.

It is appropriate to instruct the patient to rest following intra-articular injection. Cameron (1995) reviewed the evidence on steroid arthropathy and found that the greatest risk of its development is from prolonged, high-dose oral steroids in the presence of associated underlying disease. Evidence exists for injected corticosteroids to be chondroprotective rather than destructive. Patients with rheumatoid arthritis or liver disease, those taking concurrent doses of NSAIDs and those given many injections at close intervals are concluded to be genuinely at risk from steroid arthropathy.

Non-steroidal anti-inflammatory drugs

These are some of the most widely used drugs for musculoskeletal lesions as well as the symptoms of headaches, flu, colds and other minor aches and pains. However, nearly all NSAIDs have side-effects, the most notorious being gastrointestinal problems, which caution against their long-term use. NSAIDs seem to have their action within the injured tissue itself.

NSAIDs produce the following three main effects:

- *Anti-inflammatory*: they modify the inflammatory reaction by reducing vasodilatation, oedema and permeability of the post-capillary venules.
- *Analgesic*: they reduce pain by inhibiting prostaglandin formation. They are therefore most effective in treating the chemical pain produced by inflammation in which the prostaglandins sensitize the nociceptors. They have little effect in mechanical pain, which is why they are not particularly effective in treating the acute pain associated with recent disc protrusion.
- *Antipyretic*: they reduce a raised temperature, but have no effect on the normal body temperature.

NSAIDs commonly prescribed include ibuprofen, naproxen, indomethacin, piroxicam, diclofenac and aspirin.

In acute inflammatory musculoskeletal lesions, e.g. acute muscle belly lesions, acute ligament sprains and acute tenosynovitis, it is probably better to allow the first 3–5 days of the inflammatory phase to pass before using anti-inflammatory drugs such as the corticosteroids (Boruta *et al.*, 1990). If the condition is very painful, NSAIDs may be administered, or other analgesics such as paracetamol together with the physical treatments of controlled and precise mobilization, coupled with relative rest, ice, compression and elevation (RICE). In chronic inflammatory states, however, the use of corticosteroid injection is strongly indicated and most beneficial, but the patient should be instructed to rest following injection.

Sclerosant therapy (prolotherapy)

The aim of sclerosant therapy is to increase ligament or tendon mass and ligament–bone or tendon–bone strength. Experiments have shown a statistically significant increase in collagen fibril diameters (Liu *et al.*, 1983), suggesting that sclerosing solution has an influence on connective tissue at the insertion sites.

P2G

- Phenol 2% w/v.
- Dextrose 25% w/v.
- Glycerol 30% w/v.

Other sclerosant solutions include hypertonic dextrose and sodium morrhuate.

P2G causes an intense inflammatory reaction at the site of injection. The intention in producing such an intense inflammatory reaction is to stimulate the formation of scar tissue. The immature scar tissue laid down is encouraged to contract and shorten by avoiding movement and stress during the repair and remodelling phases. The intense reaction causes considerable pain, but it would not be rational to use anti-inflammatory medication following sclerosant therapy.

Unwanted side-effect of sclerosant therapy

Strong phenol penetrates the nerve endings producing a local anaesthetic effect (Goodman and Gilman, 1970) which is permanent. It is not known whether the very low concentrations used in sclerosant injections has any effect other than antiseptic.

Uses in orthopaedic medicine

- Recurrent or chronic episodes of low back pain, with or without leg pain.
- Recurrent sacroiliac joint subluxation.
- Other conditions associated with ligamentous laxity, e.g. subluxing capitate bone.

Summary of principles of orthopaedic medicine treatment applied to soft-tissue lesions

Contractile lesions

Acute muscle belly strain

Days 1–5 (daily treatment)

- RICE.
- Gentle transverse friction massage in shortened position.
- Grade A mobilization aiming to broaden fibres; no stress on the healing breach.

Days 5–10 (increasing the interval between treatment sessions)

- Increasing depth of transverse friction massage.
- Increasing range of Grade A mobilization aiming to 'nudge' pain to stress fibres sufficiently without disrupting the healing breach.

Day 10 onwards

- Continue increasing depth of transverse friction massage and range of Grade A mobilization until full painfree function is restored.
- Treating the patient in this way should avoid the need to stretch contracted scar tissue.

Chronic muscle belly strain

- Deep transverse friction massage with muscle belly in shortened position.
- Vigorous Grade A mobilization.
- No stretching until the muscle tests painfree on resisted testing.

Musculotendinous lesion

- Deep transverse friction massage is usually the treatment of choice.

Chronic tendinitis

- Cortiocosteroid injection using a peppering technique or deep transverse friction massage.
- Relative rest allowing painfree movement, but avoiding overuse activity.

A special technique, the Mills' manipulation, is applied after the transverse friction massage to a lesion of the teno-osseous junction of tennis elbow only.

Acute tenosynovitis

- Daily treatment of gentle transverse friction massage.
- Ice and relative rest.

Chronic tenosynovitis

- Corticosteroid injection using a bolus technique or deep transverse friction massage with the tendon on the stretch.
- Relative rest allowing painfree movement, but no overuse activity.

Inert tissue lesions

Acute capsulitis

- Corticosteroid injection using a bolus technique to treat the pain.

Subacute capsulitis

- Corticosteroid injection using a bolus technique or Grade B mobilization.

Acute bursitis

- Corticosteroid injection plus an appropriate volume of local anaesthetic using a peppering or bolus technique.

Chronic bursitis

- Large volume of low-dose local anaesthetic plus an appropriate amount of corticosteroid using a bolus or peppering technique.
- Relative rest allowing painfree movement, but no overuse activity.

Acute ligament sprain

Days 1–5 (daily treatment)

- RICE.
- Gentle transverse friction massage.
- Grade A mobilization to move the ligament over the underlying bone.
- Gait correction, partial weight-bearing on crutches if necessary.

Days 5–10 (increasing the interval between treatment sessions)

- Increasing depth of transverse friction massage.
- Increasing range of Grade A mobilization, aiming to 'nudge' pain to stress fibres sufficiently without disrupting the healing breach.

Day 10 onwards

- Continue increasing depth of transverse friction massage and range of Grade A mobilization until full painfree function is restored.

Chronic ligament sprain

- Deep transverse friction massage.
- Vigorous Grade A mobilization.

In a chronic sprain of the medial collateral ligament at the knee and the lateral collateral ligament at the ankle, a Grade C manipulation is used to rupture adhesions between the ligament and the bone, after the ligament has been prepared by transverse friction massage.

Ligamentous laxity

- A course of sclerosant injections.

Loose body or subluxed carpal bone

- Reduce under strong distraction and Grade A mobilization.

Spinal intra-articular displacement

Cervical intervertebral disc displacement

Acute pain

- Gentle traction and Grade A mobilization.

Subacute pain

- Mobilization under traction progressing to manipulation under traction if necessary.

Thoracic intra-articular displacement

- Manipulation.

Lumbar intervertebral disc displacement

Acute pain

- Grade A mobilization.

Subacute pain

- Manipulation.
- Traction.
- Epidural injection.

Sacroiliac joint

- Manipulation.
- Course of sclerosant injections.

References

Abenhaim, L., Bergeron, A.M. (1992) Twenty years of randomized trials of manipulative therapy for back pain: a review. *Clinical and Investigative Medicine* **15**: 527–535.

Agambar, L., Flower, R. (1990) Anti-inflammatory drugs: history and mechanism of action. *Physiotherapy* **76**: 198–202.

Akeson, W. (1990) The response of ligaments to stress modulation and overview of the ligament healing response. In: *Knee Ligaments: Structure, Function, Injury and Repair* (Daniel, D. *et al.*, eds). Raven Press, pp. 315–327.

Akeson, W., Amiel, D., La Violette, D. (1967) The connective tissue response to immobility: a study of chondroitin-4 and 6-sulfate and dermatan sulfate changes in periarticular connective tissue of control and immobilised knees of dogs. *Clinical Orthopaedics* **51**: 183–197.

Akeson, W., Woo, S.L.-Y., Amiel, D. *et al.* (1973) The connective tissue response to immobility: biochemical changes in periarticular connective tissue of the immobilised rabbit's knee. *Clinical Orthopaedics* **93**: 356–362.

Akeson, W., Amiel, D., Woo, S.L.-Y. (1980) Immobility effects on synovial joints, the pathomechanics of joint contracture. *Biorheology* **17**: 95–110.

Akeson, W., Amiel, D., Abel, M.F. *et al.* (1986) Effects of immobilisation on joints. *Clinical Orthopaedics and Related Research* **219**: 28–37.

Amis, A.A. (1985) Biomechanics of ligaments. In: *Ligament Injuries and their Treatment* (Jenkins, D.H.R. ed.). Chapman and Hall Medical, pp. 3–28.

Arem, A.J., Madden, J.W. (1976) Effects of stress on healing wounds: 1 intermittent noncyclical tension. *Journal of Surgical Research* **20**: 93–102.

Barker, M.E. (1994) Spinal manipulation: a general practice study. *Journal of Orthopaedic Medicine* **16**: 42–44.

Berger, R.G., Yount, W.J. (1990) Immediate 'steroid flare' from intra-articular triamcinolone hexacetonide injection: case report and review of the literature. *Arthritis and Rheumatism* **33**: 1284–1286.

Boruta, P.M., Bishop, J.O., Braly, W.G., Tullos, H.S. (1990) Acute lateral ankle ligament injuries: a literature review. *Foot and Ankle* **11**: 107–113.

Bowsher, D. (1988) Modulation of nociceptive input. In: *Pain Management by Physiotherapy*, 2nd edn (Wells, P.E., Frampton, V., Bowsher, D. eds). Butterworth-Heinemann, pp. 30–31.

Burke-Evans, E., Eggers, G.W.N., Butler, J.K., Blumel, J. (1960) Experimental immobilisation and remobilisation of rat knee joints. *Journal of Bone and Joint Surgery* **42-A**: 737–758.

Cameron, G. (1995) Steroid arthropathy: myth or reality? A review of the evidence. *Journal of Orthopaedic Medicine* **17**: 51–55.

Carreck, A. (1994) The effect of massage on pain perception threshold. *Manipulative Physiotherapist* **26**: 10–16.

Cohen, I.K., Diegelmann, R.F., Johnson, M.L. (1977) Effect of corticosteroids on collagen synthesis. *Surgery* **82**: 15–20.

Colachis, S.C., Strohm, B.R. (1965) A study of tractive forces and angle of pull on vertebral interspaces in the cervical spine. *Archives of Physical Medicine and Rheumatology* **46**: 820–830.

Colachis, S.C., Strohm, B.R. (1966) Effect of duration of intermittent cervical traction on vertebral separation. *Archives of Physical Medicine and Rehabilitation* **47**: 353–359.

Committee on Safety of Medicines (1995) *Tendon Damage Associated with Quinolone Antibiotics*. HMSO.

Cyriax, J. (1982) *Textbook of Orthopaedic Medicine*, vol. 1, 8th edn. Baillière Tindall.

Cyriax, J.H., Cyriax P.J. (1983) *Illustrated Manual of Orthopaedic Medicine*. Butterworths.

de Bruijn, R. (1984) Deep transverse friction: its analgesic effect. *International Journal of Sports Medicine* **5**: 35–36.

Ehrlich, H.P., Hunt, T.K. (1968) Effects of cortisone and vitamin A on wound healing. *Annals of Surgery* **167**: 324–328.

Ehrlich, P.H., Tarver, H., Hunt, T.K. (1972) Effects of vitamin A and glucocorticoids upon inflammation and collagen synthesis. *Annals of Surgery* **177**: 222–227.

Enneking, W.F., Horowitz, M. (1972) The intra-articular effects of immobilisation of the human knee. *Journal of Bone and Joint Surgery* **54**: 973–985.

Evans, P. (1980) The healing process at cellular level: a review. *Physiotherapy* **66**: 256–259.

Fowler, J.D. (1989) Wound healing: an overview. *Seminars in Veterinary Medicine and Surgery* **4**: 256–262.

Goats, G.C. (1994) Massage – the scientific basis of an ancient art: part 1. The techniques. *British Journal of Sports Medicine* **28**: 149–152.

Goldie, I.F., Reichmann, S. (1977) The biomechanical influence of traction on the cervical spine. *Scandinavian Journal of Rehabilitation Medicine* **9**: 31–34.

Goodman, L.S., Gilman, A. (1970) *The Pharmacological Basis of Therapeutics*, 4th edn. Macmillan.

Grieve, G.P. (1981) *Common Vertebral Joint Problems*. Churchill Livingstone.

Grillet, B., Dequeker, J. (1990) Intra-articular steroid injection: a risk benefit assessment. *Drug Safety* **5**: 205–211.

Hadler, N.M., Curtis, P., Gillings, D.B., Stinnett, S. (1987) A benefit of spinal manipulation as adjunctive therapy for acute low back pain: a stratified controlled trial. *Spine* **12**: 703–706.

Hardy, M.A. (1989) The biology of scar formation. *Physical Therapy* **69**: 1014–1023.

Herzog, W., Conway, P.J., Kawchuk, G.N. *et al.* (1993) Forces exerted during spinal manipulative therapy. *Spine* **18**: 1206–1212.

Hood, L.B., Chrisman, D. (1968) Intermittent pelvic traction in the treatment of the ruptured intervertebral disk. *Physical Therapy* **48**: 21–30.

Hume Kendall, P. (1955) A history of lumbar traction. *Physiotherapy* **41**: 177–179.

Hunter, G. (1994) Specific soft tissue mobilisation in the treatment of soft tissue lesions. *Physiotherapy* **80**: 15–21.

Ingham, B. (1981) Transverse friction massage for the relief of tennis elbow. *Physician and Sports Medicine* **9**: 116.

Järvinen, M.J., Lehto, M.U.K. (1993) The effects of early mobilisation and immobilisation on the healing process following muscle injuries. *Sports Medicine* **15**: 78–89.

Judovitch, B. (1952) Herniated cervical disc. *American Journal of Surgery* **84**: 646–656.

Kelly, E. (1997) The effects of deep transverse frictional massage to the gastrocnemius muscle. *Journal of Orthopaedic Medicine* **19**: 3–9.

Klaber Moffatt, J.A., Hughes, G.I., Griffiths, P. (1990) An investigation of the effects of cervical traction. Part 2: the effects on the neck musculature. *Clinical Rehabilitation* **4**: 287–290.

Kleinman, M., Gross, A.E. (1983) Achilles tendon rupture following steroid injection. *Journal of Bone and Joint Surgery* **65-A**: 1345–1347.

Kulick, M.I., Brazlow, R., Smith, S., Hentz, V.R. (1984) Injectable ibuprofen: preliminary evaluation of its ability to decrease peritendinous adhesions. *Annals of Plastic Surgery* **13**: 459–467.

LaBan, M.M., Taylor, R.S. (1992) Manipulation: an objective analysis of the literature. *Orthopaedic Clinics of North America* **23**: 451–459.

Larsson, L. (1989) Anaphylactic shock after i.a. administration of triamcinolone acetonide in a 35 year old female. *Scandinavian Journal of Rheumatology* **18**: 441–442.

Lehto, M., Duance, V.C., Restall, D. (1985) Collagen and fibronectin in a healing skeletal muscle injury. *Journal of Bone and Joint Surgery* **67-B**: 820–828.

Liu, Y.K., Tipton, C.M., Matthes, R.D. *et al.* (1983) An *in situ* study of the influence of a sclerosing solution in rabbit medial collateral ligaments and its junction strength. *Connective Tissue Research* **11**: 95–102.

Loitz, B.J., Zernicke, R.F., Vailas, A.C. *et al.* (1988) Effects of short-term immobilisation versus continuous passive motion on the biomechanical and biochemical properties of the rabbit tendon. *Clinical Orthopaedics and Related Research* **244**: 265–271.

Low, J., Reed, A. (1994) *Electrotherapy Explained: Principles and Practice.* Butterworth-Heinemann.

Marks, J.G., Cano, C., Leitzel, K., Lipton, A. (1983) Inhibition of wound healing by topical steroids. *Journal of Dermatologic Surgery and Oncology* **9**: 819–821.

Mathews, J.A. (1968) Dynamic discography: a study of lumbar traction. *Annals of Physical Medicine* **9**: 275–279.

Mathews, J.A., Hickling, J. (1975) Lumbar traction: a double-blind controlled study for sciatica. *Rheumatology and Rehabilitation* **14**: 222–225.

Melzack, R., Wall, P.D. (1988) *The Challenge of Pain*, 2nd edn. Penguin Books.

Nachemson, A. (1980) Lumbar intradiscal pressure. In: *The Lumbar Spine and Back Pain*, 2nd edn (Jayson, M.I.V. ed.). Pitman Publishing, pp. 341–358.

Norris, C.M. (1993) *Sports Injuries: Diagnosis and Management for Physiotherapists.* Butterworth-Heinemann.

Noyes, F. (1977) Functional properties of knee ligaments and alterations induced by immobilisation. *Clinical Orthopaedics and Related Research* **123**: 210–242.

O'Donaghue, C. (1994) Manipulation trials. In: *Grieve's Modern Manual Therapy*, 2nd edn (Boyling, J., Palastanga, N. eds). Churchill Livingstone, pp. 661–672.

Onel, D., Tuzlaci, M., Sari, H., Demir, K. (1989) Computed tomographic investigation of the effect of traction on lumbar disc herniations. *Spine* **14**: 82–90.

Peacock, E.E. (1966) Some biochemical and biophysical aspects of joint stiffness. *Annals of Surgery* **164**: 1–12.

Pellecchia, G.L., Hamel, H., Behnke, P. (1994) Treatment of infrapatellar tendinitis: a combination of modalities and transverse friction massage versus iontophoresis. *Journal of Sports Rehabilitation* **3**: 135–145.

Ponec, M., de Haas, C., Bachra, B.N., Polano, M.K. (1977) Effects of glucocorticoids on primary human skin fibroblasts. *Research* 117–123.

Priestley, G.C. (1978) Effects of corticosteroids on the growth and metabolism of fibroblasts cultured from human skin. *British Journal of Dermatology* **99**: 253–261.

Rang, H.P., Dale, M.M., Ritter, J.M. (1995) *Pharmacology*, 3rd edn. Churchill Livingstone.

Salter, R.B. (1989) The biologic concept of continuous passive motion of synovial joints. *Clinical Orthopaedics and Related Research* **242**: 12–25.

Sandberg, N. (1964) Time relationship between administration of cortisone and wound healing in rats. *Acta Chirurgiae Scandinavica* **127**: 446–455.

Schwellnus, M.P., Mackintosh, L., Mee, J. (1992) Deep transverse frictions in the treatment of iliotibial band friction syndrome in athletes: a clinical trial. *Physiotherapy* **78**: 564–568.

Shekelle, P.G. (1994) Spine update: spinal manipulation. *Spine* **19** 858–861.

Smyth, M.J., Wright, V. (1958) Sciatica and the intervertebral disc. *Journal of Bone and Joint Surgery* **40-A**: 1401.

Stephens, F.O., Dunphy, J.E., Hunt, T.K. (1971) Effect of delayed administration of corticosteroids on wound contraction. *Annals of Surgery* **173**: 214–218.

Stratford, P.W., Levy, D.R., Gauldie, S. *et al.* (1989) The evaluation of phonophoresis and friction massage as treatments for extensor carpi radialis tendonitis: a randomised controlled trial. *Physiotherapy Canada* **41**: 93–99.

Swezey, R.L. (1983) The modern thrust of manipulation and traction therapy. *Seminars in Arthritis and Rheumatism* **12**: 322–331.

Takai, S., Woo, S.L.-Y., Horibe, S. *et al.* (1991) The effects of frequency and duration of controlled passive mobilization on tendon healing. *Journal of Orthopaedic Research* **9**: 705–713.

Threlkeld, A.J. (1992) The effects of manual therapy on connective tissue. *Physical Therapy* **72**: 893–902.

Tipton, C.M., Vailas, A.C., Matthes, R.D. (1986) Experimental studies on the influences of physical activity on ligaments, tendons and joints: a brief review. *Acta Medica Scandinavica* **711** (suppl): 157–168.

Van Story-Lewis, P.E., Tenenbaum, H.C. (1986) Glucocorticoid inhibition of fibroblast contraction of collagen gels. *Biochemical Pharmacology* **35**: 1283–1286.

Vasseljen, O. (1992) Low level laser versus traditional physiotherapy in the treatment of tennis elbow. *Physiotherapy* **78**: 329–334.

Videman, T. (1986) Connective tissue and immobilisation: key factors in musculoskeletal degeneration? *Clinical Orthopaedics* **221**: 26–32.

Warren, C.G., Lehmann, J.F., Koblanski, J.N. (1971) Elongation of the rat tail tendon: effect of load and temperature. *Physical Medicine and Rehabilitation* **52**: 465–474.

Weiner, I.J., Peacock, E.E. (1971) Biologic principles affecting repair of flexor tendons. *Advances in Surgery* **5**: 145–188.

Wells, P. (1988) Manipulative procedures. In: *Pain Management by Physiotherapy*, 2nd edn (Wells, P.E., Frampton, V., Bowsher, D. eds). Butterworth-Heinemann, pp. 187–212.

Winter, B. (1968) Transverse frictions. *South African Journal of Physiotherapy* **24**: 5–7.

Woo, S.L.-Y. (1982) Mechanical properties of tendons and ligaments II: The relationship of immobilisation and exercise on tissue remodelling. *Biorheology* **19**: 385–408.

Woo, S.L.-Y., Matthews, J., Akeson, W., Amiel, D., Convery, R. (1975) Connective tissue response to immobility: correlative study of the biomechanical and biochemical measurements of normal and immobilised rabbit knees. *Arthritis and Rheumatism*, **18**: 257–264.

Woo, S.L.-Y., Wang, C.W., Newton, P.O., Lyon, R.M. (1990) The response of ligaments to stress deprivation and stress enhancement. In: *Knee Ligaments: Structure, Function, Injury and Repair* (Daniel, D. *et al.*, eds). Raven Press, pp. 337–349.

Woodman, R.M., Pare, L. (1982) Evaluation and treatment of soft tissue lesions of the ankle and forefoot using the Cyriax approach. *Physical Therapy* **62**: 1144–1147.

Worden, R.E., Humphrey, T.L. (1964) Effect of spinal traction on the length of the body. *Archives of Physical Medicine and Rehabilitation* **44**: 318–320.

Wright, A. (1995) Hypoalgesia post-manipulative therapy: a review of a potential neurophysiological mechanism. *Manual Therapy* **1**: 11–16.

Zusman, M. (1994) What does manipulation do? The need for basic research. In: *Grieve's Modern Manual Therapy*, 2nd edn (Boyling, J.D., Palastanga, N. eds). Churchill Livingstone, pp. 651–672.

Section 2

Practice of orthopaedic medicine

Introduction to Section 2

Section 2 adopts a regional approach, encompassing the shoulder, elbow, wrist and hand, cervical spine, thoracic spine, hip, knee, ankle and foot, lumbar spine and sacroiliac joint. The anatomy, assessment, lesions and treatment techniques are discussed in turn for each region.

Throughout this book, the anatomy will be presented on a 'need to know' basis, confining itself to what is clinically relevant in the context of orthopaedic medicine. It is not intended that, through its presentation here, anatomy can be learned afresh, but rather that it should act as a reminder of that taught so stringently at undergraduate level. It may also stimulate the reader to return to the dedicated tomes on anatomy to explore each region in greater detail in the pursuit of increased accuracy, particularly in peripheral joint lesions, and enhanced clinical effectiveness.

In the sections on treatment indications and application, the words 'may' and 'might' will be encountered. It is not intended to imply a wishy-washy attitude to practice, but rather to acknowledge the existence of options and that decisions rest with the professional on the basis of judgement. This is to balance the unavoidable 'cookbook' approach in the description of the techniques.

It is our experience with teaching orthopaedic medicine that students gain confidence and competence more rapidly if they can at first be guided step by step through the techniques with feedback on their performance. Whilst unable to provide feedback, this book panders to the need for students to check treatment techniques in the unsupervised clinical situation and self-evaluation is encouraged to help develop the skills from there.

5 The shoulder

Summary

The shoulder can be a minefield of misdiagnosis with lesions grouped under the broader, non-specific headings of 'rotator cuff syndrome', 'impingement' or 'frozen shoulder'. Knowledge of anatomy and the use of selective tension aid the incrimination of the causative structure. Palpation then identifies the specific site of the lesion to which effective treatment can be applied.

 This chapter outlines the relevant anatomy of the shoulder region with guidelines for palpation. The assessment procedure follows, incorporating the pertinent elements of the subjective and objective examination towards the identification of shoulder lesions. The lesions are discussed and treatments are suggested, based on the principles of theory and practice.

Anatomy

Inert structures

In the shoulder region, simultaneous coordinated movements occur at four articulations between the scapula, clavicle, humerus and sternum: the glenohumeral joint, acromioclavicular joint, sternoclavicular joint and scapulothoracic joint. The glenohumeral joint (shoulder joint) is the most mobile joint in the body and is the first link in a mechanical chain of levers that allows the arm to be positioned in space. Movement at the spinal joints increases the range of movement available to the glenohumeral joint (Nordin and Frankel, 1989).

 The large, flat *scapula* is suspended by its muscles against the posterolateral thoracic wall and overlies the second to seventh ribs in the neutral position. It is attached to the strut-like clavicle by the acromioclavicular joint and together they position, steady and brace the shoulder laterally, so that the arm can clear the trunk. The clavicle transmits the weight of the upper limb to the axial skeleton via the coracoclavicular and costoclavicular ligaments, and the glenohumeral joint provides the upper limb with its wide range of movement.

 The inferior junction of the medial and lateral borders of the scapula forms the *inferior angle*, which lies over the seventh rib and is crossed by latissimus dorsi. The lateral border provides the attachments of teres major below and teres minor above. The medial border is long, providing attachment for the levator scapulae and the rhomboid muscles; it joins the short superior border at the *superior angle*. The *suprascapular notch* lies at the junction of the superior border with the coracoid process. This notch is converted by the *superior transverse scapular ligament* into a foramen for the passage of the suprascapular nerve. The suprascapular vessels pass above it.

The dorsal surface of the scapula is divided by the spine of the scapula into fossae above and below. The smaller upper *supraspinous fossa* gives origin to the supraspinatus muscle and the lower, larger *infraspinous fossa* gives origin to infraspinatus. The two fossae communicate laterally at the *spinoglenoid notch* through which runs the suprascapular nerve. The costal surface shows a slight hollowing for the origin of subscapularis and its medial border is roughened for the insertion of serratus anterior.

The lateral angle of the scapula is broadened to form the pear-shaped *glenoid fossa* that articulates with the head of the humerus at the glenohumeral joint. A roughened *supraglenoid tubercle* gives origin to the long head of biceps and a roughened *infraglenoid tubercle* gives origin to the long head of triceps.

The *spine of the scapula* is subcutaneous and having arisen from the upper dorsal surface of the scapula it widens laterally, projecting forwards to form the distinctive *acromion process*. When the acromion is viewed laterally it may be observed to be flat, slightly curved or to have an anterior hook-like process. The latter two may predispose to rotator cuff pathology since they reduce the vertical dimensions of the subacromial space (Flatow *et al.*, 1994; Pratt, 1994; Hulstyn and Fadale, 1995).

The lower border of the crest of the spine of the scapula is continuous with the lateral border of the acromion and forms a useful palpable bony landmark, the *posterior acromial angle*. The anteromedial border of the acromion shows an oval facet for articulation with the clavicle at the acromioclavicular joint.

Just above the glenoid fossa, the prominent hook-like *coracoid process* springs up and forwards to lie below the outer clavicle. With the arm in the anatomical position, the coracoid points directly forwards to form a prominent palpable bony landmark.

The *clavicle* is subcutaneous, running horizontally between the acromion process of the scapula and the manubrium sterni, with which it articulates. On its lateral aspect is a small oval facet that articulates with the acromion at the acromioclavicular joint. Inferiorly and laterally is a rounded conoid tubercle from which a roughened trapezoid line runs forwards and laterally. Both give attachment to the separate parts of the coracoclavicular ligament, which firmly fastens the clavicle to the scapula via the coracoid process.

The upper part of the humerus expands to bear a head and the greater and lesser tuberosities (tubercles). The *head of the humerus* is approximately hemispherical and provides an articulating surface that is much greater than its scapular counterpart, the glenoid fossa. Surrounding the head of the humerus is a slight constriction that represents the *anatomical neck* and separates the head from the two tuberosities. The head of the humerus joins the shaft at the *surgical neck*, so called since it is the common site of fracture of the humerus.

The *greater tuberosity* is large and quadrilateral and is the most lateral palpable bony landmark at the shoulder. Projecting laterally beyond the acromion, it is covered by the deltoid muscle and is continuous with the shaft of the humerus below. Three articular facets *sit* on its superior and posterior surface for the attachment of supraspinatus, infraspinatus and teres minor. Supraspinatus inserts into the highest or superior facet, infraspinatus into the middle and teres minor into the lower or inferior facet. The sharp medial edge of the greater tuberosity forms the lateral lip of the *bicipital groove (intertubercular sulcus)* which receives the insertion of pectoralis major.

The *lesser tuberosity* is a bony projection that lies below and lateral to the coracoid process. It receives the insertion of subscapularis on its medial aspect and its sharp lateral edge forms the medial lip of the bicipital groove which receives the insertion of teres major.

The *sternoclavicular joint* is a synovial joint between the medial end of the clavicle and a notch on the superolateral aspect of the manubrium sterni. A fibrocartilaginous disc is positioned between the joint surfaces. It is an important joint since it is the point of attachment of the upper limb to the axial skeleton.

The *acromioclavicular joint* is a synovial plane joint with its articular surfaces covered with fibrocartilage. A wedge-shaped fibrocartilaginous disc drops down into the joint from the superior aspect of the joint capsule, producing a partial division of the joint. The articular facet on the lateral aspect of the clavicle is directed inferolaterally and the corresponding facet on the medial border of the acromion is directed superomedially, producing a tendency for

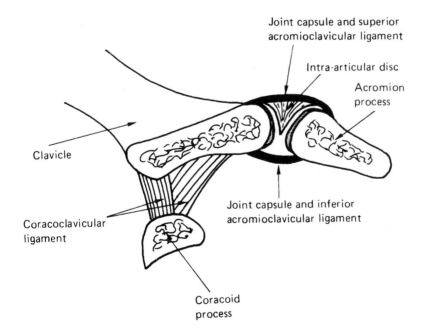

Joint capsule and superior acromioclavicular ligament

Intra-articular disc

Acromion process

Clavicle

Joint capsule and inferior acromioclavicular ligament

Coracoclavicular ligament

Coracoid process

Fig. 5.1 Acromioclavicular joint, showing intra-articular disc and ligaments. From Palastanga *et al.* (1994) with permission.

the clavicle to override the acromion. The plane of the joint tends to be variable, but may run slightly obliquely, sloping medially from superior to inferior. The joint is surrounded by a fibrous capsule that is thickened superiorly and inferiorly by the parallel fibres of the capsular ligaments running between the two bones (Fig. 5.1). The stability of the acromioclavicular joint is provided by the strong accessory coracoclavicular ligament.

The clavicle acts as a strut or brace and allows the scapula to rotate and glide forwards and backwards. The movements at the acromioclavicular joint are passive, in the same way as the sacroiliac joint. The small amounts of movement available make it impossible to determine a capsular pattern.

The *coracoclavicular ligament* is separate from the acromioclavicular joint, but in strongly binding the scapula to the clavicle via the coracoid process, it provides a stabilizing component to the joint. The ligament has two parts, the trapezoid and conoid ligaments, which are separate anatomically and functionally. The more horizontal trapezoid ligament acts as a hinge for scapular motion, whilst the more vertical conoid ligament acts as a longitudinal axis for scapular rotation. Together, the ligaments prevent medial displacement of the acromion under the clavicle.

The *glenohumeral joint* is a synovial ball-and-socket joint between the head of the humerus and the glenoid fossa of the scapula, deepened by the fibrocartilaginous glenoid labrum (Fig. 5.2). The two articular surfaces are incongruent, with the relatively large head of the humerus providing a surface area three to four times that of the glenoid fossa (Hulstyn and Fadale, 1995). The enormous range of movement is therefore at the expense of joint stability.

With no inherent bony stability available, stability is dependent primarily upon the static effects of the capsuloligamentous structures

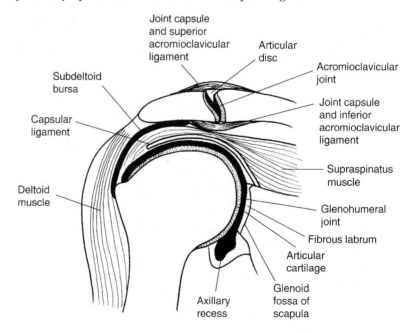

Fig. 5.2 Cross-section of glenohumeral joint showing internal structure. Adapted from Palastanga *et al.* (1994) with permission.

and the dynamic effects of the surrounding muscles. The limited joint volume and a negative intra-articular pressure provide a form of static stability. The action of muscle forces, mainly the rotator cuff, produces compression of the head of the humerus into the glenoid labrum, providing important dynamic stability and steering the joint surfaces during movement (Speer, 1995).

The *joint capsule*, lined with synovium, is thin and spacious, holding up to 30 ml of fluid or air (Cailliet, 1991). It attaches to the edge of the glenoid medially and surrounds the anatomical neck of the humerus laterally, except for its inferomedial part that descends to attach to the shaft of the humerus, approximately 1 cm below the articular margin. The inferomedial portion forms a loose axillary pouch or fold and consists of randomly organized collagen fibres (Hulstyn and Fadale, 1995). Although this arrangement facilitates movement, this part of the capsule is relatively weak as it is not supported by muscles and therefore is often subject to strain.

The capsular fibres are mainly horizontal and are reinforced anteriorly by three capsular ligaments, the *superior, middle and inferior glenohumeral ligaments*, which are only evident on the interior aspect of the capsule (Fig. 5.3). The three bands together form a Z-shape reinforcement to the anterior capsule (Kapandji, 1982). The inferior glenohumeral ligament complex plays a major stabilizing role in supporting the humeral head in a hammock or broad sling, particularly during abduction (Hulstyn and Fadale, 1995; Speer, 1995). All three bands of the glenohumeral ligaments are taut in lateral rotation and abduction stresses the middle and inferior bands. This may be significant in the development of the capsular pattern of the shoulder joint.

The rotator cuff muscles (supraspinatus, infraspinatus, teres minor and subscapularis) act as extensible ligaments to support the capsule, assisted by the long heads of triceps and biceps. Much of the capsule is less than 1 mm thick, but it is thickened to between 1 and 2 mm near its humeral attachment where it receives the rotator cuff tendon fibres (Hulstyn and Fadale, 1995).

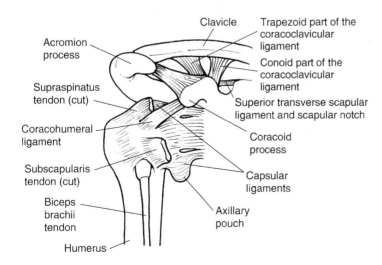

Fig. 5.3 External aspect of glenohumeral joint showing axillary pouch and capsular ligaments.

The wide range of movement available at the glenohumeral joint consists of flexion, extension, abduction, adduction, circumduction, medial and lateral rotation. The range of elevation may be up to 180° and may occur through flexion in the sagittal plane, or abduction through the frontal plane. The most functional movement is abduction in the plane of the scapula, known as scaption. This is not a fixed plane but occurs 30–40° anterior to the coronal plane of the humerus (Frame, 1991). It places deltoid and supraspinatus in an optimal position to elevate the arm (Nordin and Frankel, 1989). Abduction is accompanied by lateral rotation in the coronal plane which allows the greater tuberosity to clear the acromion; scaption does not involve this element of concomitant lateral rotation (Frame, 1991).

Elevation consists of abduction from 0 to 60° occurring at the glenohumeral joint, 60–120° occurring at the scapulothoracic joint and 120–180° occurring at the glenohumeral and scapulothoracic joints together with side flexion of the trunk to the opposite side (Kapandji, 1982). The range of lateral rotation is 80–90° and medial rotation 100–110°, with full range only achieved by taking the arm behind the back.

Rolling and translational (gliding) movements also occur and the glenohumeral joint surfaces can be separated by distraction. Muscle forces acting on the joint stabilize it and produce a combination of shearing and compression forces, maintaining the humeral head in the glenoid.

The nerve supply to the glenohumeral joint is mainly from the C5 segment.

Cameron (1995) looked at the shoulder as a weight-bearing joint. Although this joint is traditionally considered to be non-weight-bearing in character, he applied simple physical principles showing this not to be the case. With the weight of the adult arm estimated to be approximately 5 kg, forces equivalent to three times body weight are transmitted through the shoulder during simple daily activities.

The *coracoacromial ligament* is an accessory ligament of the shoulder joint, forming an osseoligamentous arch over the superior aspect of the shoulder joint and the subdeltoid bursa. It is triangular in shape and approximately 1 cm wide. Its apex attaches to the anterior aspect of the acromion and its base to the lateral aspect of the coracoid process. The coracoacromial arch is separated from the underlying tendons by the subdeltoid bursa that mechanically acts like a secondary synovial joint. The coracoacromial arch provides stability for the head of the humerus against upwards displacement and protects it from direct vertical trauma.

Numerous small bursae are associated with the shoulder joint. An anterior *subscapular bursa* lies between the tendon of subscapularis and the anterior capsule, consistently communicating with the joint. The synovial lining of the joint extends to form a sheath around the long head of biceps in the bicipital groove. A bursa, which communicates with the joint, may be present between the tendon of infraspinatus and the posterior capsule.

The *subdeltoid bursa (subacromial bursa)* is independent of the shoulder joint and normally does not communicate with it. It has a special role in the biomechanics of the shoulder joint and is frequently a cause of pain. It is a smooth synovial sac containing variable thin bands or plicae and is surrounded by fatty areolar tissue (Hulstyn and Fadale, 1995). The superficial layer of the bursa is adherent to the anterior two-thirds of the undersurface of the acromion, falling away from the posterior third. Its deep layer lies over the rotator cuff tendons and the head of the humerus (Cooper *et al.*, 1993). Medially it extends under the acromion to the acromioclavicular joint line and laterally it caps the greater tuberosity, separating it from the overlying deltoid muscle.

The *subacromial space* is sometimes considered to be a joint (Kapandji, 1982; Pratt, 1994). This is not a true articulation but it is critical to shoulder movement. As supraspinatus pulls the greater tuberosity superiorly and medially, the walls of the subdeltoid bursa glide over one another allowing the head of the humerus to slide (Netter, 1987). The subacromial space is approximately 7–14 mm deep (Frame, 1991) and is occupied by the subdeltoid bursa, the supraspinatus tendon, the superior part of the capsule of the shoulder joint and the tendon of the long head of the biceps. The tightly packed structures move constantly in relation to one another and there is the potential for friction and degeneration. Inflammation, degeneration, the shape of the acromion or degeneration of the acromioclavicular joint can all contribute to a reduction of the vertical proportions or stenosis of the subacromial space. Impingement of a painful structure in the space produces a painful arc between 60 and 120° of abduction.

Contractile structures

Four short muscles (supraspinatus, infraspinatus, teres minor and subscapularis) pass from the scapula to the head of the humerus and these are known as the rotator cuff. The rotator cuff muscles are particularly important to the function of the shoulder, working as extensible ligaments to provide dynamic stability and maintaining the head of the humerus in the glenoid fossa. Shoulder movement, particularly elevation, is governed by force couples that involve the interaction of deltoid and the rotator cuff muscles (Nordin and Frankel, 1989). The rotator cuff muscles maintain the joint's apposition, preventing excessive superior translatory movement that would lead to instability.

As the rotator cuff tendons insert into the head of the humerus they blend with the capsule of the joint forming a thickened common tendinous cuff. Fibres from subscapularis and infraspinatus interdigitate with those of supraspinatus in their deep layer, facilitating the distribution of forces directly or indirectly over a wider area (Clark and Harryman, 1992). The tendon of the long head of biceps exits the capsule through a reinforced foramen at the junction of the insertions of supraspinatus and subscapularis on to the humerus (Hulstyn and Fadale, 1995). These tendons are frequently a source of pain through degeneration and overuse.

Supraspinatus (suprascapular nerve C4–6) takes origin from the medial two-thirds of the suprascapular fossa. The fibres, which are bipennate, converge to pass under the acromion, blending with the capsule of the shoulder joint and inserting into the upper of the three facets on the greater tuberosity. As the tendon passes to its insertion it appears to be reinforced by the coracohumeral ligament that runs parallel and is firmly adherent to it (Clark and Harryman, 1992). Supraspinatus produces abduction of the glenohumeral joint but its exact role in the mechanism of shoulder movement is controversial.

Supraspinatus, together with the other rotator cuff muscles, stabilizes the head of the humerus, providing horizontal compression and reducing vertical displacement. It is considered to be responsible for initiating abduction by holding the head of the humerus down on the glenoid, before deltoid takes over at approximately 20°, to provide the force for abduction (Palastanga *et al.*, 1994; Pratt, 1994). However, both supraspinatus and deltoid have been shown to be active throughout the range of abduction with an early rise in tension in supraspinatus fixing the humeral head, and enabling deltoid to work at a better mechanical advantage (Cailliet, 1991; Frame, 1991). It may be that deltoid and supraspinatus can initiate and complete a full range of abduction independently.

Infraspinatus (suprascapular nerve C4–6) is a thick triangular muscle that takes origin from the medial two-thirds of the infraspinous fossa. Its fibres converge to form a broad, thick tendon, passing over the posterior joint capsule, with which it blends, and inserting into the middle of the three facets on the greater tuberosity of the humerus. Together with teres minor, with which it is sometimes fused, infraspinatus produces lateral rotation of the glenohumeral joint during elevation.

Teres minor (axillary nerve C5–6) takes origin from the upper two-thirds of the lateral border of the scapula, above the origin of teres major. It inserts into the lowest of the three facets on the greater tuberosity blending with the posterior capsule as it passes over it. It functions with infraspinatus to produce lateral rotation of the glenohumeral joint.

Subscapularis (upper and lower subscapular nerve C5–6) takes origin from the medial two-thirds of the subscapular fossa on the costal surface of the scapula, and inserts by a broad, thin, membranous tendon into the lesser tuberosity of the humerus. It reinforces the anterior capsule, from which it is partially separated by a bursa which communicates with the joint. It functions to produce medial rotation of the glenohumeral joint.

Trapezius (spinal accessory nerve, XI and ventral rami of C3–4) is a large, flat triangular muscle forming a trapezium with its opposite number. It has a long line of attachment from the superior nuchal line, external occipital protruberance, ligamentum nuchae and the spinous processes and intervening supraspinous ligament from C7 to T12. The upper fibres descend to the posterior border of the lateral third of the clavicle, the middle fibres pass horizontally to the medial border of the acromion and the lower fibres pass upwards to the crest of the spine of the scapula. In conjunction with other muscles, trapezius stabilizes the scapula for functional movements of the arm and the individual portions of the muscle assist other muscles in producing primary movement. The upper fibres of trapezius and levator scapulae suspend the scapula against the thoracic cage and are constantly active during ambulation (Paine and Voight, 1993). Trapezius together with serratus anterior forms a force couple to rotate the scapula on the thoracic wall (Frame, 1991).

Rhomboids, major and minor (rhomboid branch of the dorsal scapular nerve, C4–5), form a line of attachment from the lower ligamentum nuchae and the spines of C7 to T5 and pass to the medial border of the scapula, to assist in its stabilization against the thoracic cage. The rhomboids are active in scapular retraction, which is essential for overhead throwing movements and swimming strokes, e.g. crawl (Paine and Voight, 1993).

Levator scapulae (C3–5) descends from the transverse processes of the atlas and axis to the medial upper scapular border. Together with the rhomboids it controls and positions the scapula.

Latissimus dorsi (thoracodorsal nerve C6–8) has an extensive origin from the lumbar spine, lumbar fascia and thorax. The fibres converge towards the humerus, attaching to the inferior angle of the scapula as they pass by. The tendinous fibres twist through an angle of 180° before inserting into the floor of the bicipital groove. At the shoulder latissimus dorsi extends, adducts and medially rotates the humerus.

Teres major (lower subscapular nerve, C6–7) passes from the lower dorsal aspect of the scapula near the inferior angle to insert into the medial lip of the bicipital groove. It functions together with latissimus dorsi to adduct and medially rotate the humerus and together they form the posterior fold of the axilla. In conjunction with pectoralis major, teres major stabilizes the shoulder joint.

Deltoid (axillary nerve C5–6) gives the shoulder its rounded contour. The muscle has three sets of fibres which all converge to insert into the deltoid tubercle in the middle of the lateral aspect of the shaft of the humerus. The anterior fibres attach to the anterior border of the lateral third of the clavicle and assist flexion and medial rotation. The middle fibres attach to the acromion and the posterior fibres attach to the lower lip of the crest of the spine of the scapula assisting extension and lateral rotation. The direction of the muscle fibres is almost vertical and the muscle's basic action is to elevate the head of the humerus up into the overhanging coracoacromial ligament (Cailliet, 1991). Overall, deltoid is a powerful abductor of the glenohumeral joint but its function is dependent on supraspinatus and the other rotator cuff muscles.

Pectoralis major (lateral and medial pectoral nerves, clavicular part C5–6: sternocostal part C7–8, T1) is a thick triangular muscle, originating as two separate parts from the anterior chest wall to insert into the lateral lip of the bicipital groove. As the fibres cross to the arm they twist to form the anterior axillary fold. The two parts of the muscle are both powerful adductors and medial rotators of the humerus; the clavicular part produces flexion. Together with latissimus dorsi, pectoralis major acts in climbing activities and is involved in pushing and throwing.

Pectoralis minor (both pectoral nerves, C6–8) passes from the upper ribs to the coracoid process. In conjunction with other muscles that anchor the scapula, pectoralis minor protracts, depresses, rotates and tilts the scapula.

Serratus anterior (long thoracic nerve C5–7, descending on its external surface) has an extensive origin from the side of the thorax, passing round the thoracic cage to insert into the medial border of the costal surface of the scapula. It is responsible for stabilizing the scapula during elevation and protraction of the scapula in the functional activities of reaching and pushing. Loss of its nerve supply leads to winging of the scapula.

Movement of the scapula on the thoracic cage occurs at the scapulothoracic joint between two fascial planes, the most superficial of which lies between subscapularis and serratus anterior (Kapandji, 1982; Pratt, 1994). The surrounding muscles stabilize this joint and dynamically position the glenoid fossa to facilitate efficient glenohumeral movement (Paine and Voight, 1993).

Coracobrachialis (musculocutaneous nerve C5–7) originates from the tip of the coracoid process and forms a conjoint tendon with the short head of the biceps, inserting into the medial aspect of the middle of the shaft of the humerus. It adducts the humerus, its position being analogous to the adductor group of muscles at the hip.

Biceps brachii (musculocutaneous nerve C5–6) has a short head arising from the tip of the coracoid process and a long head originating within the capsule of the glenohumeral joint from the supraglenoid tubercle and adjacent glenoid labrum. The intracapsular part of the tendon is surrounded by a double sheath, an extension of the synovial lining of the glenohumeral joint (Williams *et al.*, 1989). The long head passes through the subacromial space and exits the joint behind the transverse humeral ligament. It continues on into the bicipital groove together with its synovial sheath. The two muscle bellies fuse to insert into the tuberosity of the radius. Biceps has its main effect at the elbow where it is a powerful supinator and elbow flexor. The long head exerts a stabilizing effect on the superior aspect of the shoulder joint, which may become more important if the shoulder becomes less stable (Itoi *et al.*, 1994). Its passage laterally, then turning a 90° angle into the bicipital groove, assists forward flexion of the shoulder (Cailliet, 1991).

Triceps (radial nerve C6–8) originates by three heads. The long head arises from the infraglenoid tubercle of the scapula and the glenoid labrum, where it exerts a stabilizing effect on the shoulder joint. It also assists adduction and extension movements of the humerus from the flexed position. The lateral head originates from the humerus above and lateral to the spiral groove, and the medial head from the posterior humerus below the spiral groove. The three heads come together to insert into the olecranon process. The main action of the triceps is to extend the elbow.

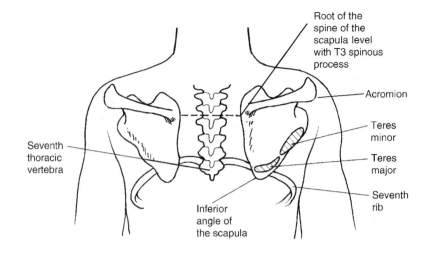

Root of the spine of the scapula level with T3 spinous process

Acromion

Teres minor

Teres major

Seventh rib

Seventh thoracic vertebra

Inferior angle of the scapula

Fig. 5.4 Posterior aspect of the shoulder.

Guide to surface marking and palpation

Posterior aspect (Fig. 5.4)

Palpate the *inferior angle of the scapula* which, in most people, can be grasped between a finger and thumb. Abducting the arm may make the inferior angle easier to locate as it advances around the chest wall.

Palpate along the medial and lateral borders of the scapula. The lower medial border is subcutaneous and more readily palpable, lying parallel to and approximately three fingers from the spinous processes. Visualize the position of *latissimus dorsi* as it crosses the inferior angle, and track the *teres major and minor* muscles that take origin from the lateral border of the scapula. Teres major originates below teres minor.

The *crest of the spine of the scapula* may be visible and is readily palpable. Feel it sloping medially down to meet the medial border of the scapula at the level of the spinous process of T3.

Palpate the lateral end of the spine of the scapula and follow the lower border round until it joins the lateral border of the acromion. A sharp 90° angle is formed here, the *posterior angle of the acromion*, which is a useful bony landmark.

Palpate the flat upper surface of the *acromion* which is subcutaneous and forms the summit of the shoulder, lying just lateral to the acromioclavicular joint. Palpate the anterior edge of the acromion with an index finger and the posterior angle with a thumb, to appreciate its width.

Lateral aspect

Palpate the lateral edge of the acromion. Note its depth and visualize the position of the subdeltoid bursa beneath it.

Follow the anterior and posterior portions of the *deltoid muscle* down on to its insertion into the deltoid tubercle.

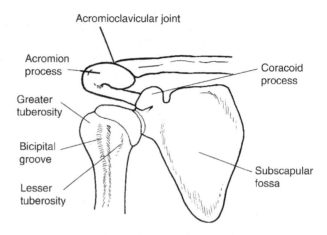

Fig. 5.5 Anterior aspect of the shoulder.

Anterior aspect (Fig. 5.5)

Palpate the *clavicle*; it is usually visible and palpable throughout its length in most people. Start at the medial end and follow the anterior curve as it lies over the first rib, then the reverse curve that produces a hollow at the lateral end of the clavicle. Below this hollow, between deltoid and pectoralis major, lies the infraclavicular fossa.

Palpate the *acromioclavicular joint* line that lies approximately 1–2 cm medial to the lateral border of the acromion. The clavicular end of the joint may project a little higher than the acromion since it overrides it slightly, and this may produce a slight step between the clavicle and acromion. The joint line should be palpable from above. Apply a downwards pressure on the lateral end of the clavicle and ask the model (or patient) to flex and extend the shoulder to feel movement at the joint.

Below the junction of the lateral third and the medial two-thirds of the clavicle, in the lateral infraclavicular fossa, feel the prominent *coracoid process* that is directed almost straightforwards with the arm resting at the side. This is covered by the anterior deltoid and deep palpation, which may be uncomfortable, is necessary. With a finger on the coracoid process, abduct the arm and the corocoid should move out from under your palpating finger.

Moving slightly downwards and laterally from the coracoid process, palpate the *lesser tuberosity* of the humerus. Immediately lateral to it is the *bicipital groove* and further laterally still, the *greater tuberosity* should be palpable.

Place the arm in the anatomical position and feel the greater tuberosity lying laterally and the lesser tuberosity lying anteriorly on either side of the bicipital groove. Relax the arm, allowing it to fall into the more functional position with some medial rotation, and feel the greater tuberosity lying more anteriorly and the lesser tuberosity medially.

The *greater tuberosity* can be easily located as it lies in line with and above the lateral epicondyle of the humerus. It can be grasped with the thumb, index and middle fingers placed on its anterior, superior and posterior surfaces. Note its width. The greater tuberosity is slightly wider from anterior to posterior than the acromion process. Try to visualize its three facets for the insertions of supraspinatus, infraspinatus and teres minor.

Palpation of the insertions of the rotator cuff tendons

To palpate *supraspinatus*, the greater tuberosity must be brought forwards from under the acromion to expose its superior facet. Position the patient sitting up at an angle of about 45° against the couch. Medially rotate and extend the arm to position it behind the back (Fig. 5.6). Palpate for the anterior edge of the acromion and locate the greater tuberosity. The tendon of supraspinatus is running directly forwards between the two bony points (remember that you have turned the greater tuberosity to lie more anteriorly). The tendon of insertion is approximately one finger's-width.

To palpate *infraspinatus*, the greater tuberosity must be brought backwards from under the acromion to expose its middle facet. Position the patient in prone lying with the weight supported on the forearms. Ensure that the elbow is placed directly below the shoulder and laterally rotate and adduct the shoulder (Fig. 5.7). Palpate for the posterior angle of the acromion and locate the greater tuberosity. The tendon of infraspinatus runs parallel to the spine of the scapula to insert into the greater tuberosity, immediately below the posterior angle of the acromion. The tendon of insertion is approximately two fingers wide. Together with the insertion of *teres minor* the tendon is three fingers wide.

To locate *subscapularis*, position the arm with the humerus in the anatomical position. Either palpate the coracoid process and move laterally and slightly downwards, or identify the bicipital groove and move directly medially to find the sharp lateral lip of the lesser tuberosity (Fig. 5.8). Follow round on to the medial aspect

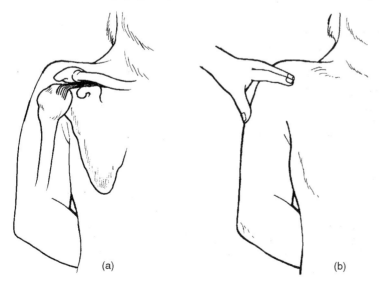

(a)   (b)

Fig. 5.6 Position of arm for palpation of the supraspinatus tendon.

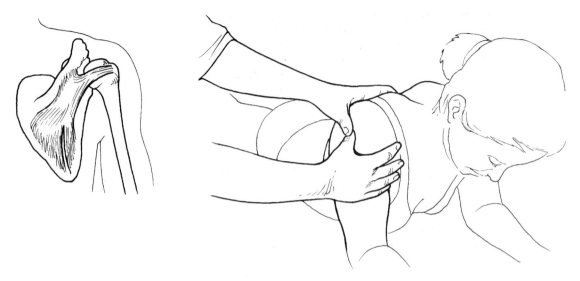

Fig. 5.7 Position of arm for palpation of the infraspinatus tendon.

of the lesser tuberosity to locate the insertion of subscapularis. The tendon itself cannot be felt and the underlying bone is tender to palpation. The tendon is approximately three fingers wide.

Commentary on the examination

The history at the shoulder is important, although it probably will not reveal a conclusive diagnosis. Cyriax (1982) considered the

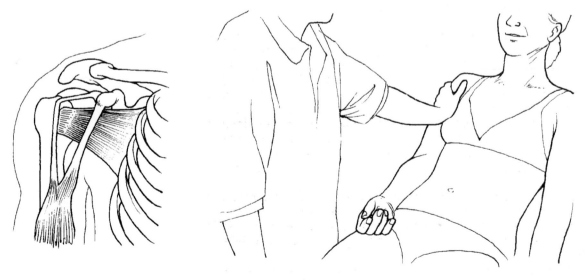

Fig. 5.8 Position of arm for palpation of the subscapularis tendon.

shoulder to be an 'honest' joint but most clues are related to the anatomy at the shoulder and are revealed in the objective examination rather than in the patient's account. Lesions may be complicated and due to a contribution of several factors. For instance, pain tends to cause immobility and it is not uncommon to find a secondary capsulitis accompanying bursitis or tendinitis.

Observation

A general observation of the patient's *face, posture and gait* will alert the examiner to abnormalities and serious illness. Acute subdeltoid bursitis produces a constant acute pain that disturbs sleep and the patient looks tired.

The acute shoulder is usually held in a position of comfort, i.e. medially rotated with the elbow flexed and supported. An alteration in the rhythmical arm swing may be obvious. The head of the humerus is so positioned in the glenoid that functional movements tend to occur in diagonal patterns and this should be evident in the arm swing during gait activity.

Due to the many anatomical components that make up the shoulder region and the interrelationship between the function of each group, lesions can be subtly complicated. Multiple lesions can exist and instability can produce secondary problems at the shoulder. In focusing on the differential diagnosis of specific lesions, orthopaedic medicine looks at common lesions at the shoulder. For more detailed coverage of shoulder instability and its relationship to shoulder lesions the reader is referred to the approach of Jenny McConnell and others.

History (subjective examination)

The *age, occupation, sports, hobbies and lifestyle* of the patient may give clues to diagnosis. The younger patient engaged in physical work or active in sport may have a minor instability problem related to overuse, producing secondary impingement. The middle-aged group may present with overuse rotator cuff lesions or chronic bursitis. In the older age group, degenerative rotator cuff lesions with secondary or idiopathic capsulitis may occur. Overuse injuries are a common cause of pain felt at the shoulder and the lifestyle of the patient can be directly responsible for the condition.

Knowledge of lifestyle is useful to advise the patient on preventing recurrence.

Shoulder injuries are common in throwing sports, swimming and all overhead activities. Tennis strokes involve rotation, abduction and elevation, leading to repetitive and stressful use of the arm in the overhead position, possibly causing impingement and instability (McCann and Bigliani, 1994).

Throwing has several different mechanisms, e.g. the straight-arm throw of the javelin, the centrifugally induced velocity of hammer throwing, the explosive push of putting the shot, or the spinning pull of the discus thrower. A 'dead arm' syndrome may be produced during the acceleration phase of throwing, when the arm becomes useless and drops down by the side. It may be associated with pins and needles and takes several minutes to recover. It is considered to be due to momentary subluxation of the glenohumeral joint associated with compression of the brachial plexus (Copeland, 1993).

The *site* of the pain does not reliably indicate the site of the lesion. The shoulder joint and its surrounding capsule, ligaments and muscles are mainly derived from the C5 segment. Lesions of any of these structures will cause the pain to be referred into the C5 dermatome which extends into the anterolateral aspect of the arm and forearm as far as the base of the thumb. The most common point of referral for these structures is to the area over the insertion of deltoid. The more irritable the lesion, the further the referral of pain into the C5 dermatome, such that the *spread* of pain will give an indication of the severity of the lesion. As a deep joint lying proximally in its dermatome, the glenohumeral joint has the potential to refer pain over a considerable distance.

The acromioclavicular joint and surrounding ligaments produce an accurate localization of pain over the joint. This is because, in contrast to the glenohumeral joint, the acromioclavicular joint is a superficial joint giving little reference.

The *symptoms and behaviour* need to be considered. The shoulder area is a point of referral of pain from other deep structures. The cervical spine in particular can refer pain to the area and visceral problems may mimic musculoskeletal lesions. The diaphragm is a C4 structure and will produce pain felt at the shoulder if affected by adjacent conditions such as pleurisy.

The *onset* of the pain may be sudden or gradual. If the onset was sudden it is important to know if there was any related trauma, with the possibility of fracture. A fall on the outstretched hand may initiate a traumatic shoulder joint capsulitis or, less commonly, chronic subdeltoid bursitis, tendon strain or acromioclavicular joint sprain. A direct blow to the shoulder area may be responsible for acromioclavicular joint sprain, but not usually tendinitis or chronic subdeltoid bursitis. An acute subdeltoid bursitis has a characteristic sudden onset with no apparent cause.

The common shoulder lesions of overuse, tendinitis, bursitis or capsulitis, present most typically with a gradual onset of pain due to overuse factors. A capsulitis may be precipitated by trauma, but this is often minor and the patient cannot recall the incident. Tendinitis may be provoked by overstretching or contraction against strong resistance. The *duration* of the symptoms gives an indication of the stage the lesion has reached in the inflammatory cycle.

Non-specific shoulder pain may be associated with nerve entrapment, which would be confirmed by signs of objective weakness but with no pain on shoulder movements (Biundo and Harris, 1993; Schulte and Warner, 1995).

The *behaviour* of the pain is relevant to diagnosis with the common lesions producing typical musculoskeletal pain on movement which is eased by rest. The patient should be asked if the pain is constant or only present on movement, giving an indication of the irritability of the lesion. Chronic overuse tendinitis or bursitis often produces a dull ache rather than a pain, although twinges of pain may be experienced if impingement occurs during movement. An acute subdeltoid bursitis produces severe pain that is constant and often unrelenting, disturbing sleep. A capsulitis shows an increasing worsening pain, referring further and further into the C5 dermatome. The inflammatory nature of the pain may be obvious in complaints of pain and stiffness on waking. 'Catching' pain may be described on activities such as reaching for a seat belt or into the back of the car, or placing an arm in a coat sleeve, and may indicate impingement of structures under the coracoacromial arch.

The behaviour can also help to assess the severity and irritability of the lesion as well as distinguish it from a lesion that is referring pain into the shoulder area. Does pain occur primarily after use, during use, or is it constant? If the patient is unable to lie on that side because the increase in pain disturbs sleep, the lesion is irritable. It may indicate a chronic subdeltoid bursitis or more commonly an irritable capsulitis. Sleeping postures may cause stress in structures, inducing microtrauma or impingement.

A loss of functional activity such as being unable to do up a bra or reach into the back pocket will indicate limitation of movement. There may be evidence of shoulder instability in patients complaining of 'clicking', 'snapping' or feeling as if the shoulder is 'coming out'. Crepitus or grating sounds may indicate degenerative changes.

To distinguish the lesion from one of cervical or thoracic origin the patient should be questioned about the presence of paraesthesia, and whether pain is increased on a cough, sneeze or deep breath. Heaviness, tiredness, puffiness, sweating or altered temperature may indicate associated or referred autonomic symptoms.

Assessment of *other joint involvement* will indicate generalized arthritis, possibly rheumatoid. It is also interesting to note if the patient has had previous shoulder problems since both 'frozen shoulder' (adhesive capsulitis) and acute subdeltoid bursitis often affect the other shoulder some years after the first incidence. In frozen shoulder the patient may complain of cervical involvement and there may be associated trigger points over the posterior aspect of the shoulder (Grubbs, 1993). This may be due to compensatory overuse of other muscles and holding the shoulder in a position of ease, or may be indicative of abnormal neural mobility.

The *past medical history* will alert the examiner to serious illness and operations encountered by the patient. The patient should be specifically asked about a history of diabetes since there is an association between diabetes mellitus and the development of a frozen shoulder (Owens-Burkhart, 1991). The examiner should be on the alert for possible contraindications to treatment.

An indication of the patient's current state of health is necessary and the patient should be asked about recent unexplained weight loss. Tumours involving the shoulder area are rare, but sarcomas may affect the shoulder girdle, though not as commonly as at the hip, pelvis and knee.

Medications currently being taken by the patient are determined to eliminate possible contraindications to treatment. The amount of analgesia required by the patient gives an indication of the severity of the lesion.

From the history, the possible diagnoses are noted. If the eventual diagnosis is one of capsulitis, three special questions asked during the history will give an indication of the severity of the lesion and act as a guideline to treatment.

> **Three questions**
>
> - **Does the pain spread below the elbow? (site and spread)**
> - **Can you lie on that side at night? (symptoms)**
> - **Is the pain constant? (behaviour)**

Inspection

The patient should undress to enable the area to be inspected in a good light. The quality of shoulder movement can be observed at this stage and hyper- or hypomobility noted. Generally speaking, the painful shoulder shows some disturbance in the normal smooth rhythm of movement. Patients with a frozen shoulder have difficulty undressing and may remark that they particularly choose clothes with buttons down the front.

A general inspection will determine any **bony deformity**. Look at the position of the cervical spine and take an overall view of the spinal curvatures in general. The general posture of the patient can be important. It has been postulated that abnormal cervical and thoracic posture, particularly an increased thoracic kyphosis, alters the resting position of the scapula and may be related to shoulder pain caused by overuse (Greenfield *et al.*, 1995).

The attitude of the shoulder should be noted. Is it higher than the other or excessively medially rotated? In a frozen shoulder, one shoulder may be held higher than the other due to pain, with the scapula elevated and retracted. The position of the scapulae should be noted. Are they more or less symmetrical, lying approximately three fingers from the midline, or are they excessively retracted or protracted? There may be evidence of winging of the scapula but this is usually more obvious on movement.

Lumps, scars, bony prominences and bruising should be observed. A prominent bump at the end of the clavicle may signify an old fracture or dislocation of the acromioclavicular joint.

Colour changes and swelling are unusual findings at the shoulder unless associated with direct trauma. *Muscle wasting* is suspected if the spine of the scapula is prominent, due to neuritis or rotator cuff rupture. The 'pop-eye' deformity of a rupture of the long head of the biceps is usually obvious, but the patient does not particularly complain of pain. In deltoid atrophy, the normal rounded contour of the shoulder may be lost, with a 'squared-off' appearance. If the shoulder is dislocated, the more common anterior dislocation shows the greater tuberosity as sitting forwards.

State at rest

Before any movements are performed, the state at rest is established to provide a baseline for subsequent comparison.

The suggested sequence for the objective examination will now be given, followed by a commentary including the reasoning in performing the movements and the significance of the possible findings.

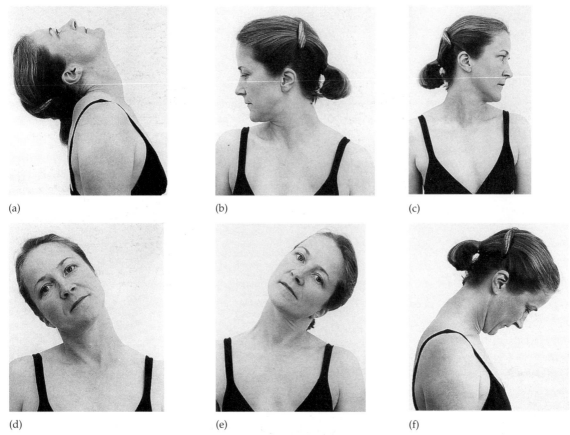

(a)

(b)

(c)

(d)

(e)

(f)

Fig. 5.9 Six active movements of the
cervical spine: (a) extension; (b, c)
rotations; (d, e) side flexions; (f) flexion.

Examination by selective tension (objective examination)

Eliminate the cervical spine:

- Active cervical extension (Fig. 5.9a)
- Active right cervical rotation (Fig. 5.9b)
- Active left cervical rotation (Fig. 5.9c)
- Active right cervical side flexion (Fig. 5.9d)
- Active left cervical side flexion (Fig. 5.9e)
- Active cervical flexion (Fig. 5.9f)

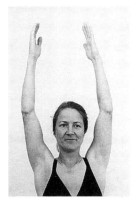

Fig. 5.10 Active shoulder elevation.

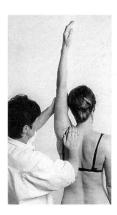

Fig. 5.11 Passive shoulder elevation.

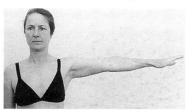

Fig. 5.12 Active elevation through abduction, looking for a painful arc.

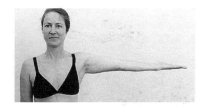

Fig. 5.13 Varying arm position to explore for a painful arc.

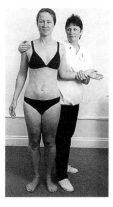

Fig. 5.14 Passive lateral rotation.

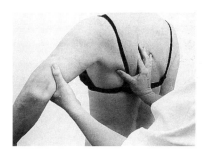

Fig. 5.15 Passive abduction.

Shoulder elevation tests:

- Active elevation through flexion (Fig. 5.10)
- Passive elevation (Fig. 5.11)
- Active elevation through abduction for a painful arc (Fig. 5.12, 5.13)

Passive glenohumeral movements:

- Passive lateral rotation (Fig. 5.14)
- Passive abduction (Fig. 5.15)
- Passive medial rotation (Fig. 5.16)

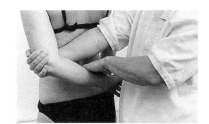

Fig. 5.16 Passive medial rotation.

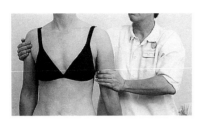

Fig. 5.17 Resisted abduction.

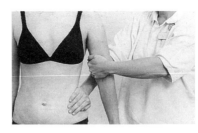

Fig. 5.18 Resisted adduction.

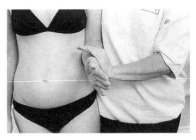

Fig. 5.19 Resisted lateral rotation.

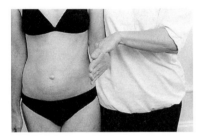

Fig. 5.20 Resisted medial rotation.

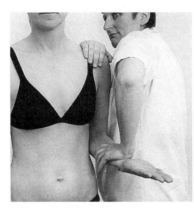

Fig. 5.21 Resisted elbow flexion.

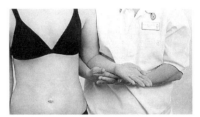

Fig. 5.22 Resisted elbow extension.

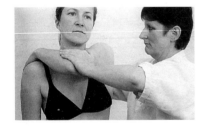

Fig. 5.23 The scarf test.

Resisted tests:

- Resisted shoulder abduction (Fig. 5.17)
- Resisted shoulder adduction (Fig. 5.18)
- Resisted shoulder lateral rotation (Fig. 5.19)
- Resisted shoulder medial rotation (Fig. 5.20)
- Resisted elbow flexion (Fig. 5.21)
- Resisted elbow extension (Fig. 5.22)

Accessory test for acromioclavicular joint or lower fibres of subscapularis:

- Passive shoulder flexion and adduction (scarf test) (Fig. 5.23)

Palpation

- Once a diagnosis has been made, the structure at fault is palpated for the exact site of the lesion

The examination of the shoulder should first exclude possible cervical lesions, therefore six active cervical movements are performed and if a pattern of signs emerges implicating the cervical spine then a full assessment of this region must be conducted.

Three elevation tests are conducted for the glenohumeral joint. Since the shoulder is considered to be an 'emotional' area, active elevation indicates the patient's willingness to move the joint. The range of movement and level of pain should then be consistent with other findings as the objective examination proceeds.

Passive elevation is added to assess pain, range of movement and end-feel. The normal end-feel of passive elevation is elastic. Any limitation of passive elevation suggests that the capsular pattern exists at the glenohumeral joint and this will be confirmed when the passive glenohumeral movements are assessed individually.

Active elevation through abduction is conducted in the coronal plane to assess for the presence of a painful arc. This involves abduction to 90° followed by lateral rotation, to enable the greater tuberosity to clear the coracoacromial arch. The test performed in this way is usually consistent with the patient's account of symptoms. However, functionally, the arm is more commonly lifted through scaption.

A painful arc is a localizing sign and indicates impingement of a painful structure in the subacromial space. Which structure, will only be revealed by completing the full examination procedure. An arc is more easily elicited on active movement as contraction of the muscle groups tends to raise the humeral head and reduce the space.

Be prepared to explore for a painful arc, especially in the light of findings later in the examination, remembering that a diagnosis is not made until the full examination has been completed. The position may be modified to place the rotator cuff tendons into a more vulnerable position for compression against the corocoacromial arch.

Elevation of the humerus through abduction in the coronal plane favours compression of the distal end of the supraspinatus tendon. Abduction with lateral rotation, palm up, brings the upper part of subscapularis to face upwards to be compressed against the arch, whilst abduction with medial rotation brings infraspinatus forwards and increases the possibility of its compression. Forward elevation in the sagittal plane combined with lateral rotation, palm-up, compresses the tendon of the long head of the biceps (Burns and Whipple, 1993).

The passive glenohumeral movements are conducted looking for pain, range of movement and end-feel. Since variation in movement between individuals is probable, movements should always be compared with the other side. However, variation between sides may exist, for example in tennis players or fast bowlers, who may have a greater range of one rotation at the expense of the other, on the dominant side. Passive lateral and medial rotation have a normal elastic end-feel, passive abduction is assessed for range of movement only, since it is not possible to appreciate the end-feel. Assessment

Capsular pattern at the glenohumeral joint:

- **Most limitation of lateral rotation**
- **Followed by limitation of abduction**
- **Least limitation of medial rotation**

of the passive glenohumeral movements may confirm the presence of the capsular pattern indicating arthritis.

As movements become limited in the capsular pattern they develop an abnormally 'hard' end-feel. The capsular pattern results in overall limitation of passive elevation. Limitation or pain at the end of range of lateral rotation only may be a sign of early capsulitis.

It may not be possible to fully assess the range of medial rotation in severe capsulitis since the accompanying limitation of abduction prevents the arm from being placed behind the patient's back. As a guide for subsequent comparison, measure the range of movement against certain landmarks that can be reached by the hand, e.g. pocket, buttock, waist, inferior angle of scapula.

Subdeltoid bursitis provides a typical example of a non-capsular pattern of movement at the shoulder. Whilst the acromioclavicular joint does not demonstrate its own capsular pattern, it produces a non-capsular pattern of movement at the glenohumeral joint.

The resisted tests are conducted looking for pain and reduced power which will indicate a muscle lesion or possible neurological involvement. The resisted tests performed in the upright position apply a degree of upwards shearing and compression to the glenohumeral joint in stabilizing the head of the humerus. For this reason the resisted tests may be accessory signs in subdeltoid bursitis, or show involvement of the joint. To confirm diagnosis, the resisted tests may be repeated in lying, with some joint distraction, where the effect of compression and shear on the joint is reduced.

Resisted abduction tests mainly supraspinatus, resisted adduction tests latissimus dorsi and the pectoral muscles, resisted lateral rotation tests infraspinatus and teres minor, resisted medial rotation tests subscapularis, resisted elbow flexion tests biceps and resisted elbow extension tests triceps.

Painful weakness on resisted testing may indicate partial rupture, but it may be difficult to decide whether a test is producing real or apparent weakness since the patient is limited from making a maximal effort by pain (Pellecchia *et al.*, 1996).

In athletes it may be difficult to produce positive findings, especially on resisted testing, as the symptoms may only be provoked during the athletic or sporting activity itself. It may be necessary for the patient to provoke the pain before the examination is carried out.

An accessory test, the 'scarf' test, as in putting a scarf over the opposite shoulder, may be performed to localize the lesion. This compresses the acromioclavicular joint or impinges the lower fibres of the subscapularis tendon against the coracoid process. It may also be positive as part of the 'muddle' of signs of a chronic subdeltoid bursitis.

Palpation is conducted for the site of the lesion, but only along the structure determined to be at fault since the shoulder is notorious for tender trigger points.

Through this scheme, a working diagnosis is established on which to base a treatment programme, with constant monitoring and reassessment. This approach is just one possible way of assessing the shoulder. Pellecchia *et al.* (1996) looked at the intertester reliability of the Cyriax evaluation and showed it to be highly reliable in the assessment of patients with shoulder pain, facilitating the identification of diagnostic categories for subjects with shoulder pain.

However, the approach does not investigate hypermobility at the shoulder with consequent instability and the reader is recommended to employ provocative instability tests as appropriate. The examination of neural structures can also be incorporated into the procedure.

Capsular lesions

The movements limited in the capsular pattern have a characteristic 'hard' end-feel, although this is less marked in the early stage, and any restriction of the glenohumeral range is consistent with an overall loss of shoulder elevation. The presence of the capsular pattern at the shoulder indicates an arthritis. Commonly this is traumatic or idiopathic arthritis (frozen shoulder), but the shoulder can be less commonly affected by degenerative osteo-arthrosis, rheumatoid arthritis or any of the spondylarthropathies.

> **Capsular pattern at the glenohumeral joint**
>
> - **Most limitation of lateral rotation.**
> - **Followed by limitation of abduction.**
> - **Least limitation of medial rotation.**

'Frozen shoulder' (adhesive capsulitis)

The term frozen shoulder is commonly used by the general public to describe any stiff or painful shoulder, but it is an overused term much criticized since it appears to avoid definite diagnosis. It is, however, an easy term to use and describes the signs and symptoms indicating involvement of the capsule of the shoulder joint, which is the key factor.

The natural history of the condition is that it follows a pattern of increasing signs and symptoms (freezing), followed by a plateau stage (frozen) before a slow, spontaneous recovery of partial or complete function (thawing). Recovery tends to occur within 1–3 years (Wadsworth, 1986). A short painful period is associated with a short recovery period and a longer painful period with a longer period of recovery (Owens-Burkhart, 1991).

Several authors have reviewed the history of the frozen shoulder (Wadsworth, 1986; Owens-Burkhart, 1991; Anton, 1993). It was first described by Duplay in 1872 and Codman was responsible for the term 'frozen shoulder' in 1934, but used the term in association with rotator cuff tendinitis. Neviaser introduced the concept of 'adhesive capsulitis' in 1945, because of the appearance of the thickened, adherent capsule that could be peeled from the bone like sticky plaster.

The cause of the condition is unknown. It is probably multifactorial, including a period of immobilization due to pain, and may include local periarticular inflammatory and degenerative changes. Association with other lesions has been reported, including cervical spine disorders, dysfunction of neural structures, thoracic spine immobility, thoracic surgery, trauma, neurological disease, reflex sympathetic dystrophy, systemic disease, in particular diabetes mellitus, and the presence of immunological factors, e.g. human leukocyte antigen (HLA)-B27 (Jeracitano *et al.*, 1992; Anton, 1993; Grubbs, 1993; Stam, 1994).

Pathology of frozen shoulder

In a review of the literature various authors observed and reported the following changes seen at arthrography, arthroscopy and surgery (Wadsworth, 1986; Owens-Burkhart, 1991; Wiley, 1991; Uhthoff and Sarkar, 1992; Anton, 1993; Grubbs, 1993; Uitvlugt *et al.*, 1993; Stam, 1994; Bunker and Anthony, 1995):

- Volumes of less than 10 ml, compared with the normal intra-articular volume of 20–30 ml, and a failure to fill the subscapularis bursa or biceps tendon sheath.
- Inflammatory changes, adhesion formation, erythematous fibrinous pannus over the synovium and loss of the redundant axillary fold.
- Fibrosis, not inflammation, with changes similar to those seen in Dupuytren's disease of the hand.
- Retraction of the capsule away from the greater tuberosity, thickening of the coracohumeral ligament and subscapularis tendon and a loss of the normal interval between the glenoid and humeral head.

Involvement of the joint capsule seems to be a common feature to all cases studied, but the above list shows that debate still continues over the nature of that involvement.

Frozen shoulder consists of a spontaneous onset of gradually increasing shoulder pain, referring to the deltoid region, and forearm if severe, with an increasing limitation of movement. The syndrome has been divided into primary or secondary types by Lundberg (1969).

- Primary frozen shoulder is idiopathic.
- Secondary frozen shoulder occurs follows a precipitating cause.

Causes may include trauma, or any condition which causes immobilization of the shoulder, e.g. neurological conditions, fracture and pain associated with bursitis or tendinitis, thyroid disease, cardiac disease, thoracic surgery, pulmonary disease, diabetes mellitus, postmenopausal hormonal changes or psychological factors such as depression, apathy and emotional stress (Owens-Burkhart, 1991, Stam, 1994).

The steroid-sensitive arthritis and traumatic arthritis described by Cyriax (1982) fit into the primary and secondary groups respectively.

Primary frozen shoulder

Cyriax (1982) called this condition 'steroid-sensitive arthritis' or 'monoarticular rheumatoid arthritis'. The condition seems particularly resistant to physical treatment, but responds well to corticosteroid injection.

The patient's condition follows a typical pattern:

- The patient is usually between 40 and 70 years old.
- Women are affected slightly more frequently than men.
- There is no reason for the onset.
- The condition progresses slowly to spontaneous recovery over 2–3 years.
- Recurrence of the condition in the other shoulder within 2–5 years is common (Cyriax, 1982).

Secondary frozen shoulder

This type of arthritis most frequently occurs secondary to trauma. The condition can be secondary to a number of conditions, some of which are listed above. A painful shoulder may be kept relatively immobile by involuntary muscle spasm, contributing to pain and stiffness, but the close proximity of other anatomical structures may also be relevant. The subdeltoid bursa, rotator cuff tendons and the long head of the biceps are all closely related to the capsule of the shoulder joint and it may be possible for changes in these structures to have a secondary effect on the capsule.

If precipitated by trauma, the incident may be minor and the initial pain usually settles. Therefore the patient may have difficulty recalling a traumatic incident or associating it with the onset of the pain. As a guideline, the condition can be divided into three stages, each of which gives an indication of the irritability of the lesion and a suggested programme of treatment. The three special questions taken from the history (see below) and the assessment of the degree of capsular pattern present give reliable diagnostic criteria.

Stage 1
After the precipitating incident, the initial pain settles. Approximately 1 week later, pain develops and gradually increases. The pain is felt over the area of deltoid, but as inflammation increases, the pain is referred further into the C5 dermatome. The extent of reference of pain indicates the degree of severity of the condition. This stage develops over several weeks and pain is the key feature, not the limited movement.

Since the shoulder joint has a wide range of movement, the early developing capsular pattern may not affect function and the patient may be oblivious to the loss of movement at this stage. Diagnosis in this early stage is not easy but it becomes conclusive once the capsular pattern of limited movement occurs. If treated early enough, it is possible to abort the progressive cycle of the condition. Unfortunately, as pain is the main feature of this stage and not loss of function, patients may not seek help for the condition early enough.

The examination of the patient provides a set of signs and symptoms that categorizes the patient as a stage 1 capsulitis and indicates a possible line of treatment.

From the history the three special questions reveal that:

- The pain is above the elbow.
- The pain is not constant.
- The patient can sleep on that side at night.

From the objective examination:

- A minor capsular pattern exists (this may involve lateral rotation only).
- The end-feel of passive movements remains relatively elastic.

The history and examination indicate a relatively non-irritable joint that will respond to corticosteroid injection or Grade B mobilization. Of course, any mobilizing technique can be applied to such a joint and the treatment programme for each individual patient is formulated based on the therapist's experience. Orthopaedic medicine treatment techniques will be described below.

Stage 2

Pain and loss of function are now the key features of the condition. The capsular pattern has developed to affect abduction and medial rotation adversely, and, subjectively, the latter is the most inconvenient functional movement for the patient to lose. As the pain gradually peaks and spreads, the patient notices that he or she is unable to reach into a back pocket or do up a bra. The limitation of lateral rotation is apparent in that the patient is unable to comb the hair.

From the history the three special questions reveal that:

- The pain spreads beyond the elbow.
- The pain is constant.
- The patient cannot sleep on that side at night.

From the objective examination:

- A full capsular pattern is present.
- The characteristic 'hard' end-feel of arthritis exists due to involuntary muscle spasm and capsular contracture.

The history and examination reveal an irritable joint. The presence of the capsular pattern is marked and the accessory glenohumeral movements will also be lost. Adhesion formation in the axillary fold, tightness in the anterior capsular ligaments and shortening of subscapularis combine to limit lateral rotation and abduction significantly, producing the capsular pattern. At this stage corticosteroid injection may be used to treat the pain and/or relatively gentle painfree mobilization may be applied to restore accessory range. The orthopaedic medicine treatment techniques will be described below.

Stage 3

If the patient progresses through the complete cycle of the condition, this represents the stage of recovery. The pain is settling and receding and full functional movement is returning. However, the end result of the condition may leave the patient with a degree of pain and some limited movement, especially lateral rotation and full elevation. Shaffer *et al.* (1992), in a long-term follow-up (average 7 years) of idiopathic frozen shoulder treated non-operatively, showed 50% of patients to have residual mild pain or stiffness of the shoulder, or both. Limitation of lateral rotation was present when restriction of movement was a feature.

Stage 3 shows similar signs and symptoms to stage 1 and the same treatment may be applied together with rehabilitation, including strengthening and stretching exercises, towards full function.

Treatment techniques for frozen shoulder

There is no standard agreed treatment for frozen shoulder. Various approaches have been advocated, including analgesic drugs, corticosteroid injections, mobilization techniques and exercises of various forms, manipulation under anaesthetic, brisement (forcible breaking of adhesions) or distension arthrography, arthroscopic distension and surgical release of adhesions (Hsu and Chan, 1991; Hulstyn and Weiss, 1993; Sharma *et al.*, 1993; Ogilvie-Harris *et al.*, 1995). The aim of treatment in each of these measures, as in the use of orthopaedic medicine techniques, is to relieve pain and restore function.

For primary frozen shoulder, i.e. steroid-sensitive arthritis, Cyriax (1982) suggested a course of intra-articular injections of corticosteroids to treat the pain. These are given over increasing intervals and, with the relief of pain, a gradual increase in movement occurs with recovery to full function.

For secondary frozen shoulder, i.e. traumatic arthritis, the practitioner has a choice of treatment dependent upon the stage of irritability and the techniques available. Those recommended in orthopaedic medicine will be described, but the reader is urged not to be limited to this choice, but to draw on experience of other mobilization techniques that can be incorporated to provide an individual treatment programme for each patient.

Injection of the glenohumeral joint (Cyriax and Cyriax, 1983; Cyriax, 1984)

Adcortyl 10 mg/ml	Total steroid	Lignocaine 1%	Total volume
2–3 ml	20–30 mg	1 ml	3–4 ml

$21G \times 1\frac{1}{2}$ (0.8 × 40 mm) or 2 in (0.8 × 50 mm) green needle

---

Position the patient either comfortably in prone lying or sitting in a chair (Figs 5.24 and 5.25). Place the patient's affected arm to rest in medial rotation across the abdomen with the elbow flexed. Stand behind the patient and place your thumb on the posterior angle of the acromion and your index or middle finger on the coracoid process. Insert the needle 1 cm below your thumb placed on the acromion and direct it forwards towards the index finger

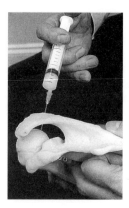

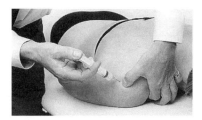

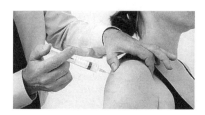

Fig. 5.24 Injection of the glenohumeral joint, prone lying.

Fig. 5.25 Injection of the glenohumeral joint, sitting.

Fig. 5.26 Injection of the glenohumeral joint, showing direction of approach and needle position.

placed on the coracoid process (Fig. 5.26). Once the needle rests against the articular surface, deliver the injection as a bolus, withdrawing slightly if there is resistance.

An explanation of the condition and prognosis is important. A review appointment is made for 7–10 days' time when a second injection may be considered. The principle is to give the next injection as the pain begins to peak, which usually occurs at increasing intervals. Generally not more than three or four injections are given in total. The patient is instructed to apply relative rest for up to 2 weeks and then to begin painfree mobilization. Injections of corticosteroid are efficacious in treating frozen shoulder providing the patients selected fulfil the diagnostic criteria based on Cyriax, described above in stages 1, 2 and 3 of the condition (Cameron, 1995).

Jacobs *et al.* (1991) looked at the effect of administrating intra-articular steroids with distension for the management of the early frozen shoulder. Fifty frozen shoulders were divided into three treatment groups: a distension group only, a steroid group only and a steroid and distension group. A total of three injections were offered at 6-week intervals using the posterior approach described above. All patients were provided with an information sheet explaining capsulitis and a home exercise programme.

All patients entered into the study showed improvement during treatment, with a decreased need for analgesia and improvement in pain symptoms. A significantly increased rate of improvement in the range of passive abduction and forward flexion occurred in the two groups treated with intra-articular corticosteroid, indicating a positive role for the use of corticosteroids in the early frozen shoulder.

Grade B mobilization

Grade B mobilization is applied to the non-irritable joint only. The aim is to relieve pain and to increase the range of movement. Heat

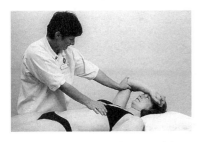

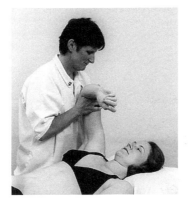

Fig. 5.27 Grade B mobilization of the glenohumeral joint.

Fig. 5.28 Returning the arm from the elevated position, with distraction for comfort.

may be used to assist the technique. The condition, prognosis and treatment are explained carefully to the patient since the recovery time may be prolonged over many months or even years, and the patient must be encouraged to continue the stretching techniques at home, eventually taking over treatment, with the therapist remaining in a supervisory role for as long as necessary.

Position the patient comfortably in lying with the arm in as much elevation as possible (Fig. 5.27). Place a hand on the sternum to stabilize the thorax and the other hand over the patient's raised elbow to apply a stretch into elevation. The principles of Grade B mobilization are applied (see Chapter 4) and the arm is returned under some distraction for comfort (Fig. 5.28).

This technique is fairly aggressive and will cause a certain amount of afterpain. Approximately 2–4 h of discomfort is acceptable and this should be explained to the patient. An increase in mobility is often reported before the reduction of pain but both are indications for continued treatment.

Distraction techniques

These are a form of Grade A mobilization since they occur within the painfree range of movement. The aim is to restore the accessory range of movement to the joint. The techniques can be applied together with Grade B mobilization in the non-irritable joint or alone in the more irritable joint. Once accessory range returns in the irritable joint and the end-feel of the limited movements regains some elasticity, the joint is deemed to be non-irritable and techniques can be progressed, adding Grade B mobilization.

Lateral distraction (Cyriax and Cyriax, 1983; Cyriax, 1984)

Position the patient comfortably in supine lying close to the edge of the couch. Place a pillow under and around the arm to support

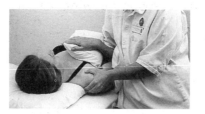

Fig. 5.29 Lateral distraction.

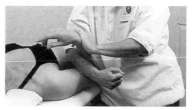

Fig. 5.30 Caudal distraction.

it in the loose packed position of adduction and some medial rotation. Place a hand into the axilla to apply the lateral distraction whilst simultaneously applying counterpressure to the patient's elbow, resting against your hip (Fig. 5.29). The distraction is held for as long as possible and repeated often.

Caudal distraction

Position the patient as above. Hook your forearm into the crook of the patient's flexed elbow (Fig. 5.30). Apply sustained and repeated caudal distractions. A 'seat belt' can be used to aid distraction techniques, but the reader is referred to courses and texts on 'seat belt therapy' for the description of its use. Other mobilizing techniques can also be incorporated into this regime.

Non-capsular lesions

Chronic subdeltoid bursitis (synonymous with subacromial bursitis)

Chronic subdeltoid bursitis is an extremely common cause of pain at the shoulder. However, it can present a challenge to diagnosis because of the muddled picture presented on examination. The bursa's intimate relationship with the capsule, the rotator cuff tendons and the biceps tendon makes it difficult to diagnose definitively and treatment response can help to confirm or refute diagnosis.

Furthermore, lesions can coexist, and a primary lesion can indirectly affect the structures closely related to it. In reviewing the anatomy it will be seen that the inner synovial aspect of the bursa is also the outer aspect of the rotator cuff, the supraspinatus tendon in particular. Therefore, they cannot be separated and inflammation of one tends to affect the other.

Prolonged inflammation can cause adhesion formation between the layers of the bursa and may produce a secondary frozen shoulder. In an unwell patient subdeltoid abscess or infective bursitis may be suspected (Ward and Eckardt, 1993).

Chronic subdeltoid bursitis has a gradual onset of pain due to the microtrauma of overuse. Together with rotator cuff lesions, chronic bursitis is a common cause of pain in athletes using the arm in the overhead position, e.g. racket sports, throwing activities of all kinds, swimming, etc. Occasionally it can be directly caused by a fall on the outstretched hand or may be due to the congenital shape of the acromion process reducing the vertical height of the subacromial space and producing impingement. Altered joint mechanics, posture, incorrect or overtraining and muscle imbalances which affect the steering mechanism of the rotator cuff tendons are all factors which may contribute to chronic bursitis at the shoulder.

The patient complains of a low-grade ache over the insertion of deltoid and may not be able to sleep on that side at night. On examination there is a non-capsular pattern of movement, often with pain felt at the end of range of passive elevation. A painful arc may be present and various resisted tests may also produce the pain. The room in the subacromial space is minimal and inflammation of the bursa causes it to become impinged under the coracoacromial arch, producing a painful arc on movement.

The application of resisted tests produces some compression of the glenohumeral joint and subacromial space. This produces a characteristic muddle of signs associated with a bursitis. The pain may be on the application of resistance, on the release of resistance or may produce several positive signs, e.g. pain on resisted abduction, lateral rotation and elbow extension. The resisted tests may not be consistent and on reassessment of the patient a completely different set of resisted tests may be present.

Treatment, ideally, consists of an injection of a large volume of low-dose local anaesthetic together with an appropriate amount of corticosteroid.

Injection of chronic subdeltoid bursitis			
Adcortyl 10 mg/ml 2 ml	Total steroid 20 mg	Lignocaine 1% 5 ml	Total volume 7 ml
21G × 1½ in (0.8 × 40 mm) green needle			

Position the patient comfortably in sitting with the arm hanging by the side. Locate the lateral border of the acromion and insert the needle just below at an oblique angle upwards with respect to the acromion (Fig. 5.31). Insert the needle and deliver the injection as a bolus, having detected the area, or areas, of less resistance. The synovial folds and adhesions within the bursa may present a resistance to the injection and it may be necessary to deliver the injection by a series of withdrawals and reinsertions. The patient is advised to maintain a period of relative rest for approximately 2 weeks following injection.

Attention should be paid to the mechanism by which the bursa becomes inflamed, as described above. An explanation is given to the patient together with restoration of balanced forces, aiming to ensure normal shoulder movement and to avoid excessive superior translation.

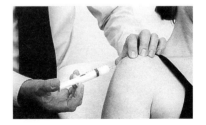

Fig. 5.31 Injection of the subdeltoid bursa.

Acute subdeltoid bursitis

This condition is a completely separate entity from chronic subdeltoid bursitis. It has a typical presentation of a sudden onset of pain for no apparent reason. The pain is felt in the shoulder area; it rapidly increases in severity and within hours the pain is referred into the whole C5 dermatome. The patient may look tired and unwell as the condition is very painful and disturbs sleep. Since the bursa is an extra-articular structure it is not protected by involuntary muscle spasm. Voluntary muscle spasm is responsible for the patient holding the arm in an antalgic position and as the patient attempts to sleep he or she loses the protective voluntary muscle spasm, waking with severe pain. Severe twinges of pain are experienced on attempted active movement, especially abduction, which compresses the inflamed bursa in the subacromial space.

On examination, a non-capsular pattern of limited movement is present. Voluntary muscle spasm is responsible for producing an empty end-feel on examination, where the examiner is aware that much more range is available, but the patient will not allow the movement to be tolerated. Usually full lateral rotation can be coaxed, especially with a little distraction applied to the joint, but the range of abduction is severely limited by pain, indicating a non-capsular pattern. Swelling and tenderness may be present along the lateral border of the acromion.

The condition is self-limiting and is usually very much better within 7–10 days, clearing completely within 6 weeks, but prone to recurrence (Cyriax, 1982). Treatment does not alter the course of the condition but should take the form of pain-relieving modalities and an explanation to the patient. The application of transcutaneous nerve stimulation and oral administration of analgesics are appropriate. Advice should also be given on sleeping position, suggesting that the arm should be well-supported by pillows, bandaged to the side or supported inside a tight-fitting t-shirt to maintain comfort when the protective muscle spasm is lost. A collar-and-cuff sling provides less support but may be used if the patient is unable to tolerate the compression of the previous suggestions.

An injection of corticosteroid is usually helpful, although it may increase the pain initially as the bursa is already swollen and very painful. The technique is the same as for chronic subdeltoid bursitis, but less volume is used.

Injection of acute subdeltoid bursitis			
Adcortyl 10 mg/ml	Total steroid	Lignocaine 1%	Total volume
2 ml	20 mg	1 ml	3 ml
21G × 1½ in (0.8 × 40 mm) green needle			

Acromioclavicular joint

The pain from the acromioclavicular joint is characteristically felt in the epaulette region of the shoulder. The onset may be precipitated by trauma – either a fall on the outstretched hand or a direct blow such as a heavy fall against the wall whilst playing squash, in a rugby tackle or at touchdown.

On examination a non-capsular pattern of painful movement is present, with pain felt at extremes of passive elevation, lateral and medial rotation. The diagnosis is confirmed by a positive scarf test reproducing the pain.

Degenerative osteoarthrosis affects the acromioclavicular joint, especially in those who have been extremely active in sport (Stenlund, 1993). Overuse can provoke a traumatic arthritis of the degenerate joint. The degenerative changes cause narrowing and osteophyte formation, which can have a secondary effect on the structures in the subacromial space.

Allman classified injuries of the acromioclavicular joint into three categories (Cailliet, 1991; Hartley, 1995):

- *Type I* injury is sprain or partial tearing of the capsular ligamentous fibres with local pain and tenderness and no joint instability.
- *Type II* injury involves tearing of capsular ligamentous fibres and minor subluxation, but as the coracoclavicular ligament remains intact, there is no instability.
- *Type III* injury is dislocation of the acromioclavicular joint with disruption of the capsule and the coracoclavicular ligaments. Treatment for type III injury is usually surgery.

Orthopaedic medicine treatment may be useful in type I and II lesions. Corticosteroid injection of the joint may be curative or, if the superior aspect of the capsular ligament is involved, it may be treated with transverse friction massage.

Injection of the acromioclavicular joint (Cyriax and Cyriax, 1983; Cyriax, 1984)

Kenalog 40 mg/ml 0.25 ml	Total steroid 10 mg	Lignocaine 1% 0.25 ml	Total volume 0.5 ml

23G × 1 in (0.6 × 25 mm) blue needle or 25G × ⅝ in (0.5 × 16 mm) orange needle

---

Position the patient comfortably in sitting or half lying and palpate the superior aspect of the joint line (Fig. 5.32). There is considerable variation in the size, shape and direction of the joint surfaces and if the joint is narrowed by degenerative changes it may be difficult to enter. The needle may have to be angled obliquely inferomedially and the presence of the articular disc may make entry difficult. Insert the needle into the joint and deliver the injection as a bolus, or pepper the superior ligament if needle entry proves to be difficult. The patient is advised to maintain a period of relative rest for approximately 2 weeks following injection.

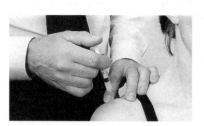

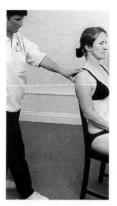

Fig. 5.32 Injection of the acromioclavicular joint.

Fig. 5.33 Transverse friction massage of the acromioclavicular joint.

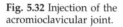

> **Transverse friction massage of the acromioclavicular capsular ligament (Cyriax and Cyriax, 1983; Cyriax, 1984)**

Stand behind the seated patient and palpate the joint line. Using an index finger reinforced by a middle finger, thumb-down on the scapula for counterpressure, direct the pressure down on to the ligament and impart the friction massage in an anteroposterior direction (Fig. 5.33).

Other mobilization techniques can be incorporated into the treatment regime for acromioclavicular strain and management may include strapping or taping the joint, particularly if the injury is type II.

Contractile lesions

The more common contractile lesions at the shoulder involve the rotator cuff tendons, particularly supraspinatus. Rotator cuff lesions can vary from simple tendinitis to degeneration and partial or complete thickness tears. The lesion may be secondary to sub-acromial impingement and may also involve the subdeltoid bursa and tendon of the long head of the biceps, which all lie in very close proximity.

Tendinitis occurs from the cumulative effects of microtrauma which has a gradual onset usually due to overuse. Single traumatic incidents may produce tendinitis, but this is unusual and the effect of trauma in this case is more likely to cause tearing of an already degenerate tendon. Pain is localized to the deltoid area and, although the patient may be aware of a vague ache, the pain is considerably increased by use and movements such as reaching, pushing and pulling – in particular those activities associated with using the hands above shoulder level.

On examination, pain is reproduced on the appropriate resisted test and there may be localizing signs of a painful arc and/or positive scarf test. Resisted abduction implicates supraspinatus, resisted lateral rotation implicates infraspinatus and teres minor and resisted medial rotation implicates subscapularis. Passive movements should be of full range with a normal end-feel, but occasionally the opposite passive movement or end-range passive elevation reproduces the pain by stretching or compressing the tendinous insertion respectively.

Simple, early tendinitis responds to conservative treatment and corticosteroid injection or transverse friction massage may be successful. However, early tendinitis may progress to degeneration, may be complicated by involvement of the nearby subdeltoid bursa or biceps tendon, or involve subtle instability or lesions of the glenoid labrum.

'Impingement syndrome' is a generic term for rotator cuff lesions encompassing all stages of tendon disease from early inflammation through degeneration and eventually partial or complete tears. Impingement may be due to subacromial space stenosis, inflammation and/or fibrosis of the contents of the space. Anatomical anomalies, particularly type III hook-shaped acromions or congenital subacromial stenosis, may predispose to impingement syndrome (Farley *et al.*, 1994; Frieman *et al.*, 1994; Burkhart, 1995).

Microtrauma of the cuff tendons may interfere with their stabilizing function, allowing the humeral head to ride higher in the glenoid, further reducing the subacromial space. Impingement may be associated with shoulder instability, degenerative changes in the acromioclavicular joint, osteophyte formation, degenerative spur formation under the acromion and thickening of the coracoacromial ligament.

The rotator cuff, especially supraspinatus, maintains the subacromial space by depressing the head of the humerus to prevent superior translation during abduction and elevation movements. Repetitive use, fatigue or overload results in cumulative microtrauma and the cuff muscles are unable to resist this superior translation, leading to subtle instability (Copeland, 1993).

Patients under 35, particularly athletes using the arm in the overhead position (e.g. swimming, tennis, squash, javelin, golf) in which large ranges of movement, forces, acceleration and repetitive movements are involved, may present with signs of impingement. This may be secondary to minor instability, possibly involving labral tears (Copeland, 1993; Jobe and Pink, 1993, 1994). Subtle or subclinical subluxation reduces the maximum congruency of the glenoid head and it appears that the supraspinatus and infraspinatus tendons are pinched in the posterosuperior labrum. The combination of instability, impingement and rotator cuff lesions should be considered in the younger athlete and the management directed at improving movement patterns to correct the instability (Iannotti, 1994).

In patients over 35, changes occur in the subacromial space which are related to degeneration and the ageing process. Fatigue and degeneration of fibres may produce muscle imbalances which lead to altered neuromuscular control and abnormal movement patterns. The humeral head is no longer effectively depressed and superior translation occurs, compromising the subacromial space (Copeland, 1993; Wilk and Arrigo, 1993; Greenfield *et al.*, 1995).

The impingement syndrome involves inflammation and oedema in the first instance and secondary thickening and fibrosis is followed by partial or full tears of the rotator cuff. The tears are usually longitudinal and on the undersurface of the tendons, which may be relatively avascular compared with the bursal surface (Cailliet, 1991; Uhthoff and Sarkar, 1992; Copeland, 1993; Fukuda *et al.*, 1994; McCann and Bigliani, 1994). Early tendon lesions may involve intrasubstance tears and calcific deposits can occur within the substance of the tendon (Meister and Andrews, 1993).

Neer (1983) was responsible for classifying the impingement syndrome into three progressive stages and provided additional evidence that impingement occurs against the anterior edge and undersurface of the anterior third of the acromion and the coracoacromial ligament. Sometimes the acromioclavicular joint is involved but not the lateral edge of the acromion.

- *Stage I* impingement involves oedema and haemorrhage, characteristically seen in younger patients. Conservative treatment at this stage usually has good results and can reverse the condition.
- *Stage II* follows repeated episodes of mechanical inflammation and the subdeltoid bursa may become thickened and fibrotic. This stage occurs in older patients and the shoulder functions well for light use, but becomes symptomatic after overuse, particularly in the overhead position. Neer recommends conservative management, with surgery only considered if the condition fails to respond to treatment after an 18-month period.
- *Stage III* involves incomplete or complete tears of the rotator cuff, biceps lesions and bone alteration of the anterior acromion and greater tuberosity. These are found almost exclusively in the over-40 age group with tears of supraspinatus occurring in a ratio of 7:1 over biceps. Stage III lesions are referred for surgical opinion. Neer also states that in his experience 95% of tears of the cuff are initiated by impingement wear rather than circulatory impairment or trauma, although trauma may enlarge an existing tear.

Dalton (1994) reports that an area of hypovascularity in supraspinatus, 1 cm from its insertion, has been both proposed and disputed. A critical zone of vascular ischaemia has been proposed, existing between the supraspinatus tendon and the coracohumeral ligament, where degeneration and tears usually occur (Cailliet, 1991). The critical zone is said to vary from being ischaemic when the vascular anastomosis is constricted, to hyperaemic when it is allowed to flow freely. The vessels are elongated when the arm is hanging by the side and compressed when the rotator cuff tendons contract to produce movement, both potentially causing relative ischaemia. Hyperaemia is said to occur only when the arm is passively supported at rest.

Clark and Harryman (1992), however, studied cadaver shoulders aged between 17 and 70 years and found no avascular area in supraspinatus. The blood vessels in the deeper tendon layers were found to be small compared with those in the superficial layers. There was no associated evidence of degeneration and the authors concluded that the blood supply was adequate for the metabolic needs of the tissue.

The aim of treatment for rotator cuff tendinitis is to relieve pain and to restore full functional movement to the shoulder. The cause of the lesion should be determined and factors such as instability and muscle imbalance should be addressed, with the rehabilitation of movement patterns to ensure restoration of the dynamic stabilizing function of the rotator cuff. Excessive superior and anterior translation should be prevented, to avoid the long-term complications of impingement which may eventually lead to surgery.

Supraspinatus tendinitis

A lesion in supraspinatus produces pain on resisted abduction. A painful arc or pain at the end of range of passive elevation localizes the lesion to the distal end of the tendon, usually at the teno-osseous junction. If pain is produced on resisted abduction only, without this localizing sign, the lesion is probably at the musculotendinous junction. Either way, palpation will confirm the exact site of the lesion.

Injection of the teno-osseous junction of supraspinatus (Cyriax and Cyriax, 1983; Cyriax, 1984)			
Kenalog 40 mg/ml	**Total steroid**	**Lignocaine 1%**	**Total volume**
0.25 ml	10 mg	0.75 ml	1 ml
25G × ½ in (0.5 × 16 mm) orange needle or 23G × 1 in (0.6 × 25 mm) blue needle			

Position the patient in sitting at an angle of 45°, medially rotating the shoulder and placing the arm behind the back to expose the

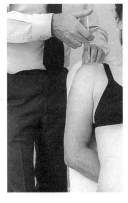

Fig. 5.34 Injection of the supraspinatus tendon.

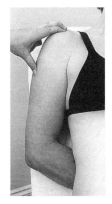

Fig. 5.35 Transverse friction massage of the supraspinatus tendon, teno-osseous site.

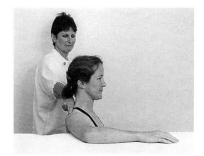

Fig. 5.36 Transverse friction massage of the supraspinatus tendon, musculotendinous junction.

tendon insertion (Fig. 5.34). Insert the needle perpendicular to the teno-osseous junction and deliver the injection using a peppering technique. The patient is advised to maintain a period of relative rest for approximately 2 weeks following injection.

Transverse friction massage of supraspinatus (Cyriax and Cyriax, 1983; Cyriax, 1984)

Teno-osseous junction
Position the patient as above. Stand at the side of the patient and identify the area of tenderness. Place an index finger, reinforced by the middle finger on to the tendon and direct the pressure down on to the insertion (Fig. 5.35). Deliver the friction massage transversely across the fibres, keeping the index finger parallel to the anterior edge of the acromion process. The supraspinatus tendon is approximately one finger wide (1 cm). Maintain the technique for 10 min after the numbing effect has been achieved. Relative rest is advised where functional movements may continue, but no overuse or stretching until painfree on resisted testing.

Musculotendinous junction of supraspinatus
Position the patient in sitting with the shoulder abducted to 90° and supported comfortably on the couch. Stand on the opposite side of the patient but facing forwards with your arm straight across and behind the patient's shoulders. Locate the musculotendinous junction in the 'V' created by the clavicle and the acromion process (Fig. 5.36). Using the middle finger reinforced by the index finger, direct the pressure down on to the tendon and deliver the friction massage by rotating the forearm. The friction is delivered for 10 min after a numbing effect has been achieved. Relative rest is advised where functional movements may continue, but no overuse or stretching until painfree on resisted testing.

Infraspinatus and teres minor

A lesion in infraspinatus and teres minor produces pain on resisted lateral rotation. A painful arc and pain at the end of range of passive elevation indicate that the lesion lies at the distal end of the tendon, usually at the teno-osseous junction. If no arc is present the lesion is often a little further proximally in the body of the tendon. Palpation will confirm the exact site of the lesion.

Injection of the teno-osseous junction of infraspinatus (Cyriax and Cyriax, 1983; Cyriax, 1984)

Kenalog 40 mg/ml	Total steroid	Lignocaine 1%	Total volume
0.25 ml	10 mg	0.75 ml	1 ml

23G × 1 in (0.6 × 25 mm) or 23G × 1¼ in (0.6 × 30 mm) blue needle or
21G × 1½ in (0.8 × 40 mm) green needle

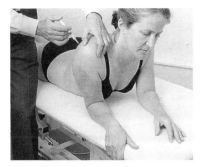

Fig. 5.37 Injection of the infraspinatus tendon.

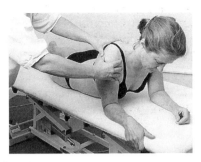

Fig. 5.38 Transverse friction massage of the infraspinatus tendon.

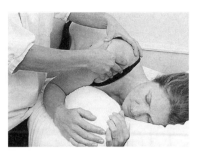

Fig. 5.39 Alternative position for transverse friction massage of the infraspinatus tendon.

Position the patient in prone lying propped up on the elbows. Laterally rotate and adduct the affected arm to expose the greater tuberosity. Locate the area of tenderness over the greater tuberosity, which now lies adjacent to the posterior angle of the acromion (Fig. 5.37). Insert the needle and deliver the injection by a peppering technique to the whole extent of the lesion, which may be up to 2–3 cm wide. The patient is advised to maintain a period of relative rest for approximately 2 weeks following injection.

> **Transverse friction massage of infraspinatus (Cyriax and Cyriax, 1983; Cyriax, 1984)**

Position the patient as above. Locate the area of tenderness and place a thumb on the area parallel to the direction of the tendon fibres; reinforce this with the other thumb (Fig. 5.38). Standing back to apply body weight, press down on to the tendon and deliver a transverse sweep across the fibres aiming to touch the posterior angle of the acromion with each stroke. The infraspinatus is two fingers (2 cm) wide; if teres minor is involved the sweep should cover a width of three fingers (3 cm). Ten minutes' friction is delivered after achieving the numbing effect. Relative rest is advised where functional movements may continue, but no overuse or stretching until painfree on resisted testing.

If the lesion lies in the body of the tendon, the technique for friction massage is the same, but applied a little more proximally at the site of the lesion, identified by palpation.

The patient position for both the injection and friction massage technique is a little uncomfortable, but can be varied to suit patient comfort (Fig. 5.39).

Subscapularis tendinitis

A lesion in subscapularis produces pain on resisted medial rotation. A painful arc indicates a lesion in the upper fibres; a positive scarf test indicates a lesion in the lower fibres. Palpation will confirm the exact site of the lesion, which may cover a large area of tendon, i.e. approximately three fingers (3 cm) wide.

Injection of subscapularis (Cyriax and Cyriax, 1983; Cyriax, 1984)			
Kenalog 40 mg/ml 0.25 ml	Total steroid 10 mg	Lignocaine 1% 0.75 ml	Total volume 1 ml
23G × 1 in (0.6 × 25 mm) or 23G × 1¼ in (0.6 × 30 mm) blue needle			

Position the patient in sitting with the arm supported to allow the humerus to rest in the anatomical position. Locate the lesser tuberosity and deliver the injection by peppering technique to the full width of the lesion (Fig. 5.40). The patient is advised to maintain a period of relative rest for approximately 2 weeks following injection.

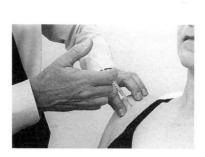

Fig. 5.40 Injection of the subscapularis tendon.

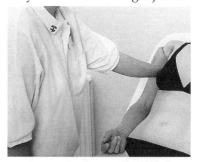

Fig. 5.41 Transverse friction massage of the subscapularis tendon.

Transverse friction massage of subscapularis (Cyriax and Cyriax, 1983; Cyriax, 1984)

Position the patient as above and locate the area of tenderness (upper fibres, lower fibres or both) on the medial aspect of the lesser tuberosity (Fig. 5.41). Place the thumb perpendicular to the direction of the fibres, parallel to the shaft of the humerus and directed laterally; deliver the friction massage in a superoinferior direction transversely across the fibres. The subscapularis may be approximately three fingers wide (3 cm). Ten minutes' friction massage is delivered after the numbing effect is achieved. Relative rest is advised where functional movements may continue, but no overuse or stretching until painfree on resisted testing.

The therapist's position can be varied to give better access to the tendon (Fig. 5.42).

Tendinitis of the long head of the biceps

In its position in the subacromial space, the tendon of the long head of biceps may be involved in an impingement syndrome. It will

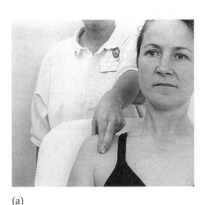 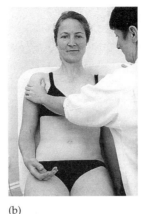

(a)   (b)

Fig. 5.42 (a, b) Alternative positions for transverse friction massage of the subscapularis tendon.

produce pain felt at the shoulder on resisted elbow flexion. With the former lesion, a painful arc is usually present on forwards flexion of the shoulder, with a straight arm and the palm uppermost.

Injection of the long head of the biceps in the bicipital groove			
Kenalog 40 mg/ml	Total steroid	Lignocaine 1%	Total volume
0.25 ml	10 mg	1 ml	1.25 ml
23G × 1 in (0.6 × 25 mm) or 33G × 1¼ in (0.6 × 30 mm) blue needle			

Position the patient in sitting with the arm supported so that the humerus rests in the anatomical position. Locate the bicipital groove and slide the needle in parallel to the groove (Fig. 5.43). Deliver the injection by a bolus technique alongside the tendon. The patient is advised to maintain a period of relative rest for approximately 2 weeks following injection.

Transverse friction massage of the long head of the biceps (Cyriax and Cyriax, 1983; Cyriax, 1984)

Position the patient as above and place a thumb parallel to the tendon in the groove, fingers wrapped around the arm for counterpressure (Fig. 5.44). Deliver the friction massage by alternately rotating the arm into medial and lateral rotation. Alternatively, the therapist may hold the patient's arm stationary and deliver the friction by abducting and adducting the thumb. Relative rest is advised where functional movements may continue, but no overuse or stretching until painfree on resisted testing.

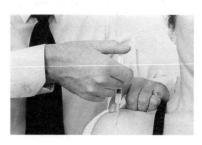

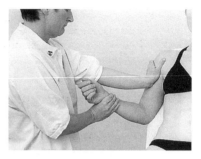

Fig. 5.43 Injection of the long head of biceps tendon.

Fig. 5.44 Transverse friction massage of the long head of biceps tendon.

General note on injection techniques at the shoulder

Hollingworth *et al.* (1983) compared two methods of corticosteroid injection with local anaesthetic to various shoulder joint or tendon lesions. One method was injection accurately placed anatomically into the lesion, based on diagnosis by selective tension, and the other involved injection into the trigger point or the point most tender to palpation. The anatomical injection group gave 60% success compared with the tender or trigger point group, which gave 20% success.

References

Anton, H.A. (1993) Frozen shoulder. *Canadian Family Physician* **39**: 1773–1777.

Biundo, J.J., Harris, M.A. (1993) Peripheral nerve entrapment, occupation-related syndromes and sports injuries, and bursitis. *Current Opinion in Rheumatology* **5**: 224–229.

Bunker, T.D., Anthony, P.P. (1995) The pathology of frozen shoulder. *Journal of Bone and Joint Surgery,* **77-B**: 677–683.

Burkhart, S.S. (1995) Congenital subacromial stenosis. *Journal of Arthroscopic and Related Surgery* **11**: 63–68.

Burns, W.C., Whipple, T.L. (1993) Anatomic relationships in the shoulder impingement syndrome. *Clinical Orthopaedics and Related Research* **294**: 96–102.

Cailliet, R. (1991) *Shoulder Pain*, 3rd edn. F.A. Davis.

Cameron, G. (1995) The shoulder is a weight bearing joint: implications for clinical practice. *Journal of Orthopaedic Medicine* **17**: 46–50.

Clark, J.M., Harryman, D.T. (1992) Tendons, ligaments and capsule of the rotator cuff. *Journal of Bone and Joint Surgery* **74-A**: 713–725.

Cooper, D.E., O'Brien, S.J., Warren, R.F. (1993) Supporting layers of the glenohumeral joint. An anatomic study. *Clinical Orthopaedics and Related Research* **289**: 144–155.

Copeland, S. (1993) Throwing injuries of the shoulder. *British Journal of Sports Medicine* **27**: 221–227.

Cyriax, J. (1982) *Textbook of Orthopaedic Medicine*, vol. 1, 8th edn. Baillière Tindall.

Cyriax, J. (1984) *Textbook of Orthopaedic Medicine*, vol. 2, 11th edn. Baillière Tindall.

Cyriax, J., Cyriax, P. (1983) *Illustrated Manual of Orthopaedic Medicine*. Butterworths.

Dalton, S.E. (1994) The conservative management of rotator cuff disorders. *British Journal of Rheumatology* **33**: 663–667.

Farley, T.E., Neumann, C.H., Steinbach, L.S., Petersen, S.A. (1994) The coracoacromial arch – MR evaluation and correlation with rotator cuff pathology. *Skeletal Radiology* **23**: 641–645.

Flatow, E.L., Soslowsky, L.J., Ticker, J.B. *et al.* (1994) Excursion of the rotator cuff under the acromion. *American Journal of Sports Medicine* **22**: 779–788.

Frame, M.K. (1991) Anatomy and biomechanics of the shoulder. In: *Clinics in Physical Therapy, Physical Therapy of the Shoulder* (Donatelli, R.A. ed.). Churchill Livingstone, pp. 1–18.

Frieman, B.G., Albert, T.J., Fenlin, J.M. (1994) Rotator cuff disease – a review of diagnosis, pathophysiology and current trends in treatment. *Archives of Physical Medicine and Rehabilitation* **75**: 604–609.

Fukuda, H., Hamada, K., Nakajima, T., Tomonaga, A. (1994) Pathology and pathogenesis of the intratendinous tearing of the rotator cuff viewed from en bloc histologic sections. *Clinical Orthopaedics and Related Research* **304**: 60–67.

Greenfield, B., Catlin, P.A., Coats, P.W. *et al.* (1995) Posture in patients with shoulder overuse injuries in healthy individuals. *Journal of Orthopaedic and Sports Physical Therapy* **21**: 287–295.

Grubbs, N. (1993) Frozen shoulder syndrome – a review of the literature. *Journal of Orthopaedic and Sports Physical Therapy* **18**: 479–487.

Hartley, A. (1995) *Practical Joint Assessment, Upper Quadrant*, 2nd edn. Mosby.

Hollingworth, G.R., Ellis, R., Hattersley, T.S. (1983) Comparison of injection techniques for shoulder pain – results of a double blind, randomised study. *British Medical Journal* **287**: 1339–1341.

Hsu, S.Y.C., Chan, K.M. (1991) Arthroscopic distension in the management of frozen shoulder. *International Orthopaedics* **15**: 79–83.

Hulstyn, M.J., Fadale, P.D. (1995) Arthroscopic anatomy of the shoulder. *Orthopaedic Clinics of North America* **26**: 597–612.

Hulstyn, M.J., Weiss, A. (1993) Adhesive capsulitis of the shoulder. *Orthopaedic Review* **22**: 425–433.

Iannotti, J.P. (1994) Evaluation of the painful shoulder. *Journal of Hand Therapy* **7**: 77–83.

Itoi, E., Newman, S.R., Kuechle, D.K. *et al.* (1994) Dynamic anterior stabilisers of the shoulder with the arm in abduction. *Journal of Bone and Joint Surgery* **76-B**: 834–836.

Jacobs, L.G.H., Barton, M.A.J., Wallace, W.A. *et al.* (1991) Intra-articular distension and steroids in the management of capsulitis of the shoulder. *British Medical Journal* **302**: 1498–1501.

Jeracitano, D., Cooper, R., Lyon, L.J., Jayson, M.I.V. (1992) Abnormal temperature control suggesting sympathetic dysfunction in the shoulder skin of patients with frozen shoulder. *British Journal of Rheumatology* **31**: 539–542.

Jobe, F.W., Pink, M. (1993) Classification and treatment of shoulder dysfunction in the overhead athlete. *Journal of Orthopaedic and Sports Physical Therapy* **18**: 427–432.

Jobe, F.W., Pink, M. (1994) The athlete's shoulder. *Journal of Hand Therapy* **7**: 107–110.

Kapandji, I.A. (1982) *The Physiology of the Joints, Upper Limb*, 5th edn. Churchill Livingstone.

Lundberg, B.J. (1969) The frozen shoulder. *Acta Orthopaedic Scandinavica: With Supplements* **119**: 1–59.

McCann, P.D., Bigliani, L.U. (1994) Shoulder pain in tennis players. *Sports Medicine* **17**: 53–64.

Meister, K., Andrews, J.R. (1993) Classification and treatment of rotator cuff injuries in the overhead athlete. *Journal of Orthopaedic and Sports Physical Therapy* **18**: 413–421.

Neer, C.S. (1983) Impingement lesions. *Clinical Orthopaedics and Related Research* **173**: 70–77.

Netter, F.H. (1987) Musculoskeletal system part I. *Ciba Collection of Medical Illustrations*, vol. 8. Ciba-Giegy.

Nordin, M., Frankel, V.H. (1989) *Basic Biomechanics of the Musculoskeletal System*, 2nd edn. Lea & Febiger.

Ogilvie-Harris, D.J., Biggs, D.J., Fistsialos, D.P., MacKay, M. (1995) The resistant frozen shoulder, manipulation versus arthroscopic release. *Clinical Orthopaedics and Related Research* **319**: 238–248.

Owens-Burkhart, H. (1991) Management of frozen shoulder. In: *Clinics in Physical Therapy, Physical Therapy of the Shoulder* (Donatelli, R.A., ed.). Churchill Livingstone, pp. 91–116.

Paine, R.M., Voight, M. (1993) The role of the scapula. *Journal of Orthopaedic and Sports Physical Therapy* **18**: 386–391.

Palastanga, N., Field, D., Soames, R. (1994) *Anatomy and Human Movement*, 2nd edn. Butterworth-Heinemann.

Pellecchia, G.L., Paolino, J., Connell, J. (1996) Intertester reliability of the Cyriax evaluation in assessing patients with shoulder pain. *Journal of Orthopaedic and Sports Physical Therapy* **23**: 34–38.

Pratt, N.E. (1994) Anatomy and biomechanics of the shoulder. *Journal of Hand Therapy* **7**: 65–76.

Schulte, K.R., Warner, J.J.P. (1995) Uncommon causes of shoulder pain in the athlete. *Orthopaedic Clinics of North America* **26**: 505–528.

Shaffer, B., Tibone, J.E., Kerlan, R.K. (1992) Frozen shoulder – a long term follow-up. *Journal of Bone and Hand Surgery* **74-A**: 738–746.

Sharma, R.K., Bajekal, R.A., Bhan, S. (1993) Frozen shoulder syndrome. *International Orthopaedics* **17**: 275–278.

Speer, K.P. (1995) Anatomy and pathomechanics of shoulder instability. *Clinics in Sports Medicine* **14**: 751–760.

Stam, H.W. (1994) Frozen shoulder – a review of current concepts. *Physiotherapy* **80**: 588–598.

Stenlund, B. (1993) Shoulder tendinitis and osteoarthrosis of the acromioclavicular joint and their relation to sports. *British Journal of Sports Medicine* **27**: 125–130.

Uhthoff, K.J., Sarkar, K. (1992) Periarticular soft tissue conditions causing pain in the shoulder. *Current Opinion in Rheumatology* **4**: 241–246.

Uitvlugt, G., Detrisac, D.A., Johnson, L.J. *et al.* (1993) Arthroscopic observations before and after manipulation of frozen shoulder. *Journal of Arthroscopic and Related Surgery* **9**: 181–185.

Wadsworth, C.T. (1986) Frozen shoulder. *Physical Therapy* **66**: 1878–1883.

Ward, W.G., Eckardt, J.J. (1993) Subacromial/subdeltoid bursa abscesses, an overlooked diagnosis. *Clinical Orthopaedics and Related Research* **288**: 189–194.

Wiley, A.M. (1991) Arthroscopic appearance of frozen shoulder. *Journal of Arthroscopic and Related Surgery* **7**: 138–143.

Wilk, K.E., Arrigo, C. (1993) Current concepts in the rehabilitation of the athletic shoulder. *Journal of Orthopaedic and Sports Physical Therapy* **18**: 365–378.

Williams, P.L, Warwick, R., Dyson, M., Bannister, L.H. (1989) *Gray's Anatomy*, 37th edn. Churchill Livingstone.

6 The elbow

Summary

Tennis elbow is the most commonly encountered elbow problem in clinical practice and probably presents the greatest challenge. This chapter suggests an approach to its management, as well as addressing other common and more unusual lesions.

To aid diagnosis and accurate treatment, the chapter begins by outlining the relevant anatomy and provides guidelines for palpation. A commentary on the history and objective sequence follows, leading to discussion of the lesions which may be encountered, with suggestions for their effective treatment and management.

Anatomy

Inert structures

Anatomically the elbow consists of two articulations, the elbow joint proper and the superior radioulnar joint, both contained within the same joint capsule.

The *elbow joint* proper is a synovial hinge joint between the distal end of the humerus, comprising the capitulum and trochlea, and the proximal ends of the radius and ulna. The articular capsule surrounds the articular margins. In common with other synovial hinge joints, the relatively weak articular capsule is reinforced by strong collateral ligaments.

The *capitulum* is roughly hemispherical in shape and articulates with the radial head. The *trochlea* is pulley or spool-shaped and extends from the anterior aspect of the distal end of the humerus to the olecranon fossa posteriorly. It articulates with the trochlear notch of the ulna.

On the distal, anterior surface of the humerus sit the *radial and coronoid fossae* accommodating the rims of the radial head and coronoid process of ulna in full flexion. The *olecranon fossa* of the humerus accepts the olecranon process of the ulna in full extension.

The proximal end of the radius consists of a head, neck and tuberosity. The radial head is cup-shaped superiorly for articulation with the capitulum. The periphery of the head is an articulating surface for the superior radioulnar joint, articulating with the inner surface of the annular ligament. The *radial tuberosity* gives insertion to the biceps tendon.

At the proximal end of the ulna is the massive hook-shaped *olecranon process*. Anteriorly, the coronoid process arises with the radial notch on its medial side for articulation with the radius at the superior radioulnar joint. The elbow joint itself permits flexion and extension coupled with a small amount of adjunct rotation (Williams *et al.*, 1989). About 160° of passive flexion exists as the bones become almost parallel and the radial and coronoid fossae allow for extra functional movement by accommodating to the flexor muscle bulk. The normal end-feel of elbow flexion is soft due to approximation of the flexor muscles. Passive extension is achieved by locking the olecranon into the olecranon fossa; it corresponds to a 180° angle and has a hard end-feel due to bone contact.

The elbow joint receives a nerve supply from the musculocutaneous, median and radial nerves anteriorly, and the ulnar and radial nerves posteriorly (C5–8).

The *superior radioulnar joint* is a uniaxial pivot joint permitting the movements of pronation and supination. These movements occur between the circumference of the radial head in the fibro-osseous ring created by the annular ligament and the radial notch of the ulna. The annular ligament is covered internally by a thin layer of articular cartilage.

Movement occurring at the superior and inferior radioulnar joints is rotation of the radius around the ulna to produce pronation and supination. The range of passive pronation is approximately 85° and passive supination 90°, normally with an elastic end-feel.

The *carrying angle (cubitus valgus)* is evident in the anatomical position. The medial end of the distal humerus projects more distally and anteriorly than the lateral, pushing the ulna laterally to produce this valgus angle. It is approximately 10–15° in men and 20–25° in women (Palastanga *et al.*, 1994).

The *cubital fossa* is situated on the front of the elbow. Its proximal border is an imaginary line drawn between the two epicondyles of the humerus, its lateral border is brachioradialis and its medial border is pronator teres. On the floor of the fossa lies supinator and biceps and the roof is formed by the overlying skin and fascia. The contents of the cubital fossa from lateral to medial are the tendon of the biceps in the centre, the brachial artery and the median nerve.

Contractile structures

Biceps brachii (musculocutaneous nerve C5–6) has two heads of origin. The muscle ends in a stout tendon which attaches to the posterior aspect of the radial tuberosity. As the tendon passes to its insertion it twists so that its anterior surface comes to rest laterally. The tendon is separated from the anterior aspect of the radial tuberosity by the subtendinous bicipital bursa. Biceps is a powerful elbow flexor. Its secondary action is to assist supinator in supination of the forearm, particularly with the elbow joint in 90° of flexion, but it has no supinating action in the extended elbow.

Brachialis (musculocutaneous nerve C5–6) takes origin from the anterior aspect of the lower half of the shaft of the humerus and inserts into the coronoid process of the ulna. As it crosses the elbow joint some of its deep fibres insert into the capsule of the elbow joint. Its action is to flex the elbow in either pronation or supination.

Brachioradialis (radial nerve C5–7) passes from the upper two-thirds of the lateral supracondylar ridge of the humerus to the distal end of the radius just above the styloid. It flexes the elbow, being most effective in the mid pronation–supination position.

Triceps (radial nerve C6–8) has three heads of origin above the elbow with its tendon inserting into the olecranon process. It is the major forearm extensor and is involved in pushing and thrusting activities as well as raising body weight on semiflexed elbows, as in getting up from a chair.

Pronator teres (median nerve C6–7) has two heads of origin: a humeral head from just above the medial epicondyle, the coronoid process and from the common flexor tendon, and an ulnar head from the medial side of the coronoid process. It passes down and laterally to insert into a roughened area along the lateral aspect of the shaft of the radius. Its main action is to pronate the forearm, especially against resistance.

Pronator quadratus (median nerve C8, T1) binds the lower parts of the radius and ulna and is the principal pronator of the forearm.

Supinator (posterior interosseous nerve C5–6) has its proximal attachment from the supinator crest of the ulnar, lateral epicondyle of the humerus and the radial collateral and annular ligaments. It wraps round to insert into the proximal third of the radius and supinates the forearm, bringing the palm of the hand to face upwards, whatever the degree of flexion at the elbow.

Extensor carpi radialis longus (radial nerve C6–7) takes its main origin from the lower third of the lateral supracondylar ridge and some origin from the common extensor tendon. It passes to the radial side of the base of the second metacarpal.

Extensor carpi radialis brevis (posterior interosseous nerve C7–8) takes its main origin from the lateral epicondyle via the common extensor tendon and inserts into the radial side of the base of the third metacarpal. It is very commonly involved in tennis elbow.

Extensor carpi radialis longus and brevis extend the wrist and produce radial deviation. They work synergistically with the finger flexor tendons by holding the wrist in extension, allowing the finger flexors to form an effective grip (Palastanga *et al.*, 1994).

Other muscles which take origin from the common extensor tendon and also responsible for wrist extension are extensor digitorum, extensor digiti minimi and extensor carpi ulnaris (which also produces ulnar deviation). All of these muscles are supplied by the posterior interosseous nerve (C7–8).

Flexor carpi radialis (median nerve C6–7) arises from the medial epicondyle via the common flexor tendon and becomes tendinous above the wrist, before passing through its own lateral compartment under the flexor retinaculum. It inserts into the bases of the second and third metacarpals.

Palmaris longus (median nerve C7–8), often absent, arises from the medial epicondyle via the common flexor tendon and passes over, not under, the flexor retinaculum and attaches to this and the palmar aponeurosis.

Flexor digitorum superficialis (median nerve C7–8, T1) lies in a slightly deeper plane than the above flexor muscles and has a humeral head from the medial epicondyle via the common flexor tendon, and a small radial head. It divides to pass under the flexor retinaculum before entering the fingers to attach to the middle phalanx of each.

Flexor carpi ulnaris (ulnar nerve C7–8) has two heads of origin: a small humeral head from the medial epicondyle via the common flexor origin and an ulnar head from the ulna. It passes over the retinaculum into the pisiform.

Guide to surface marking and palpation

Lateral aspect (Fig. 6.1)

Palpate the *lateral supracondylar ridge*, which is a subcutaneous sharp ridge, giving part origin to extensor carpi radialis longus and brachioradialis.

The lateral supracondylar ridge terminates in the *lateral epicondyle*, a small bony projection which you will palpate more easily if the elbow is flexed.

Visualize the small facet on the anterolateral aspect of the lateral epicondyle which gives origin to the *common extensor tendon* of the superficial wrist extensor muscles. This facet is approximately the size of the patient's little finger nail.

Palpate the *head of the radius* on the lateral side of the extended forearm; it is located in a posterior depression just distal to the

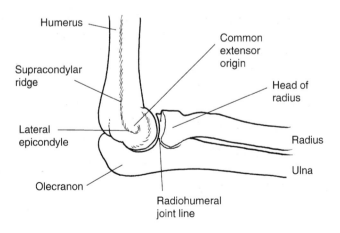

Fig. 6.1 Lateral aspect of the elbow in flexion.

lateral epicondyle. Confirm the correct position by rotating the forearm to feel the radial head move under your finger.

Move proximally a short distance to palpate the *radiohumeral joint line*, just above the radial head. Here the gap between the head of the radius and the capitulum of the humerus should be obvious; flex your elbow and feel the joint open. Flexion past 45° tightens the joint capsule, making the joint line less obvious.

Identify *brachioradialis*, the most superficial forearm muscle on the lateral side of the forearm, by flexing the elbow against resistance in the mid pronation–supination position.

Medial aspect (Fig. 6.2)

Palpate the *medial supracondylar ridge* which ends in the rounded knob of the *medial epicondyle*. Identify the medial epicondyle, which is subcutaneous and most easily felt with the elbow in extension. Palpate the anterior aspect of the medial epicondyle, which provides the attachment for the *common flexor tendon* of the superficial wrist flexor muscles.

Visualize the position of the superficial wrist flexor muscles by placing the thenar eminence of one hand on to the opposite medial epicondyle and spread the digits down the forearm to represent the following tendons (Fig. 6.3):

- Thumb: pronator teres.
- Index: flexor carpi radialis.
- Middle: palmaris longus.
- Ring: flexor digitorum superficialis (deeper than the others and not so obvious).
- Little: flexor carpi ulnaris.

Anterior aspect

It is not possible to palpate the joint line of the elbow anteriorly because of the position of the flexor muscles, but it can be visualized by drawing a line joining points 1 cm below the lateral epicondyle and 2 cm below the medial epicondyle (Palastanga *et al.*, 1994).

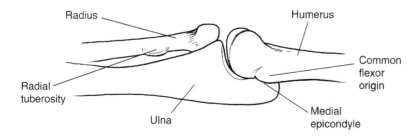

Fig. 6.2 Medial aspect of the elbow in extension.

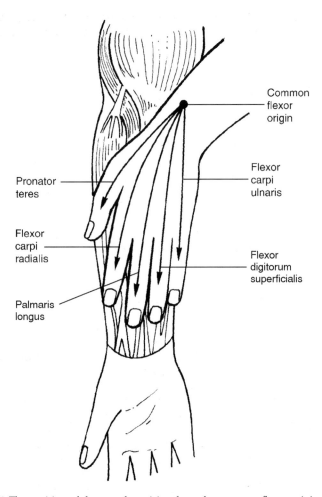

Fig. 6.3 The position of the muscles arising from the common flexor origin.

Locate the ***tuberosity of the radius*** by flexing the elbow to make the tendon of the biceps more obvious. Follow the tendon down to its insertion on to the radial tuberosity. The tendon of the biceps will be easily palpable as it passes deep into the cubital fossa, but the tuberosity may not feel distinct to the palpating finger, although it is tender to deep palpation.

Place the arm in the anatomical position of elbow extension and supination and note the obvious valgus angle, known as the ***carrying angle***. It should be symmetrical bilaterally.

Posterior aspect

Palpate the proximal surface of the ***olecranon***, the point of the elbow, which is subcutaneous and most easily palpated when the elbow is flexed. The olecranon gives insertion to triceps and a subcutaneous bursa, the olecranon bursa, lies under the loose skin at the back of the elbow.

Commentary on the examination

Observation

Before proceeding with the history, a general observation of the patient's *face, posture and gait* will alert the examiner to abnormalities and serious illness. The acute elbow is usually held in a position of flexion and a degree of supination, and medial rotation at the shoulder, with the patient nursing the arm in a position of comfort.

Lesions commonly found at the elbow are due to overuse when abnormalities of posture are not usually observed.

History (subjective examination)

The *age, occupation, sports, hobbies and lifestyle* of the patient may give an indication of the nature of the onset and cause of the injury, and will alert the examiner to possible postural or overuse problems. It may also give an indication of whether the source of the problem is in the cervical spine.

Age may be relevant, as certain conditions affect particular age groups, e.g. in children, conditions such as 'pulled elbow' (a subluxation of the small radial head in the relatively immature annular ligament) which affects children in the 1–4-year age group. Degenerative osteoarthrosis generally affects the elderly, with rheumatoid arthritis involving the elbow at any age. Loose bodies can occur in adolescents, associated with osteochondritis dissecans, or in the middle-aged/elderly group associated with degenerative changes in the articular cartilage. The overuse lesions of tennis and golfer's elbow tend to be a problem of middle age as the ageing process causes the tendinous material to become less extensible and more prone to injury.

The elbow joint and surrounding structures are situated within the C5–7 and T1 dermatomes. However, the *site* of pain is usually well-localized, indicating a less severe, superficial lesion. A *spread* of pain would indicate greater inflammation and possibly referral of pain from a deeper more proximal structure.

The patient may report local tenderness with an olecranon bursitis or, more commonly, with a tennis or golfer's elbow, which may produce a diffuse reference of pain into the forearm, as well as point tenderness over either the lateral or medial epicondyle respectively.

The *onset* of the symptoms may be sudden, due to trauma, or gradual, due to overuse or arthritis. If the onset is traumatic in nature the mechanism of injury should be deduced. Acute injuries include dislocations and fractures of the radial head, olecranon and distal humerus (Safran, 1995).

Hyperextension injuries may cause a capsulitis, or a fall on the outstretched hand may cause fracture (e.g. supracondylar, distal radius or ulna) and/or dislocation. The possible neurovascular complications, secondary to trauma, should be kept in mind.

A sudden onset of pain associated with locking of the elbow could indicate a loose body.

The *duration* of the symptoms may be long-standing. The commonest lesions at the elbow are due to chronic overuse and result in the enthesiopathies tennis elbow (lateral epicondylitis) and golfer's elbow (medial epicondylitis). The common tendons of the forearm flexors and extensors are susceptible to excessive use because they function across two joints. The causative factors may be intrinsic overload, from the force of muscle contraction; extrinsic overload, through excessive joint torque forces stressing the connective tissue, stretching and eventually disrupting it, or a combination of intrinsic and extrinsic forces (Safran, 1995).

These overuse injuries are often associated with the middle-aged racquet sports player or individuals participating in throwing activities. Throwing motions may produce a valgus stress on the medial elbow and compressive forces at the lateral elbow. Such repetitive actions may result in microtrauma to the joint or surrounding tissues (Nicola, 1992).

Climber's elbow affects brachialis, as climbing involves the use of the semiflexed pronated forearm (Safran, 1995). Overuse may cause friction between the radial tuberosity and the biceps tendon, resulting in inflammation of the biceps subtendinous bursa, or an overuse lesion in the tendon itself.

The duration of symptoms indicates the stage of the lesion in the inflammatory process. The common presentation of tennis or golfer's elbow is pain of weeks' or even months' duration, whilst the less common loose body has recurrent episodes of twinging, often resolving spontaneously. Arthritis is characterized by recurrent episodes of exacerbation of pain.

The *symptoms and behaviour* need to be considered. The behaviour of the pain indicates the nature of the lesion: mechanical lesions are eased by rest and aggravated by repeated movements, particularly those involved in the mechanism of the lesion. For example, tennis elbow gives an increase of pain on gripping activities – simple things such as lifting a cup or pulling up bedclothes. Patients often report that knocking the lateral aspect of the elbow can give excruciating pain and it is very tender to touch. Other symptoms described by the patient could include twinges of pain with locking of the elbow, usually just short of full extension, which would indicate a possible loose body. A twinge of pain in the forearm on gripping is also associated with a tennis elbow, causing the patient to drop the object and giving an apparent feeling of muscle weakness.

Paraesthesia may be indicative of nerve involvement and the exact location of these symptoms should be ascertained. Paraesthesia may be referred distally from the cervical spine, but as the ulnar nerve lies in an exposed location behind the medial epicondyle, it is occasionally subject to direct trauma.

Both the posterior interosseous nerve (passing between the two heads of supinator) and the median nerve (passing between the two heads of pronator teres) are susceptible to muscular compression. This may complicate the clinical presentation of either tennis or golfer's elbow and may be a reason for a poor response to treatment directed at the more common musculoskeletal problem.

An indication of *past medical history, other joint involvement* and *medications* will establish whether contraindications to treatment exist, or that the lesion is part of an ongoing inflammatory arthritis.

Inspection

An inspection is conducted in standing with the upper limb resting in the anatomical position, if this can be achieved. Assess the overall posture from above down, looking for any *bony deformity*, noting the position of the head, the lordosis in the cervical spine and the position of both shoulders. Assess the carrying angle in the

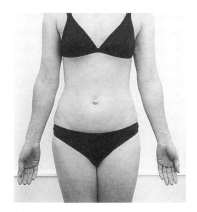

(a)

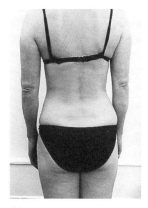

(b)

Fig. 6.4 (a, b) Inspection of the elbow.

anatomical position, comparing it with the other side for symmetry (Fig. 6.4a,b).

Inspect for *colour changes*, including contusions and abrasions which are associated with direct trauma. These may be located at the point of the elbow or over either epicondyle. Bruising over the biceps or triceps muscles can occur in contact sports where a direct blow is possible. Abrasions may be a site of entry for bacteria, with septic olecranon bursitis being a possible result of such infection.

Muscle wasting may be evident in the forearm if a patient has a long or recurrent history of tennis elbow. Other muscle wasting would be unusual and would probably be a neurological sign associated with cervical pathology.

Swelling is usually associated with trauma. It may be diffuse, engulfing the elbow area, in which case the elbow will be fixed in the position of ease, to accommodate the swelling with minimal pain. The dimples seen at the back of a flexed elbow are obliterated if swelling is present, as here the capsule is lax and usually accommodates excess fluid.

Immediate swelling indicates bleeding and possibly a haemarthrosis. Swelling developing 6–24 h after trauma indicates synovial irritation and capsular involvement. Local swellings are associated with direct trauma. A localized soft, boggy, fluctuating swelling may be seen over the point of the elbow and is indicative

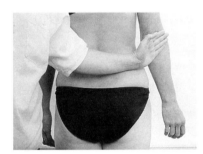

Fig. 6.5 Palpation for heat.

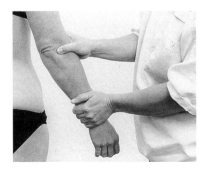

Fig. 6.6 Palpation for synovial thickening.

of an olecranon bursitis. Occasionally patients complain of swelling over the lateral epicondyle in tennis elbow, but this is not always evident clinically.

Palpation

Since the elbow is a peripheral joint, the joint is palpated for signs of activity. *Heat* indicates an active inflammation (Fig. 6.5), as does *synovial thickening* which is most easily palpable over the radial head in the more chronic state (Fig. 6.6). *Swelling* is usually most apparent in the dimples at the back of the elbow and may be palpated in that area. Other swellings such as nodules or associated with olecranon bursitis can also be palpated to assess whether they are hard or soft.

State at rest

Before any movements are performed, the state at rest is established to provide a baseline for subsequent comparison.

The suggested sequence for the objective examination will now be given, followed by a commentary including the reasoning in performing the movements and the significance of the possible findings.

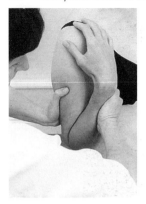

Fig. 6.7 Passive elbow flexion.

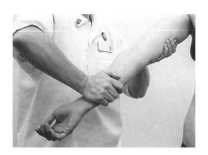

Fig. 6.8 Passive elbow extension.

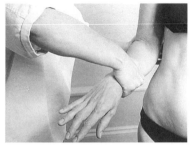

Fig. 6.9 Passive pronation.

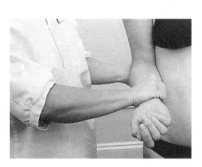

Fig. 6.10 Passive supination.

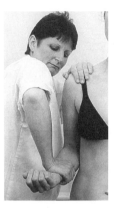

Fig. 6.11 Resisted elbow flexion.

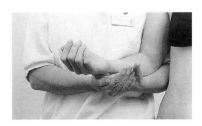

Fig. 6.12 Resisted elbow extension.

Examination by selective tension (objective examination)

Elbow and superior radioulnar joints:

- Passive elbow flexion (Fig. 6.7)
- Passive elbow extension (Fig. 6.8)
- Passive pronation of the superior radioulnar joint (Fig. 6.9)
- Passive supination of the superior radioulnar joint (Fig. 6.10)
- Resisted elbow flexion (Fig. 6.11)
- Resisted elbow extension (Fig. 6.12)

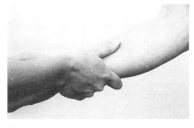

(a)

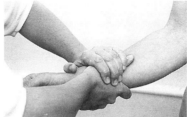

(b)

Fig. 6.13 (a–c) Hand and body positioning for resisted pronation and supination.

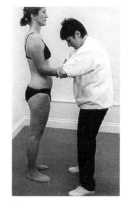

(c)

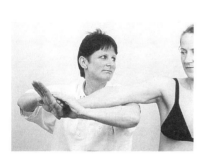

Fig. 6.14 Resisted wrist extension.

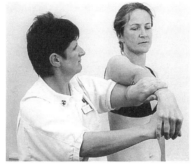

Fig. 6.15 Resisted wrist flexion.

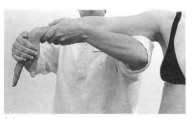

(a)

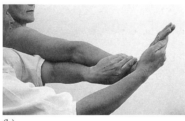

(b)

Fig. 6.16 Examples of further provocative tests: (a) resisted wrist extension from the flexed position; (b) resisted wrist flexion from the extended position.

- Resisted pronation (Fig. 6.13a,b,c)
- Resisted supination (Fig. 6.13a,b,c)

Provocative tests for epicondylitis:

- Resisted wrist extension for tennis elbow (Fig. 6.14 and 6.16a)
- Resisted wrist flexion for golfer's elbow (Fig. 6.15 and 6.16b)

Palpation

- Once a diagnosis has been made, the structure at fault is palpated for the exact site of the lesion

The elbow joint and the superior radioulnar joint are assessed by four passive movements looking for pain, range and end-feel. In the normal patient, passive flexion has a 'soft' end-feel and passive extension has a 'hard' end-feel. At the superior radioulnar joint, passive pronation and supination have an 'elastic' end-feel. The signs elicited will establish whether or not the capsular pattern exists.

A loose body in the elbow joint produces a non-capsular pattern of movement with either limitation of passive flexion or extension, but not both. The limited movement has an abnormal 'springy' end-feel.

The resisted tests are conducted for the muscles around the elbow, looking for pain and power. Resisted elbow flexion tests biceps and resisted elbow extension tests triceps. Resisted pronation tests pronator quadratus and pronator teres, but since pronator teres takes origin from the common flexor tendon, this may be an accessory sign in golfer's elbow. Resisted supination tests biceps, since it is assessed with the elbow flexed, and supinator.

Two provocative resisted tests are conducted at the wrist to assess the common extensor and common flexor tendons for epicondylitis. Resisted wrist extension and resisted wrist flexion are assessed with the elbow joint fully extended. To provoke pain, further provocative tests can be applied for lateral epicondylitis (tennis elbow), e.g. passive wrist flexion, resisted wrist extension from the flexed position, resisted radial deviation and resisted middle finger extension. For medial epicondylitis (golfer's elbow) resisted wrist flexion can be assessed from the extended position.

> **Capsular pattern of the elbow joint**
> - **More limitation of flexion than extension**
>
> **Capsular pattern of the superior radioulnar joint**
> - **Pain at the end of range of both rotations**

Capsular lesions

The capsular pattern indicates the presence of arthritis in the joint which, at the elbow, is frequently rheumatoid arthritis. Degenerative osteoarthrosis is of itself symptom-free, but traumatic arthritis may be secondary to overuse or trauma of a restricted joint. Treatment of choice is a corticosteroid injection into the elbow joint complex.

Injection of the elbow joint complex			
Adcortyl 10 mg/ml	Total steroid	Lignocaine 1%	Total volume
2 ml	20 mg	1 ml	3 ml
$25G \times \frac{5}{8}$ in (0.5 × 16 mm) orange needle			

Sit the patient with the elbow flexed to approximately 45° and the forearm pronated (Fig. 6.17). Locate the radiohumeral joint line on the posterolateral aspect of the upper forearm. Insert the needle between the head of the radius and the capitulum (Fig. 6.18). Once intra-articular, deliver the injection as a bolus. The patient is advised to maintain a period of relative rest for approximately 2 weeks following injection.

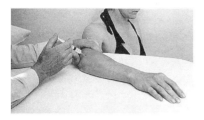

Fig. 6.17 Injection of the elbow joint complex.

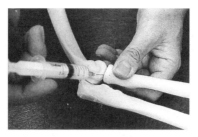

Fig. 6.18 Injection of the elbow joint, showing direction of approach and needle position.

Traumatic arthritis can be treated with other physiotherapeutic modalities.

Non-capsular lesions

Loose body

Osteochondritis dissecans occurs in adolescents and can give rise to loose-body formation, particularly with activities such as gymnastics, throwing and racket sports. Repeated compressive forces cause microtrauma between the radial head and capitulum and focal degeneration results in fragmentation and the formation of loose bodies (Ho, 1995; Patten, 1995). Surgical removal is advisable in this age group.

Loose bodies can also be encountered in the middle-aged/elderly group. Characteristically, the patient complains of a history of twinging pain, with the elbow giving way under pressure or locking, usually just short of full elbow extension. The history alone may be the only diagnostic evidence available since the loose body may spontaneously reduce. Sometimes diagnostic imaging may be necessary to identify and localize loose bodies before arthroscopic removal (Ho, 1995).

On examination, a non-capsular pattern may exist with either a small degree of limitation of flexion or extension, but not both. The end-feel to the limited movement is abnormally springy.

The treatment of choice to reduce a loose body is strong traction together with Grade A mobilization, theoretically aiming to shift the loose body to another part of the joint and to restore full, painfree movement.

There are two possible manoeuvres, both working towards elbow extension. The choice of starting manoeuvre is random and sometimes it may be necessary to try both and repeat the most successful, although sometimes one manoeuvre is sufficient. As with all mobilization techniques, the patient is reassessed after every manoeuvre and a decision made about the next, based on the outcome.

Mobilization for loose body in the elbow joint

Towards extension and supination
Position the patient against the raised head of the couch, with the arm resting against a pillow. Use a butterfly grip with the thumbs placed on the flexor surface of the forearm, over the radius (Fig. 6.19). Face the direction of the supination movement and lift the

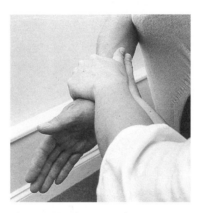

Fig. 6.19 Hand position for mobilization for loose body in the elbow joint, towards extension and supination.

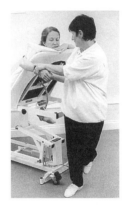

Fig. 6.20 Body position for mobilization for loose body in the elbow joint, towards extension and supination: step forwards.

leg farthest from the patient off the ground, leaning out to establish traction with straight arms. Step forwards, taking the elbow joint towards extension (not full range), whilst simultaneously rotating the forearm with several flicking movements towards supination (Fig. 6.20). The manoeuvre is easier to perform if you begin the rotation from a position of some pronation.

Towards extension and pronation
The patient's position is the same. Face the movement of pronation, placing the thumbs on the extensor surface of the forearm, over the radius (Fig. 6.21). Establish the traction as above and step backwards, simultaneously rotating the forearm with several flicking movements towards pronation (Fig. 6.22). The manoeuvre is easier to perform if you begin the rotation from a position of some supination.

The patient may need to be reviewed to assess the success of the treatment. Generally speaking, the manoeuvre is usually successful, but there are no guarantees that the condition will not recur. Occasionally the patient may present with a history of the condition only and treatment may be experimental. Excessive recurrences of the condition may need referral for surgery.

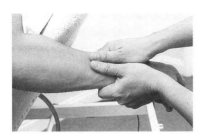

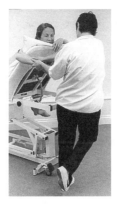

Fig. 6.21 Hand position for mobilization for loose body in the elbow joint, towards extension and pronation.

Fig. 6.22 Body position for mobilization for loose body in the elbow joint, towards extension and pronation: step backwards.

Olecranon bursitis

Swelling and inflammation of the olecranon bursa can occur due to repeated pressure and friction, or to direct trauma of the bursa. The bursa is the most vulnerable structure to trauma on the posterior surface of the elbow and septic bursitis is not uncommon (Nicola, 1992; Hoppmann, 1993). The patient may present with an obvious swelling over the olecranon which is boggy and fluctuating. Provided sepsis is not present, conservative management includes aspiration, ice and non-steroidal anti-inflammatory drugs (Nicola, 1992). Any physiotherapeutic modality may be applied and corticosteroid injection may be given.

Pulled elbow

This condition occasionally presents to the general practitioner's surgery or the casualty department. Typically the child is aged between 1 and 4 years old and has a sudden onset of pain in the arm, followed by a reluctance to use the arm. The child is unhappy and holds the arm in elbow flexion and pronation. The arm is painfree provided it is not moved.

There may be a history of the child stumbling or falling or it may occur if the child grabs the cot rails or other stationary object whilst falling. Frequently the child is accompanied by a guilty parent, if pulling a resistant toddler or lifting the child by the arms and swinging them in play was the cause.

The mechanism is thought to be a distal subluxation of the radial head into the annular ligament (Hardy, 1978; Kohlhaas and Roeder, 1995), however, X-rays taken before and after reduction show no evidence of displacement (Hardy, 1978).

Reduction of a pulled elbow involves supporting the child's elbow with one hand, feeling the radial head and providing counter-pressure to axial compression. Quickly pronate the forearm through a small range whilst maintaining axial compression until a click is felt. The reduction is confirmed by immediate use of the arm by the child, to the subsequent relief of the parent.

Adeniran and Merriam (1994) reported a case of 'pulled elbow' in a 21-year-old woman, as an exception to the usual age group of the condition. Spontaneous reduction occurred as the patient was positioned into supination for X-ray.

Contractile lesions

Tennis elbow (lateral epicondylitis)

Tennis elbow is the term commonly applied to a strain of the wrist extensor muscles at the site of their common origin from the anterolateral aspect at the lateral epicondyle of the humerus. It most commonly involves the extensor carpi radialis brevis tendon. It is by far the most common lesion treated at the elbow and is seven times more common than golfer's elbow (medial epicondylitis) (Coonrad and Hooper, 1973; Gellman, 1992). The condition may be resistant to treatment and is prone to recurrence.

Tennis elbow was first described in 1898 by Runge as *writer's cramp* (Gellman, 1992; Verhaar *et al.*, 1993). Of all diagnosed cases, 35–64% are associated with work-related activities, with tennis players representing 8% of the total diagnosed. However, competitive tennis players are susceptible to tennis elbow, 50% of them experiencing at least one episode (Noteboom *et al.*, 1994). Altered biomechanics, particularly of the backhand stroke, predisposes tennis players to the condition (Schnatz and Steiner, 1993).

The condition occurs in middle age (Ernst, 1992; Katarincic *et al.*, 1992), with incidence of the condition peaking between the ages of 35 and 54 and with a duration of an average episode of between 6 months and 2 years (Assendelft *et al.*, 1996). It affects the dominant arm most commonly, with epidemiological studies showing a prevalence of 1% in men and 4% in women (Verhaar *et al.*, 1993; Noteboom *et al.*, 1994).

The patient complains of a gradually increasing pain felt on the lateral aspect of the elbow and forearm, sometimes referred to the wrist and into the dorsum of the hand. The condition is so common that patients often make the diagnosis for themselves. There is a constant ache which is aggravated by repeated gripping actions, together with rotation of the forearm. The gripping action is often related to occupational or sporting activities and rarely is tennis elbow related to direct trauma or a traumatic incident.

Point tenderness is present over the lateral epicondyle and the patient will often experience excruciating pain when the elbow is knocked. An apparent muscle weakness may be reported, as pain is often accompanied by a severe twinge which causes the patient to drop relatively light objects (e.g. coffee cup).

On examination there is usually a full range of painfree movement at the elbow joint. Pain on resisted extension of the wrist is pathognomonic of the condition. Passive wrist flexion stretches the common extensor tendon and other resisted tests which may be positive include resisted radial deviation and resisted extension of the middle digit, which implicates extensor carpi radialis brevis through its insertion into the base of the third metacarpal.

Mills' sign is sometimes used to confirm diagnosis. The forearm is fully pronated and the wrist joint flexed. Whilst maintaining this position, passive elbow extension is performed and a positive sign is elicited if pain is reproduced at the lateral side of the elbow (Noteboom *et al.*, 1994; Sölveborn *et al.*, 1995).

Mechanism of tennis elbow

The normal ageing process causes degenerative changes in collagen fibres and ground substance similar to the changes seen when tissues are immobilized (Akeson *et al.*, 1968). Degeneration and relative avascularity of the tendon make it susceptible to microtrauma through overuse activity.

The repeated gripping action may initially produce traction of the common extensor origin causing microtrauma and inflammation (Foley, 1993). Microscopic and macroscopic tears occur at the common extensor origin, with the development of fibrous scar tissue and contracture. Eventually, degenerative foci and calcification can occur (Coonrad and Hooper, 1973; Ernst, 1992; Gellman, 1992; Noteboom *et al.*, 1994).

Initial inflammatory changes may produce a characteristic tendinitis, but as the chronic condition develops, the degenerative features of tendinosis are thought to become paramount. This degenerative condition of the tendon is considered to be similar to the ongoing degenerative tendinosis seen in the Achilles tendon and rotator cuff tendons (Bennett, 1994).

Chard *et al.* (1994) conducted histological studies of normal and biopsy tendon specimens (rotator cuff tendinitis and lateral epicondylitis) to determine the mechanisms involved in tendon degeneration. The major mechanism of tennis elbow or rotator cuff tendinitis was not inflammation, but a sequence of degenerative changes which increased with age, although chronic traction is believed to have an effect. The tendons studied were considered to have an area of relative avascularity which seemed to predispose them to degeneration.

The sequence of degeneration included changes in the blood vessel walls and fibroblasts and alteration in the gel-to-fibre ratio, with glycosaminoglycans replacing collagen fibres. This led to lack of maintenance of collagen turnover, loss of the wavy configuration of collagen fibres and transformation of the fibroblasts into chondrocyte-type cells, with subsequent cartilage formation, calcification and eventual bone formation. It would seem that as the degenerative process progresses the tendon fibroblasts undergo fibrocartilaginous change, ultimately to convert the tendon to bone.

Palpation determines the site of the lesion. Of the cases of tennis elbow encountered, 90% involve the teno-osseous junction of the

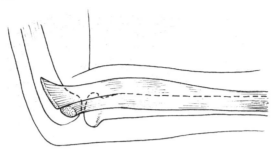

Fig. 6.23 Four possible sites of tennis elbow: (a) teno-osseous junction (enthesis); (b) supracondylar ridge; (c) body of the common extensor tendon; (d) the muscle bellies.

common extensor tendon. The remaining 10% involve the body of the tendon, the extensor carpi radialis longus attachment on the supracondylar ridge or the muscle bellies (Fig. 6.23) (Cyriax, 1982).

Treatment of tennis elbow

Treatment of tennis elbow should always look to address the causative factors. A full explanation should be given so that the patient is responsible for modifying activities to give treatment, whatever the choice, the best possible opportunity. Lifting should be performed with a supination action rather than pronation (Gellman, 1992), and various counterforce elbow or forearm supports are available to alter the stress on the common extensor origin or to rest the wrist to avoid strain. Patient and therapist can discuss the best choice for the individual patient.

Four possible sites:

- Teno-osseous junction (enthesis) – *mainly extensor carpi radialis brevis*
- Supracondylar ridge – *origin of extensor carpi radialis longus*
- Body of the common extensor tendon
- The muscle bellies.

Tendinitis at the teno-osseous junction of the common extensor tendon (the enthesis), principally extensor carpi radialis brevis

This is the most common type of tennis elbow lesion (Cyriax, 1982; Cyriax and Cyriax, 1983). Pain is localized to the common extensor tendon, the teno-osseous junction on the anterolateral aspect of the lateral epicondyle of the humerus. This facet faces mainly anteriorly and is approximately the size of the patient's little finger nail.

The choice of treatment may be corticosteroid injection or Mills' manipulation.

Injection of tennis elbow, teno-osseous site			
Kenalog 40 mg/ml	Total steroid	Lignocaine 1%	Total volume
0.25 ml	10 mg	0.75 ml	1 ml
25G × $\frac{5}{8}$ in (0.5 × 16 mm) orange needle			

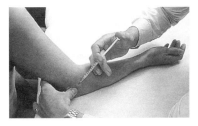

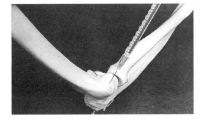

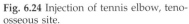

Fig. 6.24 Injection of tennis elbow, teno-osseous site.

Fig. 6.25 Injection of tennis elbow, teno-osseous site, showing direction of approach and needle position.

The aim of the corticosteroid injection is to reduce inflammation in the scar tissue. If the theory is correct, that the initial inflammatory process of tennis elbow is rapidly superseded by degeneration, corticosteroid injection would seem to be most appropriate in the early stages of the condition. The evidence would seem to support this (see below). Once rendered painfree, the patient, through normal movement, will encourage alignment of fibres and mobility of the scar.

Support the patient with the forearm resting on a pillow, the elbow flexed to approximately 90° and fully supinated (Fig. 6.24). Identify the area of tenderness over the teno-osseous junction of the common extensor tendon with the anterolateral aspect of the lateral epicondyle. Insert the needle from an anterior direction, perpendicular to the facet, and deliver the injection by a peppering technique (Fig. 6.25). The patient is advised to maintain a period of relative rest for approximately 2 weeks following injection.

Sölveborn *et al.* (1995) conducted a study of 109 cases of tennis elbow treated with a single corticosteroid injection (10 mg triamcinolone) together with local anaesthetic. Bupivacaine (a long-acting local anaesthetic) was compared with lignocaine (a short-acting local anaesthetic). An impressive improvement was reported 2 weeks after the injection, with the patients treated with bupivacaine showing a significantly better outcome. However, at 3 months, the results in both groups showed deterioration and relapse, with patients seeking other treatments.

Assendelft *et al.* (1996), on reviewing the literature, determined that the existing evidence on effectiveness, optimal timing of injections, composition of injection fluid and adverse effects of injections is not conclusive, although they appear to be safe and effective in the short term (2–6 weeks). Three injections seem to be the recommended maximum in several reviews, with post-injection pain and subcutaneous atrophy being the adverse side-effects. Corticosteroid injections are relatively easy to administer and cheap, and specialist referral is not necessary.

An alternative treatment to corticosteroid injection is to aim to elongate the scar tissue by rupturing adhesions within the teno-osseous junction, thus making the area mobile and painfree. This is achieved by a Mills' manipulation, which must be followed by stretching exercises to maintain the lengthening achieved. Before the Mills' manipulation can be performed, the teno-osseous junction must be prepared by deep transverse friction massage to mobilize the tendon and numb it, in preparation for the manipulative technique.

G. Percival Mills described this technique for the treatment of tennis elbow in the *British Medical Journal* (1928). On examining patients with tennis elbow, he found that on combined pronation and wrist and finger flexion, the elbow joint could not achieve full extension. He suggested that forcing the restricted movement (now known as Mills' manipulation) could be curative.

Mills' manipulation (Cyriax and Cyriax, 1983; Cyriax, 1984)

Position the patient comfortably with the elbow fully supinated and in 90° of flexion. Locate the anterolateral aspect of the lateral epicondyle and identify the area of tenderness (Fig. 6.26). Apply

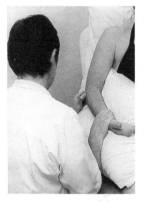

Fig. 6.26 Transverse friction massage of tennis elbow, teno-osseous site.

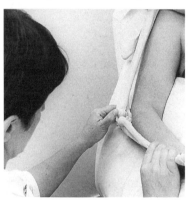

Fig. 6.27 Transverse friction massage of tennis elbow, teno-osseous site, showing site of anterolateral facet on the lateral epicondyle of the humerus, and the direction of application.

friction massage with the side of the thumb tip, applying the pressure in a posterior direction on to the teno-osseous junction (Fig. 6.27). Maintain this pressure whilst imparting transverse friction massage in a direction, towards your fingers which should be positioned on the other side of the elbow, for counterpressure. Friction massage is delivered for 10 min after the numbing effect has been achieved, to prepare the tendon for the manipulation.

The Mills' manipulation is performed immediately after the transverse friction massage, providing the patient has a full range of passive elbow extension. If the patient has limitation of passive elbow extension, the manipulative thrust will affect the elbow joint, rather than the common extensor tendon, possibly causing a traumatic arthritis.

Position the patient on a chair with a back rest. Stand behind the patient:

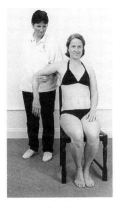

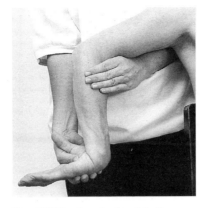

Fig. 6.28 Mill's manipulation, starting position.

Fig. 6.29 The thumb placed in the palm, forearm pronated and wrist maintained in full flexion.

- Support the patient's arm under the crook of the elbow with the shoulder joint abducted to 90° and medially rotated. The forearm will automatically fall into pronation (Fig. 6.28).
- Place the thumb of your other hand in the web space between the patient's thumb and index finger and fully flex the patient's wrist and pronate the forearm (Fig. 6.29).
- Move the hand supporting the crook of the elbow on to the posterior surface of the elbow joint and, whilst maintaining full wrist flexion and pronation, extend the patient's elbow until you feel all the slack has been taken up in the tendon.
- Step sideways to stand behind the patient's head, taking care to prevent the patient from leaning away either forwards or sideways, which would reduce the tension on the tendon (Fig. 6.30).
- Apply a minimal-amplitude, high-velocity thrust (Grade C manipulation) by simultaneously side-flexing your body away from your arms, and pushing smartly downwards with the hand over the patient's elbow.

This manoeuvre is usually conducted once only at each treatment session since it is not a comfortable procedure for the patient and the effects of treatment often become fully apparent over the following few days. Between sessions the patient is instructed to continue stretching the tendon to maintain length and mobility.

Verhaar *et al.* (1996) conducted a prospective randomized trial of 106 patients with tennis elbow. They compared the effects of corticosteroid injections with Cyriax physiotherapy, i.e. deep transverse friction massage followed by Mills' manipulation. Both groups showed significant improvement at 6 weeks, with the injection group demonstrating better results. However, at 1-year follow-up, there was no significant difference between the groups, with 17 patients in the injection group and 14 patients in the physiotherapy group going on to eventual surgery. There were no adverse side-effects from either group. The authors reached the conclusion that, although corticosteroid injections alleviate pain in

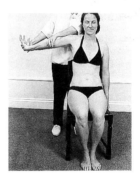

Fig. 6.30 Positioning of hand on posterior aspect of extended elbow for application of the Grade C manipulation.

the short term, they do not address the cause of the condition. Since corticosteroid injection is more time-efficient than physiotherapy (three visits maximum for the injection group; 12 visits for the physiotherapy group), it was considered to be the more effective treatment in the short term. However, the effect of corticosteroid injection on healing at different stages is uncertain.

The resistant tennis elbow

The short-term relief gained from either injection or physiotherapy is an indication that the causative factors and ideal treatment for tennis elbow still elude us. Injection or physiotherapy seem to work well for uncomplicated tennis elbow of recent onset. The chronic nature of the condition, however, means that most of us do not see patients until the condition is well-established. The disappointing results and recurrence of symptoms indicate that there may be one or more components involved in tennis elbow.

The gradual onset of tennis elbow means that problems can coexist within the elbow joint and surrounding neural structures. Pain may restrict the range of active movement and the relative immobilization may produce an associated capsular pattern in the elbow joint. Similarly, dysfunction at one site can cause dysfunction at others and adverse neural tension can be a primary cause or associated cause with tennis elbow (Yaxley and Jull, 1993). A cervical lesion can refer pain into the forearm and mimic tennis elbow, or cervical syndromes can coexist with a lesion at the elbow.

Nerve entrapment at the elbow may be a complication (Noteboom *et al.*, 1994; Hartley, 1995). The radial nerve divides into its terminal branches at the elbow and the posterior interosseous nerve passes between the deep and superficial head of supinator. The upper edge of the superficial head of supinator is a thickened fibrous band forming a firm arch known as the arcade of Frohse, which provides a possible site for nerve entrapment.

The musculotendinous, neural, neurological and articular components should be assessed in the resistant tennis elbow, although there is little evidence in the literature to confirm that addressing all possible components gives any better results.

Transverse friction massage of the origin of extensor carpi radialis longus from the supracondylar ridge (Cyriax and Cyriax, 1983; Cyriax, 1984)

Transverse friction massage is the only effective treatment at this site. Position the patient with the elbow supported in 90° of flexion and the forearm in supination. Sit facing the patient and place the pad of your thumb against the lower third of the lateral supracondylar ridge (Fig. 6.31). Direct the pressure back against the ridge and impart the transverse friction in a superoinferior direction. Relative rest is advised where functional movements may continue, but no overuse or stretching until painfree on resisted testing.

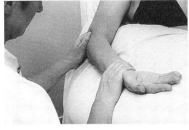

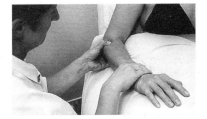

Fig. 6.31 Transverse friction massage of tennis elbow, supracondylar ridge.

Fig. 6.32 Transverse friction massage of tennis elbow, body of the tendon.

Transverse friction massage of the body of the common extensor tendon (Cyriax and Cyriax, 1983; Cyriax, 1984)

This variety of tennis elbow is not so common. The area of tenderness is located in the region of the radial head. Injection of the tendon is controversial and treatment is preferably by transverse friction massage.

Position the patient with the forearm supported in pronation and flexion (Fig. 6.32). Locate the body of the tendon over the radial head. Impart deep transverse friction massage across the fibres for 10 min after some numbing has taken effect. Relative rest is advised where functional movements may continue, but no overuse or stretching until painfree on resisted testing.

Transverse friction massage of the muscle bellies (Cyriax and Cyriax, 1983; Cyriax, 1984)

The lesion is in the bellies of the common extensor muscles lying deep to the brachioradialis. Treatment by transverse friction massage is usually successful.

Position the patient with the forearm supported with the elbow flexed to 90° and the forearm in the mid-position (Fig. 6.33). Palpate

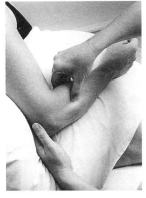

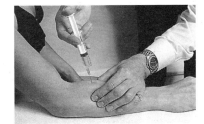

Fig. 6.33 Transverse friction massage of tennis elbow, muscle bellies.

Fig. 6.34 Injection of tennis elbow, muscle bellies.

for the site of the lesion deep to brachioradialis. Grasp the affected muscle fibres between a finger and thumb and impart the friction massage by a pinching pressure applied up and down in a superoinferior direction. Relative rest is advised where functional movements may continue, but no overuse or stretching until painfree on resisted testing.

Injection of the bellies of the extensor muscles

The muscle bellies can be injected using a large-volume low-dose local anaesthetic, i.e. 5 ml of 0.5% lignocaine or procaine, infiltrating the area of the lesion using a peppering technique (Fig. 6.34). The large volume of local anaesthetic spreads the fibres of the muscle bellies aiming to disrupt the adhesions.

Golfer's elbow (medial epicondylitis)

Although not as common as tennis elbow, golfer's elbow has a similar presentation, aetiology, disease process and management.

The patient presents with a gradual onset of pain on the medial aspect of the arm. This may radiate distally, but in general it does not project as far as the pain seen in tennis elbow. The pain is aggravated by use and the elbow is often stiff after rest. Onset of symptoms may be associated with occupational overuse, sporting activities, e.g. tennis, bowling, archery, or hobbies, e.g. knitting or needlework (Rayan, 1992; Kurvers and Verhaar, 1995). The motion of throwing may cause golfer's elbow as it produces a valgus stress at the elbow which has to be supported by the flexor muscles (Ho, 1995).

The tendons involved in medial epicondylitis control movement at two joints and are susceptible to overuse through overload. Stretching, valgus forces and intrinsic forces from muscle contraction all contribute to the condition (Safran, 1995). In the degenerative process of golfer's elbow tendinosis is evident rather than the acute inflammatory changes of tendinitis (Bennett, 1994; Patten, 1994).

Golfer's elbow, generally speaking, is a less complicated condition to treat than tennis elbow, but coexistent ulnar neuritis (cubital tunnel syndrome) may produce medial elbow pain with tenderness and paraesthesia in the distribution of the ulnar nerve (Kurvers and Verhaar, 1995; O'Dwyer and Howie, 1995). Some cases of medial epicondylitis come to surgery, involving incision of the flexor tendons around the medial epicondyle, denervation of the epicondyle and transposition of the ulnar nerve.

There are two sites for the lesion: teno-osseous site and musculotendinous site.

Treatment of golfer's elbow

Teno-osseous site (enthesis)

The common flexor tendon takes origin from the anterior aspect of the medial epicondyle. Palpation will identify the site of the lesion.

Treatment may be by either corticosteroid injection or transverse friction massage.

Injection of golfer's elbow, teno-osseous site (Cyriax and Cyriax, 1983; Cyriax, 1984)

Kenalog 40 mg/ml	Total steroid	Lignocaine 1%	Total volume
0.25 ml	10 mg	0.75 ml	1 ml

25G $\times \frac{5}{8}$ in (0.5 $\times$ 16 mm) orange needle or 23G $\times$ 1 in (0.6 $\times$ 25 mm) blue needle

---

Position the patient with the elbow supported in extension and fully supinated. Locate the anterior aspect of the medial epicondyle and identify the area of tenderness. Insert the needle perpendicular to the facet and deliver the injection by a peppering technique (Fig. 6.35). Bear in mind the position of the ulnar nerve behind the medial epicondyle. The patient is advised to maintain a period of relative rest for approximately 2 weeks following injection.

Transverse friction massage of golfer's elbow, teno-osseous site (Cyriax and Cyriax, 1983; Cyriax, 1984)

Position the patient as above and locate the area of tenderness on the anterior aspect of the medial epicondyle (Fig. 6.36). Using an index finger reinforced by the middle finger, and thumb for counterpressure, impart the friction massage by applying the pressure down on to the anterior aspect and sweeping transversely across the fibres (Fig. 6.37). Ten minutes' deep friction massage is delivered after the numbing effect has been achieved. Relative rest

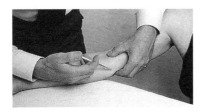

Fig. 6.35 Injection of golfer's elbow, teno-osseous site.

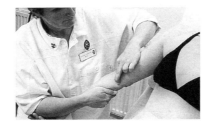

Fig. 6.36 Transverse friction massage of golfer's elbow, teno-osseous site.

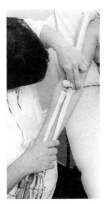

Fig. 6.37 Transverse friction massage of golfer's elbow, teno-osseous site, to give an indication of the direction of application.

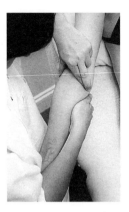

Fig. 6.38 Transverse friction massage of golfer's elbow, musculotendinous junction.

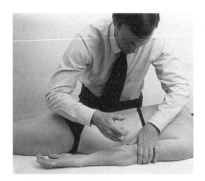

Fig. 6.39 Injection of biceps insertion.

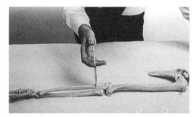

Fig. 6.40 Injection of biceps insertion, showing direction of approach and needle position.

is advised where functional movements may continue, but no overuse or stretching until painfree on resisted testing.

Musculotendinous site

> **Transverse friction massage of golfer's elbow, musculotendinous site**

Transverse friction massage is considered to be the most effective treatment here (Cyriax and Cyriax, 1983; Cyriax, 1984). Position yourself and the patient as above and, using the index finger, move 1 cm distally to palpate the musculotendinous junction at the inferior edge of the medial epicondyle (Fig. 6.38). Maintain the pressure against the bone and impart the friction massage transversely across the fibres for 10 min after the numbing effect has been achieved. Relative rest is advised where functional movements may continue, but no overuse or stretching until painfree on resisted testing.

Biceps

At the elbow, the lesion lies either in the muscle belly or at the insertion on to the radial tuberosity. The patient complains of pain at the elbow on resisted elbow flexion and resisted supination of the flexed elbow. Passive stretching into elbow extension can also cause pain.

Excessive friction may cause inflammation of the subtendinous biceps bursa and differential diagnosis from bicipital tendinitis may be difficult. A muddled presentation of signs is found, confirming the diagnosis of bursitis. Pain may be reproduced on resisted elbow flexion, passive elbow extension and passive elbow pronation, as the bursa is squeezed against its insertion.

An injection of corticosteroid is the treatment of choice for the insertion of biceps, since the tendon of insertion lies deeply.

Injection of the insertion of biceps at the radial tuberosity (Cyriax and Cyriax, 1983; Cyriax, 1984)

Kenalog 40 mg/ml	Total steroid	Lignocaine 1%	Total volume
0.25 ml	10 mg	0.75 ml	1 ml

23G × 1 in (0.6 × 25 mm) blue needle

Position the patient in prone lying in the anatomical position. Without changing the position of the glenohumeral joint, carefully pronate the extended forearm. Insert the needle between the radius and ulna approximately 2 cm distal to the radiohumeral joint line until the resistance of the tendon insertion is felt (Fig. 6.39). Deliver the injection by a peppering technique to the tendon and adjacent area if the bursa is also involved (Fig. 6.40). The patient is advised to maintain a period of relative rest for approximately 2 weeks following injection.

Transverse friction massage of the insertion of biceps at the radial tuberosity (Cyriax and Cyriax, 1983; Cyriax, 1984)

Position the patient with the elbow joint flexed to 90° and supinated. With your thumb, locate the insertion of biceps at the radial tuberosity and apply pressure against it, deeply and laterally. Wrap your fingers around the forearm to provide counterpressure. Deliver the transverse fiction massage by alternately rotating the patient's forearm between pronation and supination whilst maintaining the pressure against the radial tuberosity.

If the lesion lies in the muscle belly, the general principles of treatment can be applied (see Chapter 4).

Triceps

Distal rupture of the triceps tendon due to forced overload into extension is uncommon. A triceps muscle lesion is also rare, but would present with posterior elbow pain, increased by resisted elbow extension. The general principles of treatment would be applied.

References

Adeniran, A., Merriam, W.F. (1994) Pulled elbow in an adult. *Journal of Bone and Joint Surgery* **76-B**: 848–849.

Akeson, W.H., Amiel, D., La Violette, D., Secrist, D. (1968) The connective tissue response to immobility: an accelerated ageing response. *Experimental Gerontology* **3**: 289–301.

Assendelft, W.J.J., Hay, E.M., Adshead, R., Bouter, L.M. (1996) Corticosteroid injections for lateral epicondylitis: a systematic overview. *British Journal of General Practice* **46**: 209–216.

Bennett, J.B. (1994) Lateral and medial epicondylitis. *Hand Clinics* **10**: 157–163.

Chard, M.D., Cawston, T.E., Riley, G.P. *et al.* (1994) Rotator cuff degeneration and lateral epicondylitis: a comparative histological study. *Annals of the Rheumatic Diseases* **53**: 30–34.

Coonrad, R.W., Hooper, W.R. (1973) Tennis elbow: its course, natural history, conservative and surgical management. *Journal of Bone and Joint Surgery* **55-A**: 1177–1182.

Cyriax, J. (1982) *Textbook of Orthopaedic Medicine*, vol. 1, 8th edn. Baillière Tindall.

Cyriax, J. (1984) *Textbook of Orthopaedic Medicine*, vol. 2. 11th edn. Baillière Tindall.

Cyriax, J., Cyriax, P. (1983) *Illustrated Manual of Orthopaedic Medicine*. Butterworths.

Ernst, E. (1992) Conservative therapy for tennis elbow. *British Journal of Clinical Practice* **46**: 55–57.

Foley, A.E. (1993) Tennis elbow. *American Family Physician* **48**: 281–288.

Gellman, H. (1992) Tennis elbow (lateral epicondylitis). *Orthopedic Clinics of North America* **23**: 75–82.

Hardy, R.H. (1978) Pulled elbow. *Journal of the Royal College of General Practitioners* **28**: 224–226.

Hartley, A. (1995) *Practical Joint Assessment, Upper Quadrant*, 2nd edn. Mosby.

Ho, C.P. (1995) Sports and occupational injuries of the elbow: MR imaging findings. *American Journal of Roentgenology* **164**: 1465–1471.

Hoppmann, R.A. (1993) Diagnosis and management of common tendinitis and bursitis syndromes. *Journal of the South Carolina Medical Association* 531–535.

Katarincic, J.A., Weiss, A-P.C., Akelman, E. (1992) Lateral epicondylitis (tennis elbow): a review. *Rhode Island Medicine* **75**: 541–544.

Kohlhaas, A.R., Roeder, J. (1995) Tee shirt management of nursemaid's elbow. *American Journal of Orthopedics* **24**: 74.

Kurvers, H., Verhaar, J. (1995) The results of operative treatment of medial epicondylitis. *Journal of Bone and Joint Surgery* **77-A**: 1374–1379.

Mills, G.P. (1928) Treatment of tennis elbow. *British Medical Journal* **1**: 12–13.

Nicola, T.L. (1992) Elbow injuries in athletes. *Primary Care* **19**: 283–302.

Noteboom, T., Cruver, R., Keller, J. *et al.* (1994) Tennis elbow: a review. *Journal of Orthopaedic and Sports Physical Therapy* **19**: 357–366.

O'Dwyer, K.J., Howie, C.R. (1995) Medial epicondylitis of the elbow. *International Orthopaedics* **19**: 69–71.

Palastanga, N., Field, D., Soames, R. (1994) *Anatomy and Human Movement*, 2nd edn. Butterworth-Heinemann.

Patten, R.M. (1995) Overuse syndromes and injuries involving the elbow: MR imaging findings. *American Journal of Roentgenology* **164**: 1205–1211.

Rayan, G.M. (1992) Archery-related injuries of the hand, forearm and elbow. *Southern Medical Journal* **85**: 961–964.

Safran, M.R. (1995) Elbow injuries in the athlete. *Clinical Orthopaedics and Related Research* **310**: 257–277.

Schnatz, P., Steiner, C. (1993) Tennis elbow: a biomechanical and therapeutic approach. *Journal of the American Osteopathic Association* **93**: 778–788.

Sölveborn S.-A., Buch, F., Mallmin, H., Adalberth, G. (1995) Cortisone injection with anaesthetic additives for radial epicondylalgia (tennis elbow). *Clinical Orthopaedics and Related Research* **316**: 99–105.

Verhaar, J., Walenkamp, G., Kester, A. *et al.* (1993) Lateral extensor release for tennis elbow. *Journal of Bone and Joint Surgery* **75-A**: 1034–1043.

Verhaar, J.A.N., Walenkamp, G.H.I.M., van Mameren, H. *et al.* (1996) Local corticosteroid injection versus Cyriax-type physiotherapy for tennis elbow. *Journal of Bone and Joint Surgery* **78-B**: 128–132.

Williams, P.L., Warwick, R., Dyson, M., Bannister, L.H. (1989) *Gray's Anatomy*, 37th edn. Churchill Livingstone.

Yaxley, G.A., Jull, G.A. (1993) Adverse neural tension in the neural system. A preliminary study of tennis elbow. *Australian Physiotherapy* **39**: 15–22.

7 The wrist and hand

Summary

Repetitive strain injury and work-related upper limb disorder have done much to focus the clinician on the differential diagnosis and causative factors of pain in the wrist and hand.

This chapter takes a pragmatic approach to the identification of specific lesions and suggests localized treatment, which may form a component of overall management. The detailed but relevant anatomy that forms a basis for accurate treatment is presented. Treatment for individual lesions is discussed, with emphasis on the application of principles to less commonly encountered lesions.

Anatomy

Inert structures

The *distal radioulnar joint* is a pivot joint between the head of the ulna and the ulnar notch of the radius. Mechanically linked to the superior radioulnar joint, it is responsible for the movements of pronation (85°) and supination (90°).

A *triangular fibrocartilaginous disc* closes the distal radioulnar joint inferiorly. It lies in a horizontal plane, its apex attaching to the ulnar styloid and its base to the lower edge of the ulnar notch of the radius. The disc articulates with the lunate when the hand is in ulnar deviation. It adds to the stability of the joint and acts as an articular cushion for the ulnar side of the carpus, absorbing compression, traction and shearing forces, but is prone to degenerative changes (Livengood, 1992; Rettig, 1994; Wright *et al.*, 1994; Steinberg and Plancher, 1995).

The movements of pronation and supination rotate the radius around the ulna. Supination is stronger, hence the thread of nuts and screws which are tightened by supination in right-handed people.

There are two rows of carpal bones; on the palmar aspect, from the radial to the ulnar side they are:

scaphoid, lunate, triquetral, pisiform
trapezium, trapezoid, capitate, hamate.

The carpal bones all articulate with their neighbours, except pisiform, which is a separate bone situated on the front of the triquetral. The intercarpal joints are all supported by intercarpal ligaments.

The *wrist joint* proper is a biaxial, ellipsoid joint between the distal end of the radius and the articular disc, and the proximal row of carpal bones. However, the so-called wrist joint complex includes the *midcarpal joint* and has mobility as well as stability, which is important for the function of the hand. Movements are extension (passive, 85°), flexion (passive, 85°), ulnar deviation (passive, 45°) and radial deviation (passive, 15°). The close-packed position of the wrist joint is full extension.

The joints are surrounded by a fibrous capsule, lined with synovial membrane and reinforced by collateral ligaments. Both collateral ligaments pass from the appropriate styloid process to the carpal bones on the medial and lateral side of the carpus. A fibrocartilaginous *meniscus* projects into the joint from the ulnar collateral ligament.

The *metacarpophalangeal joints* are ellipsoid; the *interphalangeal joints* are hinge joints. Both are supported by palmar and collateral ligaments and the extensor tendons and digital expansions support the dorsal surfaces of the joints.

Flexor tendons are contained within fibrous sheaths which have thickened areas known as pulleys which may provide a restriction, producing 'trigger finger' (see below). At the wrist and in the hand, the tendons are contained within synovial sheaths (Williams *et al.*, 1989).

The *flexor retinaculum*, a strong fibrous band, creates a fibro-osseous passage, *the carpal tunnel*, through which pass the flexor tendons of the digits, the median nerve and vessels. The flexor retinaculum has four points of attachment: the pisiform and hook of hamate medially and the tuberosity of the scaphoid and ridge of trapezium laterally. Its attachment on to the trapezium splits to form a separate compartment for the tendon of flexor carpi radialis. The *median nerve* enters the carpal tunnel deep to palmaris longus. It shares its compartment of the carpal tunnel with the nine tendons of flexor digitorum superficialis and profundus and flexor pollicis longus. On leaving the carpal tunnel it supplies the thenar muscles before dividing into four or five digital branches.

The *trapeziofirst-metacarpal joint* is a saddle joint with a loose articular capsule and extensive joint surfaces giving it a wide range of movement. The first metacarpal has been rotated medially for the movement of opposition. This makes the description of the movements somewhat complicated since there are two possible combinations of terminology:

- Flexion and extension occur in a plane parallel to the palm of the hand, whilst abduction and adduction occur in a plane at right angles to the palm of the hand.
- Flexion and extension occur in a plane at right angles to the palm, whilst abduction and adduction occur in a plane parallel to the palm of the hand.

Acknowledgement of these two combinations of movement is necessary to understand the capsular pattern. It is important to use one terminology or the other consistently and the former option is used throughout this text.

The close-packed position of the trapeziofirst-metacarpal joint is strong opposition, when great force is transmitted to the joint. The functionally opposed thumb is subjected to compressive stresses which make the joint vulnerable to degenerative osteoarthrosis.

The *radial artery* passes under abductor pollicis longus and extensor pollicis brevis, crossing the snuffbox obliquely towards the first dorsal interosseous muscle. Its position should be acknowledged so that it can be avoided when injecting the trapeziofirst-metacarpal joint.

Contractile structures

Flexor carpi radialis (median nerve C6–7) is the most lateral superficial flexor tendon. It passes through its own fibro-osseous compartment on the lateral side of the carpal tunnel, to insert into the base of the second and third metacarpals.

Palmaris longus (median nerve C7–8) passes over, not under, the flexor retinaculum, to attach to the distal part of the flexor retinaculum and the palmar aponeurosis.

Flexor digitorum superficialis (median nerve C7–8, T1) lies medial to palmaris longus, but is not as visible because it lies on a slightly deeper plane. In the carpal tunnel the four tendons are contained within the same synovial sheath, with tendons to the third and fourth fingers lying superficial to those to the second and fifth. The tendons divide to provide a passage for flexor digitorum profundus, before continuing on to insert either side of the middle phalanx.

Flexor carpi ulnaris (ulnar nerve C7–8) is the most medial superficial flexor tendon and can be easily traced on to its insertion into pisiform. The tendon sends slips on as the pisohamate and pisofifth-metacarpal ligaments. The pisohamate ligament converts the space between pisiform and the hamate into a tunnel (tunnel of Guyon) for the passage of the ulnar vessels and nerves.

Flexor pollicis longus (median nerve C8, T1) passes through the lateral side of the carpal tunnel and inserts into the palmar aspect of the base of the distal phalanx of the thumb.

Flexor digitorum profundus (medial part supplied by the ulnar nerve; lateral part supplied by the median nerve C8, T1) divides into four tendons which lie deep to superficialis in the carpal tunnel. They pass through the tunnels created by superficialis and attach to the distal phalanx of each finger.

The *lumbricals* are four small muscles which arise from the flexor digitorum profundus tendons and pass to the radial side of the dorsal digital expansions of each finger. With attachments that link flexor and extensor tendons, they function by flexing the metacarpophalangeal joints and extending the interphalangeal joints. The first two lumbricals are supplied by the median nerve, the third and fourth by the ulnar nerve, C8, T1.

Extensor carpi radialis longus (radial nerve C6–7) and *extensor carpi radialis brevis* (posterior interosseous nerve C7–8) pass deep to the tendons of abductor pollicis longus and extensor pollicis brevis, under the extensor retinaculum, to attach to the radial side of the base of the second and third metacarpals respectively.

Extensor digitorum (posterior interosseous nerve C7–8) divides into four tendons which pass under the extensor retinaculum to insert into the dorsal digital expansions of the fingers.

Extensor digiti minimi (posterior interosseous nerve C7–8) inserts into the dorsal digital expansion of the little finger.

Extensor carpi ulnaris (posterior interosseous nerve C7–8) lies in a groove between the head of the ulna and the styloid process, under the extensor retinaculum. It attaches to the medial side of the base of the fifth metacarpal.

Abductor pollicis longus and *extensor pollicis brevis* (posterior interosseous nerve C7–8) become tendinous and superficial in the lower forearm where they cross the tendons of extensor carpi radialis longus and brevis at the intersect point, a site of potential friction. They occupy the same synovial sheath in the first compartment of the extensor retinaculum and form the lateral border of the anatomical snuffbox. The abductor inserts into the base of the first metacarpal and the extensor into the base of the proximal phalanx. Abductor pollicis longus has been considered both anatomically and functionally as a radial deviator of the wrist (Elliott, 1992a).

Extensor pollicis longus (posterior interosseous nerve C7–8) deviates around the ulnar side of the dorsal tubercle of the radius, to pass to the base of the distal phalanx of the thumb. It forms the medial border of the anatomical snuffbox.

Extensor indicis (posterior interosseous nerve C7–8) joins the ulnar side of the extensor digitorum tendon, passing to the index finger.

The *dorsal interossei* (ulnar nerve C8, T1) are four bipennate muscles arising from adjacent sides of the metacarpal bones and inserting into the dorsal digital expansion and base of the proximal phalanx of the appropriate finger. They are responsible for abducting the fingers from the midline of the middle finger.

The *palmar interossei* (ulnar nerve C8, T1) are four smaller muscles originating from the palmar aspect of the metacarpal bones and inserting into the dorsal digital expansions of the appropriate finger. They are responsible for adducting the fingers towards the middle finger.

Guide to surface marking and palpation

Palmar aspect (Fig. 7.1)

Look for three creases (not distinct in everyone) on the palmar aspect of the lower forearm. The distal wrist crease joins pisiform and the tubercle of the scaphoid, the bones at the heel of the hand (Backhouse and Hutchings, 1990), marking the proximal border of the flexor retinaculum. The middle crease joins the two styloid processes, marking the position of the wrist joint line whilst the

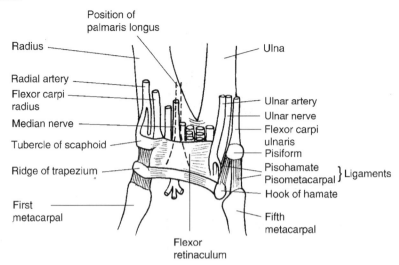

Fig. 7.1 Palmar aspect of the wrist showing position of the flexor retinaculum, its adjacent tendons and nerves.

proximal crease (if present) marks the proximal extent of the flexor tendon sheaths.

Consider the position of the bones which make up the two rows of carpal bones (Fig. 7.2). From the radial to the ulnar side, an easy way to remember the order is:

simply *l*earn *t*he *p*arts *t*hat *t*he *c*arpus *h*as	*s*caphoid, *l*unate, *t*riquetral, *p*isiform *t*rapezium, *t*rapezoid, *c*apitate, *h*amate

Palpate the ***radial and ulnar styloid processes*** at the wrist; the radial styloid extends slightly more distally than the ulnar styloid.

Palpate ***pisiform***, the pea-shaped sesamoid bone, which lies at the base of the hypothenar eminence, giving insertion to flexor carpi ulnaris.

Move a thumb approximately 1.5 cm distally and diagonally from pisiform, in the direction of the web between the thumb and index finger. Lying roughly in line with the ring finger is the ***hook of hamate***. Palpate deeply and tenderness will confirm its presence.

Radially deviate the wrist to make the ***tuberosity (tubercle) of the scaphoid*** more prominent. It lies at the base of the thenar eminence, close to the tendon of flexor carpi radialis.

Move a thumb from the tuberosity of the scaphoid, diagonally and distally approximately 1 cm, to lie in line with the index finger, and feel the ***ridge (tubercle) of trapezium*** through the bulk of the thenar eminence. It is best felt with the wrist joint in extension and is tender to deep palpation.

Joining the four points described above – pisiform, hook of hamate, tuberosity of scaphoid and ridge of trapezium – gives the position of the ***flexor retinaculum***, which is approximately the size of the width of your thumb (Fig. 7.1).

Identify the superficial forearm flexor tendons as they cross the palmar aspect of the wrist from the radial to ulnar side. ***Flexor carpi***

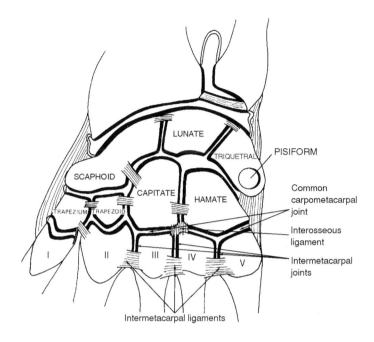

Fig. 7.2 Bones of the hand. Adapted from Palastanga *et al.* (1994) with permission.

radialis is the most lateral and **palmaris longus** passes over the flexor retinaculum and can be brought into prominence by opposing the thumb and little finger with the wrist flexed. **Flexor digitorum superficialis**, lying in a deeper plane, may not be readily palpable, but *flexor carpi ulnaris* can be followed down to its insertion on to the pisiform.

Palpate for the **radial pulse** on the palmar aspect of the lower radius lateral to flexor carpi radialis. The **ulnar pulse** can be palpated on the lower ulna, lateral to flexor carpi ulnaris.

Consider the position of the **median nerve** as it enters the carpal tunnel deep to palmaris longus. If palmaris longus is absent, oppose the thumb and little finger and the midline crease produced gives the position of the median nerve.

Dorsal aspect (Fig. 7.3)

Pronate the forearm and the **head of the ulna** can be seen as a rounded elevation in the distal forearm. Palpate anterior to the head of the ulna and feel the tendon of **extensor carpi ulnaris** in the groove between the head of the ulna and the **styloid process**.

Palpate the **inferior radioulnar joint** line, which lies approximately 1.5 cm laterally from the ulnar styloid. Confirm its presence by

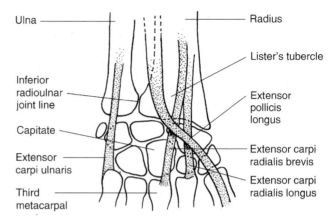

Fig. 7.3 Dorsal aspect of the wrist.

passively gliding the head of the ulna on the radius and feeling the joint line.

On the lower end of the radius, palpate the **dorsal tubercle (of Lister)** lying roughly in line with the index finger. The tubercle is grooved on either side by the passing tendons. **Extensor carpi radialis longus and brevis** pass on its lateral side, whilst **extensor pollicis longus** passes on its medial side, then taking a 45° turn laterally, and can be traced to its insertion into the base of the distal phalanx of the thumb.

The **capitate** is the largest carpal bone and is roughly the size of the patient's thumb nail. It is wider dorsally and is peg-shaped. It is situated in the centre of the carpus, articulating mainly with the third metacarpal distally, the trapezoid laterally, the hamate medially and the concavity formed by the scaphoid and lunate proximally (Williams *et al.*, 1989; Steinberg and Plancher, 1995). Run your finger proximally down the shaft of the third metacarpal with the wrist in slight flexion and drop over the end into the shallow depression to locate the position of the capitate.

Palpate the insertions of **extensor carpi radialis longus and brevis** on to the radial side of the base of the second and third metacarpals respectively. Place the wrist in flexion with the thumb relaxed to allow the tendon of extensor pollicis longus to fall out of the way. The extensor carpi radialis brevis is probably the easier of the two to feel. Palpate the insertion of extensor carpi ulnaris on to the medial side of the base of the fifth metacarpal.

Lateral aspect (Fig. 7.4)

Pronate the forearm and make a fist. The fleshy elevation seen at the distal end of the radius is formed by **abductor pollicis longus** *and extensor pollicis brevis* as they wind around the lower radius, crossing over the tendons of extensor carpi radialis longus and brevis at the intersection.

Locate the *anatomical snuffbox* (by extending the thumb) which is bordered by the tendons of abductor pollicis longus and extensor pollicis brevis laterally and by extensor pollicis longus medially. Palpate the *radial styloid* at the proximal end of the anatomical snuffbox and the trapeziofirst-metacarpal joint at the distal end.

Locate the tendons of abductor pollicis longus and extensor pollicis brevis; sometimes a V-shaped gap may be appreciated between the two.

Move the wrist into ulnar deviation and the scaphoid can be palpated; it moves with the hand, whereas the radial styloid does not. The scaphoid can be grasped between your thumb posteriorly in the base of the snuffbox and your index finger anteriorly.

Palpate the trapezium distal to scaphoid, lying at the base of the first metacarpal.

Palpate the *trapeziofirst-metacarpal joint* line by running a thumb down the shaft of the first metacarpal into the anatomical snuffbox. Flex and extend the joint to check its location.

Palpate the *first dorsal interosseous* in the web between index finger and thumb; it can be made more prominent by resisting abduction of the index finger.

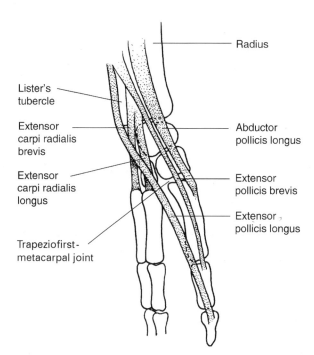

Fig. 7.4 Tendons on the lateral aspect of the wrist.

Commentary on the examination

Observation

Before proceeding with the history, a general observation of the patient's *face, posture and gait* will alert the examiner to serious abnormalities or injuries. The painful hand may be held in an antalgic position, resting with the fingers parallel to each other and in a degree of flexion, the thumb in a neutral position. Possibly, the arm swing may be absent from the gait pattern and the hand held stiffly against the side. Difficulty with fine movement may be observed during undressing, indicating a problem with dexterity.

History (subjective examination)

The *age, occupation, sports, hobbies and lifestyle* of the patient may give an indication of the cause and a possible diagnosis, since most problems in the lower forearm involve arthritis, trauma or overuse.

The *site* of pain is usually well-localized by the patient, with little *spread*, since these are peripheral joints and structures lying at the end of their respective dermatomes, with little scope for reference. The presence of paraesthesia or any apparent reference of pain may suggest a more proximal lesion, and all proximal joints must be examined, including the cervical spine. A fractured scaphoid gives localized pain and point tenderness in the anatomical snuffbox whilst X-ray investigation may not show evidence of the fracture for several weeks (Livengood, 1992).

The *onset* of the symptoms may be due to trauma, overuse or arthritis. If the onset is traumatic in nature, the possibility of fracture should be eliminated. Frequently, a direct injury involving a fall on the outstretched hand may cause fracture of the scaphoid or subluxation of the capitate or lunate bones, and may also cause a traumatic arthritis with soft-tissue swelling and contusion. Indirect injury may also occur from a rotational force or maximal effort in racket sports (Rettig, 1994), e.g. the return of service that eliminated Boris Becker from the 1996 Wimbledon championships.

Most injuries at the wrist and hand develop from repetitive overuse. Tendinitis may result from frequent overstretching or unaccustomed activity. An overuse syndrome occurs when the level of repeated microtrauma exceeds the tissue's ability to adapt (Rettig, 1994). Tensional overload or abnormal shear stresses can cause microtrauma at any point in the musculotendinous or ligamentous unit. The syndromes of carpal tunnel and de Quervain's (see below) may be associated with more proximal lesions, such as nerve entrapment, pathoneurodynamics or lesions of the cervical spine.

A hyperextension injury to the thumb is a relatively common sporting injury, producing a traumatic arthritis in either the trapeziofirst-metacarpal joint or the metacarpophalangeal joint. This may occur in skiing ('skier's thumb') or sports which involve ball-catching, e.g. volleyball or netball, goal-keepers.

Arthritis in the hand may be inflammatory, degenerative or traumatic. Rheumatoid arthritis is common in the smaller joints and therefore readily affects the joints of the wrist and hand where deformity is characteristic; it is usually bilaterally symmetrical. Any synovial space can be involved, including the tendon sheaths and bursae, as well as the joints. Juvenile chronic arthritis has less symmetrical joint involvement than adult rheumatoid arthritis.

Primary degenerative osteoarthrosis affects the trapeziofirst-metacarpal joints and the distal interphalangeal joints. These joints are subjected to stress in the functional position and are used through all extremes of range, predisposing them to primary arthritis. Secondary degenerative osteoarthrosis can affect any joint.

The *duration* of symptoms indicates the stage of the lesion in the inflammatory process. Overuse syndromes have a gradual onset with symptoms present for many months. Rheumatoid and degenerative osteoarthrosis tends to have periods of remission and exacerbation whilst traumatic lesions may be of fairly short duration.

The *symptoms and behaviour* need to be considered. The behaviour of the pain indicates the nature of the lesion, with mechanical lesions eased by rest and aggravated by activity. Overuse lesions are worsened by repetition of the mechanism of trauma. The nature of the pain is also important; is it localized or vaguely diffuse, deep or superficial, sharp, burning, aching, constant or intermittent, getting worse or better, or staying the same?

The other symptoms described by the patient could include paraesthesia. An accurate description of these associated symptoms is relevant to the source of pressure or nerve entrapment. The distribution of pins and needles and whether or not they possess edge and/or aspect helps to determine their origin. Stiffness of the hand may be relevant to arthritis or ligamentous lesions and it is therefore appropriate to know the daily pattern of the symptoms. Heat, coldness, sweating, dryness and other sensory changes may also be relevant, suggesting the vasomotor changes of Raynaud's disease or reflex sympathetic dystrophy.

An indication of *past medical history, other joint involvement and medications* will establish whether contraindications to treatment techniques exist.

Inspection

Fracture or dislocation commonly occurs with a fall on the outstretched hand and shows obvious **bony deformity** and **swelling**. Subluxation, e.g. of the capitate, may be seen as a bump on the dorsum of the hand with the wrist in flexion.

If an extensor tendon is avulsed or torn from the distal phalanx, a mallet finger occurs with flexion of the distal interphalangeal joint.

This can be associated with sporting injuries or simply occur if the finger is forcibly caught whilst making the bed, for example. Deformities of the fingers are commonly associated with rheumatoid arthritis or may result from forced hyperextension injuries, as in wicket keepers, for example. A bony swelling of the distal interphalangeal joint is a characteristic deformity known as a Heberden's node, associated with primary degenerative osteo-arthrosis.

Degenerative osteoarthrosis of the trapeziofirst-metacarpal joint produces a capsular pattern which may draw the thumb into a position of flexion and medial rotation with bony osteophytes obvious at the base of the thumb. Dupuytren's contracture is a deformity with contraction of the palmar fascia, causing flexion of the ring and little finger. Clubbed fingers may be indicative of systemic disease.

Colour changes, which may indicate circulatory involvement, should be further investigated by palpating for the arterial pulses. The fingers in particular can give clues to serious underlying pathology and the colour and shape of the fingers and nails should be noted. Bruising may be apparent, resulting from direct trauma and may be associated with abrasions on the palm due to a fall on the outstretched hand.

Muscle wasting may be obvious in the flattening of the thenar muscles, producing the ape-like hand with the thumb moving back in line with the other fingers. This indicates involvement of the median nerve in the carpal tunnel or possibly cervical nerve root pressure. Similarly, the ulnar nerve or lower cervical nerve root compression involves the hypothenar eminence and if the intrinsic muscles are involved, a claw hand develops. Involvement of the radial nerve affects the wrist extensors and produces a dropped wrist.

Swelling indicates active inflammation and the wrist may be fixed in the mid-position due to the presence of a joint effusion. Contusions with swelling are due to direct trauma. Excessive friction of the skin causes callus and blister formation, e.g. rowing and gymnastics. Ganglia are mucus-filled cysts, which are commonly seen around the wrist, particularly on the dorsum of the hand. They are common between the second and fourth decades of life (Smith and Wernick, 1994) and if symptomatic may be burst or require surgical excision. Rheumatoid nodules may be present.

Palpation

Since these are peripheral joints, palpation for signs of activity is conducted. Temperature changes are assessed and *heat* indicates an active inflammation, whilst cold may indicate circulatory problems (Fig. 7.5). *Synovial thickening* is usually palpated on the dorsum of the wrist (Fig. 7.6). *Swelling* is usually observed around the wrist where it may be fusiform, unilateral or bilateral. Other swellings such as nodules or ganglia can be palpated to assess whether they are hard or soft.

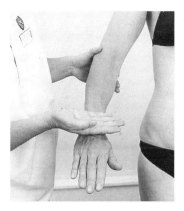

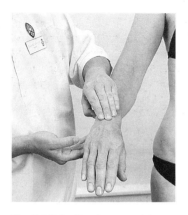

Fig. 7.5 Palpation for heat.

Fig. 7.6 Palpation for synovial thickening.

State at rest

Before any movements are performed, the state at rest is established to provide a baseline for subsequent comparison.

The suggested sequence for the objective examination will now be given, followed by a commentary including the reasoning in performing the movements and the significance of the possible findings.

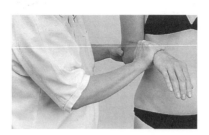

Fig. 7.7 Passive pronation.

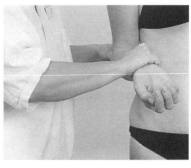

Fig. 7.8 Passive supination.

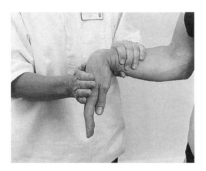

Fig. 7.9 Passive flexion.

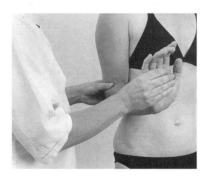

Fig. 7.10 Passive extension.

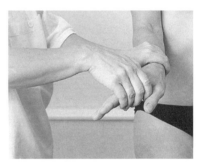

Fig. 7.11 Passive ulnar deviation.

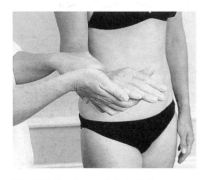

Fig. 7.12 Passive radial deviation.

Examination by selective tension (objective examination)

Inferior radioulnar joint:

- Passive pronation (Fig. 7.7)
- Passive supination (Fig. 7.8)

Wrist joint:

- Passive flexion (Fig. 7.9)
- Passive extension (Fig. 7.10)
- Passive ulnar deviation (Fig. 7.11)
- Passive radial deviation (Fig. 7.12)

The wrist and hand 197

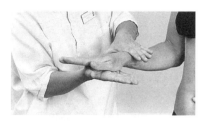

Fig. 7.13 Resisted flexion.

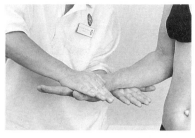

Fig. 7.14 Resisted extension.

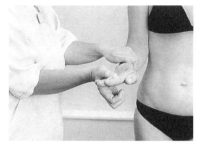

Fig. 7.15 Resisted ulnar deviation.

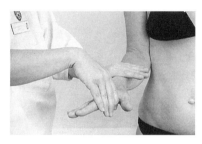

Fig. 7.16 Resisted radial deviation.

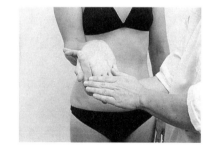

Fig. 7.17 Passive extension and adduction of the thumb.

- Resisted flexion (Fig. 7.13)
- Resisted extension (Fig. 7.14)
- Resisted ulnar deviation (Fig. 7.15)
- Resisted radial deviation (Fig. 7.16)

Trapeziofirst-metacarpal joint:

- Passive extension and adduction (Fig. 7.17)
- Resisted flexion (Fig. 7.18)

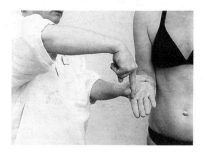

Fig. 7.18 Resisted thumb flexion.

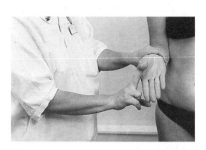

Fig. 7.19 Resisted thumb extension.

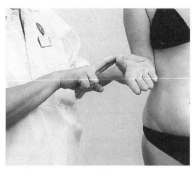

Fig. 7.20 Resisted thumb abduction.

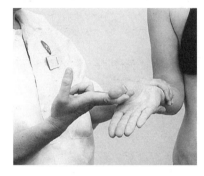

Fig. 7.21 Resisted thumb adduction.

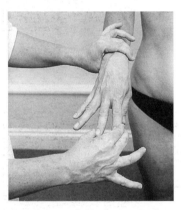

Fig. 7.22 Resisted finger abduction for palmar interossei.

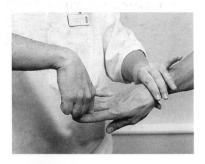

Fig. 7.23 Resisted adduction for dorsal interossei.

- Resisted extension (Fig. 7.19)
- Resisted abduction (Fig. 7.20)
- Resisted adduction (Fig. 7.21)

Interossei:

- Resisted finger abduction (Fig. 7.22)
- Resisted finger adduction (Fig. 7.23)

Palpation

- Once a diagnosis has been made, the structure at fault is palpated for the exact site of the lesion

Fingers:

- Passive and resisted testing of the fingers is not performed routinely, but is included if appropriate

The inferior radioulnar joint gives pain felt at the wrist and is assessed using two passive movements, passive pronation and supination, looking for pain, range of movement, end-feel and the presence of the capsular pattern. Both rotations normally have an elastic end-feel.

The wrist joint is then assessed by four passive movements, looking for pain, range of movement and end-feel. Passive flexion normally has an elastic end-feel due to tissue tension and passive extension a hard end-feel, whilst both deviations normally display an elastic end-feel. The presence of the capsular pattern indicates the existence of arthritis, the non-capsular pattern may be due to a subluxed capitate or collateral ligament strain.

The contractile structures at the wrist are then assessed by resisted tests looking for pain and power. A positive finding requires palpation of the appropriate anatomical structure to establish the exact site of the lesion.

The trapeziofirst-metacarpal joint is assessed by passive application of one combined movement, passive extension and adduction, to test the movements most limited in the capsular pattern.

The contractile structures around the thumb are assessed by resisted tests looking for pain and power. Resisted flexion assesses flexor pollicis longus, resisted extension assesses extensor pollicis longus and brevis, resisted abduction assesses abductor pollicis longus and resisted adduction assesses adductor pollicis.

The interossei are assessed by two resisted tests looking for pain and power. Resisted finger abduction assesses the dorsal interossei and resisted finger adduction assesses the palmar interossei.

Passive and resisted movements of the fingers are not part of the routine examination, but included if necessary. Passive movements may establish the capsular patterns described below.

Capsular lesions

The presence of the capsular pattern at the joints indicates arthritis. Rheumatoid arthritis more readily affects the smaller joints and is seen as symmetrical involvement of the joints in the wrist and hand with deformity characteristic of the condition. Primary degenerative osteoarthrosis affects the trapeziofirst-metacarpal and distal interphalangeal joints more readily. The thumb may be flexed towards the palm of the hand by the contracted anterior joint capsule and the distal interphalangeal joint may show the characteristic Heberden's nodes. Trauma may produce traumatic arthritis and fracture of a carpal bone should be eliminated.

Arthritis in the wrist and hand responds to corticosteroid injection. An alternative treatment for the trapeziofirst-metacarpal joint is described.

Capsular pattern of the inferior radioulnar joint:

- Pain at the end of range of both rotations

Capsular pattern of the wrist joint:

- Equal limitation of flexion and extension
- Eventual fixation in the mid position

Capsular pattern of the trapeziofirst-metacarpal joint:

- Most limitation of extension

Capsular pattern of the metacarpophalangeal joints:

- Limitation of radial deviation and extension
- Joints fix in flexion and drift into ulnar deviation

Capsular pattern of the interphalangeal joints:

- Equal limitation of flexion and extension

Lower radioulnar joint

The lower radioulnar joint is most commonly affected by rheumatoid arthritis.

Capsular pattern
• Pain at end of range of both rotations

Injection of the lower radioulnar joint (Cyriax and Cyriax, 1983; Cyriax, 1984)			
Kenalog 40 mg/ml 0.25 ml	Total steroid 10 mg	Lignocaine 1% 0.75	Total volume 1 ml
23G × 1 in (0.6 × 25 mm) blue needle			

Position the patient with the forearm supported in full pronation. Identify the inferior radioulnar joint line and insert the needle, which may need to be angled, into the joint (Fig. 7.24). Give the injection as a bolus once intracapsular. The patient is advised to maintain a period of relative rest for approximately 2 weeks following injection.

Wrist joint

The wrist joint is most commonly affected by rheumatoid arthritis and traumatic arthritis.

Capsular pattern
• Equal limitation of flexion and extension
• Eventual fixation in the mid-position

Injection of the wrist joint			
Adcortyl 10 mg/ml 2 ml	Total steroid 20 mg	Lignocaine 1% 1 ml	Total volume 3 ml
23G × 1 in (0.6 × 25 mm) blue needle			

Position the patient with the wrist supported and the forearm in full pronation (Fig. 7.25). Locate a point of entry (Fig. 7.26) which may be at either side of the extensor carpi radialis brevis tendon.

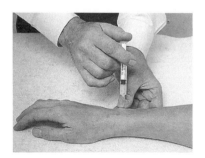

Fig. 7.24 Injection of the lower radioulnar joint.

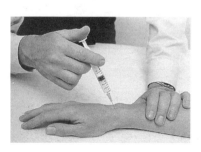

Fig. 7.25 Injection of the wrist joint.

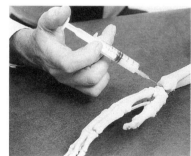

Fig. 7.26 Injection of the wrist joint showing direction of approach and needle position.

Give the injection as a bolus once the needle is intracapsular. Alternatively in the rheumatoid wrist or if degeneration is sufficient to prevent access to the joint, make two or three needle insertions and pepper the area of synovial thickening with a series of withdrawals and reinsertions. This technique is not comfortable for the patient. The patient is advised to maintain a period of relative rest for approximately 2 weeks following injection.

Trapeziofirst-metacarpal joint

The patient complains of pain and tenderness at the base of the thumb and on using the thumb under compression, e.g. writing, gripping. It is a condition common in middle-aged women (Livengood, 1992) and X-ray confirms the diagnosis. An axial compression test applies longitudinal pressure down the shaft of the first metacarpal to grind the articular surfaces together. If positive, it confirms the diagnosis of arthritis and differentiates the condition from de Quervain's tenosynovitis (see below).

Confirmation of the capsular limitation can be made by asking the patient to put the hands into the prayer position and spreading the thumbs, comparing the two sides.

> **Capsular pattern**
>
> - **Most limitation of extension**

> **Injection of the trapeziofirst-metacarpal joint (Cyriax and Cyriax, 1983; Cyriax, 1984)**
>
> | Kenalog 40 mg/ml | Total steroid | Lignocaine 1% | Total volume |
> |---|---|---|---|
> | 0.25 ml | 10 mg | 0.25 ml | 0.5 ml |
>
> 25G $\times \frac{5}{8}$ in (0.5 $\times$ 16 mm) orange needle

Position the patient with the hand resting comfortably. The patient can apply a degree of distraction to the affected thumb (Fig. 7.27). Identify the joint line by running your thumb down the first metacarpal into the anatomical snuffbox to locate the joint line. Insert the needle into the joint and give the injection as a bolus (Fig.

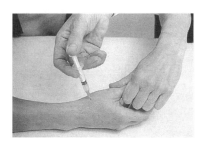

Fig. 7.27 Injection of the trapeziofirst-metacarpal joint.

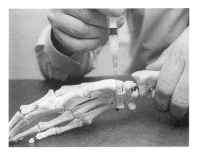

Fig. 7.28 Injection of the trapeziofirst-metacarpal joint showing direction of approach and needle position.

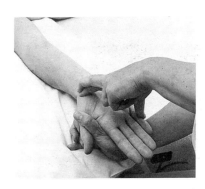

Fig. 7.29 Transverse friction massage of the anterior capsular ligament of the trapeziofirst-metacarpal joint.

7.28). Alternatively, if the thenar eminence is flattened, identify the joint line anteriorly. In either case, osteophyte formation may make the injection difficult. The patient is advised to maintain a period of relative rest for approximately 2 weeks following injection.

Transverse friction massage to the anterior capsular ligament of the trapeziofirst-metacarpal joint (Cyriax and Cyriax, 1983; Cyriax, 1984)

Place the thumb comfortably into the testing position for the capsular pattern (see above). Apply deep transverse friction massage with the thumb or index finger reinforced by the middle finger (Fig. 7.29). Direct the friction massage down on to the anterior capsular ligament and apply the sweep transversely across the fibres. Maintain the technique for 10 min after achieving a numbing effect. The principles for stretching capsular adhesions can be applied, e.g. Grade B mobilization, and distraction is a useful technique to apply to this joint.

Capsular pattern

- **Equal limitation of flexion and extension**

Finger joints

Injection of the finger joints

Kenalog 40 mg/ml 0.25 ml	Total steroid 5–10 mg	Lignocaine 1% 0.25 ml	Total volume 0.5 ml

$25G \times \frac{5}{8}$ in (0.5 × 16 mm) orange needle

Identify the affected joint. With knowledge of the position of the tendons and ligaments around it, find a point of convenient access, usually on the dorsal aspect to one side of the digital expansions. Angle the needle obliquely and, once intra-articular, give the injection as a bolus. The patient is advised to maintain a period of relative rest for approximately 2 weeks following injection.

Non-capsular lesions

Subluxed carpal bone

The capitate is particularly prone to dorsal subluxation or displacement because it is peg-shaped, with its dorsal surface slightly wider than its palmar surface. The lunate sits between scaphoid and triquetral, and the lower end of the radius and the articular disc, and may displace anteriorly when the wrist is forced into extension (Norris, 1993).

Either bone may displace, but commonly it is the capitate. The mechanism of injury involves a fall on the outstretched hand or repeated compression through the extended wrist, as occurs in gymnastics, for example, causing the capitate to displace dorsally.

The patient may complain of pain and limited movement and may be concerned about the bump seen on the dorsum of the hand. Occasionally a subluxed capitate may have been present for a long duration when there is less chance of successful relocation.

On examination there is a non-capsular pattern. Passive extension is painful and the range of movement is limited by a bony block. Passive flexion can usually achieve full range, but the patient experiences pain at the end of range. A bony bump may be obvious on passive flexion, but this should not be confused with the base of the third metacarpal which is also prominent. Diagnosis is dependent upon the appropriate history and the presence of the non-capsular pattern.

The principle of treatment applied here is to relocate the carpal bone under strong traction by a thrust applied to the capitate. This is a mobilization technique performed under strong traction, not a manipulation at the end of range. The technique for the capitate mobilization will be explained below, but this can be adapted if another carpal bone is displaced.

Reduction of the capitate

Locate the capitate by running a thumb down the shaft of the third metacarpal to its base and on to the adjacent displaced capitate (Fig. 7.30 a,b). Place one thumb, reinforced by the other, on top of the

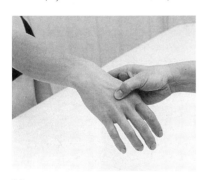

(a)

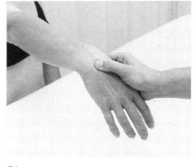

(b)

Fig. 7.30 (a, b) Palpating for the capitate bone at the base of the third metacarpal.

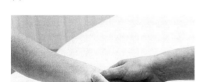

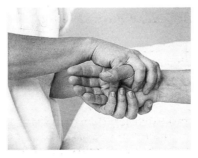

Fig. 7.31 Thumb position for the reduction of the capitate.

Fig. 7.32 Finger position for the reduction of the capitate.

capitate (Fig. 7.31), and wrap your fingers comfortably around the patient's thenar and hypothenar eminences (Fig. 7.32).

Placing your little finger into the web between the patient's thumb and index finger will prevent you from flexing the wrist during the technique.

Position the patient's proximal row of carpal bones level with the edge of the couch. Instruct an assistant to fix this proximal row of carpal bones with the web of the hand parallel to the edge of the couch and reinforced with the other hand, to give counterpressure (Fig. 7.33).

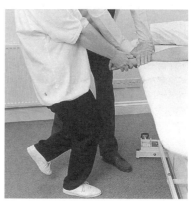

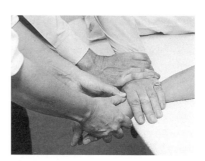

Fig. 7.33 Assistant's hand position for the reduction of the capitate.

Fig. 7.34 Body position for the reduction of the capitate.

Place your feet directly under the patient's hand and lean back to apply strong traction (Fig. 7.34). Allow this traction to establish for a few seconds to separate the two rows of carpal bones. Apply a sharp thrust downwards on the capitate to assist its relocation.

Re-examine the patient to assess the results and repeat if necessary.

If pain persists after relocation, the ligaments surrounding the capitate may be treated with deep transverse friction massage (Fig. 7.35 a,b). Recurrent subluxation of a carpal bone may require a course of sclerosant therapy to stabilize the support of the surrounding

Fig. 7.35 Transverse friction massage of the capitate ligaments: (a) horizontal for vertical fibres and (b) vertically for horizontal fibres.

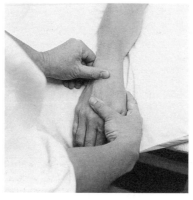

(a)

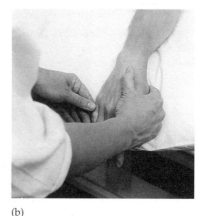

(b)

ligaments, although opinions vary on the success of this technique in this instance.

Collateral ligaments at the wrist joint

The collateral ligaments may be sprained by a traumatic over-stretching of the joint in the appropriate direction to stress the ligament, or by repetitive microtrauma due to overuse. The patient complains of localized pain and stretching the ligament by passive movement in the opposite direction reproduces the pain. The ligament is tender to palpation.

Radial collateral ligament sprain produces pain on passive ulnar deviation and a sprained ulnar collateral ligament produces pain on passive radial deviation. Either lesion may be treated by applying the principles of corticosteroid injection using a peppering technique, or deep transverse friction massage having placed the hand in a suitable position to gain access to the ligament (Figs 7.36–7.39).

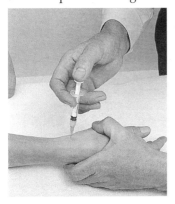

Fig. 7.36 Injection of the radial collateral ligament.

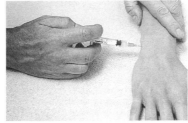

Fig. 7.37 Injection of the ulnar collateral ligament.

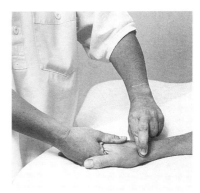

Fig. 7.38 Transverse friction massage of the radial collateral ligament.

The patient is advised to maintain a period of relative rest for approximately 2 weeks following injection.

Injection of the collateral ligaments			
Kenalog 40 mg/ml 0.25 ml	Total steroid 10 mg	Lignocaine 1% 0.25 ml	Total volume 0.5 ml
25G × ⅝ in (0.5 × 16 mm) orange needle			

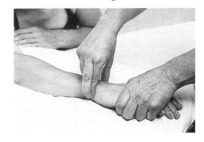

Fig. 7.39 Transverse friction massage of the ulnar collateral ligament.

Carpal tunnel syndrome

The mechanism of the lesion is uncertain, but involves some compression of the median nerve in the carpal tunnel. Mechanical and vascular factors are believed to be involved, with inflammation increasing the size of structures lying within the tunnel, causing swelling and compression, with scarring affecting the perineural vasculature (Anderson and Tichenor, 1994). Wallerian degeneration and intraneural fibrosis eventually produce an irreversible blockade (Ditmars, 1993). The muscles of the thenar eminence may be affected by denervation, abductor pollicis brevis in particular, causing the thumb to fall back into line with the other digits and flattening of the thenar eminence.

Anything which reduces the already tight space in the tunnel compresses the nerve. Intrinsic factors include inflammation and swelling of any structure within the tunnel, or reduction of the size of the tunnel itself: tenosynovitis, hypothyroidism, diabetes mellitus, pregnancy and obesity, rheumatoid arthritis and acromegaly (Kumar and Clark, 1994). External factors include trauma, pressure, repetitive occupational or leisure activities, repeated gripping or squeezing, excessive vibration from heavy machinery, keyboard use, knitting, wood working, using power tools or racket sports. It occurs more commonly in women, between the ages of 40 and 60 (Norris, 1993).

The presenting symptoms and signs of carpal tunnel syndrome are variable. The patient usually complains of an aching, burning sensation, with tingling or numbness of the finger tips. Paraesthesia is experienced in the radial three and a half digits on the palmar surface. A total of 70% of patients experience numbness at night and 40% complain of pain radiating proximally into the lower forearm with simultaneous paraesthesia felt in the fingers (Smith and Wernick, 1994). The symptoms may wake the patient at night and he or she may gain relief by shaking or rubbing the hands (Cailliet, 1990). The patient may complain of a loss of dexterity and sensitivity with clumsiness of hand function.

On examination flattening of the thenar eminence may be observed. Objective sensory loss may be found in prolonged cases of compression with weakness of the thenar muscles, especially abductor pollicis brevis, if the motor branch is involved.

Tinel's sign and Phalen's test are usually used to confirm diagnosis, although it should be recognized that these tests are not perfect diagnostic indicators. False-negative and false-positive rates have been reported of between 25 and 50%. Nerve conduction studies show diminished nerve velocity across the wrist in 90% of patients who go on to have proven nerve compression at surgery (Smith and Wernick, 1994).

Tinel's sign for median nerve compression in the carpal tunnel involves tapping the flexor retinaculum. It is positive if pins and needles are elicited in the radial three and a half digits (Hoppenfeld, 1976; Hartley, 1995).

Phalen's test applies compression to the median nerve in the carpal tunnel, achieved by maintaining maximum wrist flexion. The test is positive if pins and needles are reproduced. A normal hand would develop tingling if this position were maintained for 10 min or more; a patient with carpal tunnel syndrome will report the onset of pain, numbness and tingling within 1–2 min. If symptoms are not reproduced within 3 min the test may be considered to be negative (Hoppenfeld, 1976; Cailliet, 1990; Vargas Busquets, 1994; Hartley, 1995).

Examination of the cervical spine and neural tension testing should be conducted if there is any suspicion that the lesion lies more proximally.

Treatment of carpal tunnel syndrome

The causative factors should be discussed with the patient and attempts made to avoid repetitive actions. Symptomatic relief may be gained from a corticosteroid injection. The patient may be fitted with a wrist support splint to wear at night, to avoid flexion. If injection is unsuccessful or relief is short-term only, surgical release of the flexor retinaculum may be considered.

Injection of the carpal tunnel (Cyriax and Cyriax, 1983; Cyriax, 1984)		
Kenalog 40 mg/ml 0.5 ml	**Total steroid**	**Total volume**
	20 mg	0.5 ml
23G × 1 in or $1\frac{1}{4}$ in (0.6 × 25/30 mm) blue needle		

Position the patient with the wrist supported in extension. Choose a point of entry between the proximal and middle wrist creases on the ulnar side of palmaris longus. If palmaris longus is absent, oppose the thumb and little finger to produce a midline crease as a guide and keep to the ulnar side. Angle the needle parallel to and between the flexor tendons, until it is under the flexor retinaculum, and give the injection as a bolus within the tunnel (Fig. 7.40). Be careful to check that there is no paraesthesia before injecting to avoid injury to the median nerve. The patient is advised to maintain a period of relative rest for approximately 2 weeks following injection.

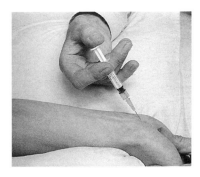

Fig. 7.40 Injection of the carpal tunnel.

Fibrocartilage tears and meniscal lesions

A triangular fibrocartilaginous disc is related to the distal radioulnar joint inferiorly and a fibrocartilaginous meniscus projects into the wrist joint from the ulnar collateral ligament. These intra-articular structures are prone to degenerative changes, tears and occasionally displacement. Trauma, such as a fall on the outstretched hand or repetitive joint overloading, can cause degeneration and tears. Central or radial tears are the most common (Rettig, 1994).

A mechanical lesion involving tear or displacement of any part of the intra-articular complex presents with pain and clicking felt on the ulnar side of the wrist. On examination the clicking may be appreciated by the examiner palpating the wrist whilst simultaneously pronating and supinating the forearm. Passive ulnar deviation may reproduce the pain and point tenderness may be felt just distal to the ulnar styloid. To confirm diagnosis of a mechanical lesion of the intra-articular complex, axial compression is applied to the ulnar side of the wrist whilst the wrist is passively circumducted.

Treatment may involve strong distraction to reduce possible displacement, or the patient may be referred for arthroscopy and excision.

Trigger finger or thumb

Trigger finger or thumb is a snapping phenomenon producing a painful catch as a flexor tendon is caught at a thickened pulley of the sheath during flexion and then released during forced extension (Smith and Wernick, 1994; Murphy *et al.*, 1995). Palmar trauma or irritation can cause thickening of the tendon, sheath or annular pulley and a palpable nodule may exist. Some 35% of cases involve the flexor pollicis longus tendon and 50% involve the middle or ring finger flexor tendons (Smith and Wernick, 1994). The condition may be secondary to systemic disease such as rheumatoid arthritis or diabetes mellitus.

Treatment by corticosteroid injection may be curative, restoring painless, smooth full range of movement to the digit (Murphy *et al.*, 1995).

Injection of trigger finger or thumb			
Kenalog 40 mg/ml 0.25 ml	Total steroid 10 mg	Lignocaine 1% 0.25 ml	Total volume 0.5 ml
25G × $\frac{5}{8}$ in (0.5 × 16 mm) orange needle			

Identify the area of thickening and deliver the injection by a peppering technique. The patient is advised to maintain a period of relative rest for approximately 2 weeks following injection.

Contractile lesions

Tendinitis at the teno-osseous junction of a tendon and tenosynovitis affecting the tendon in its sheath, as it runs under either the flexor or extensor retinacula, are common lesions found at the wrist and hand. Overuse is the most likely cause of the lesion, which may be a simple tendinitis or tenosynovitis of a single unit, or part of an overall more complex syndrome known as repetitive strain injury or work-related upper limb disorder.

Tendinitis at the teno-osseous junction can be treated by injection using a peppering technique or transverse friction massage.

Tenosynovitis can be treated by graded transverse friction massage applied with the tendon on a stretch to restore the gliding function of the tendon sheath, or corticosteroid injection delivered between the tendon and its sheath. All sites are subjected to relative rest from overusing factors following treatment.

Common contractile lesions will be discussed.

De Quervain's tenosynovitis

This condition, originally described in 1895, is a commonly seen tenosynovitis involving the tendons of abductor pollicis longus and extensor pollicis brevis in the first extensor compartment at the wrist (Elliott, 1992a; Livengood, 1992; Rettig, 1994; Klug, 1995).

Uncomplicated inflammation of the shared synovial sheath is known as de Quervain's tenosynovitis. If the shared sheath is thickened due to scarring associated with chronic inflammation it becomes stenotic (Marini *et al.*, 1994); it is then known as de Quervain's stenosing tenosynovitis. Occasionally a ganglion is associated with the condition, especially if it is chronic (Tan *et al.*, 1994; Klug, 1995).

Females are more commonly affected and the condition may be bilateral in up to 30% of patients (Klug, 1995). Onset is occasionally due to direct trauma but more usually due to repetitive occupational or leisure activities. Shea *et al.* (1991) reported a case of de Quervain's tenosynovitis associated with repeated gear-shifting in a mountain bike rider. Gout or rheumatoid arthritis may be associated conditions and Chen and Eng (1994) described a case of early tuberculous tenosynovitis mimicking de Quervain's tenosynovitis.

Pain is felt on the radial side of the wrist with point tenderness over the radial styloid. Pain is aggravated by movements into ulnar deviation, forced flexion/adduction of the thumb and wringing movements of the hand, especially into ulnar deviation. Crepitus may be audible during movements of the wrist.

On examination a local, thickened swelling may be obvious, especially to palpation (Anderson and Tichenor, 1994), with the pain reproduced on resisted thumb abduction and extension. Passive movements of the thumb also reproduce the pain as the tendon is pushed or pulled through the thickened, inflamed sheath.

The axial grind test for arthritis of the trapeziofirst-metacarpal joint should be negative in de Quervain's tenosynovitis.

Finkelstein's test, grasping the patient's thumb and placing the hand into ulnar deviation produces excruciating pain over the radial styloid. If positive it is pathognomonic of de Quervain's tenosynovitis (Shea *et al.*, 1991; Livengood, 1992; Elliott 1992b; Rettig, 1994).

The treatment of choice for de Quervain's stenosing tenosynovitis is a corticosteroid injection. Weiss *et al.* (1994) compared the use of corticosteroid and lignocaine to splinting alone and established better results in the injection group. If the symptoms are not completely cleared, the injection may be repeated.

Injection for de Quervain's tenosynovitis

Kenalog 40 mg/ml	Total steroid	Lignocaine 1%	Total volume
0.25 ml	10 mg	0.75 ml	1 ml

$25G \times \frac{5}{8}$ in (0.5 × 16 mm) orange needle

Position the patient with the forearm supported in the mid-pronation–supination position. Identify the tendons of abductor pollicis longus and extensor pollicis brevis and the V-shaped gap between them at the base of the first metacarpal. With the tendons under some tension, insert the tip of the needle into the V-shaped gap. Passively place the thumb into adduction and ulnar deviation and slide the needle between and parallel to the two tendons (Fig. 7.41). Give the injection as a bolus into the shared sheath. If the injection has been correctly placed a slight swelling will be seen around the tendons. The patient is advised to maintain a period of relative rest for approximately 2 weeks following injection.

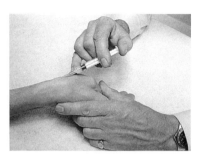

Fig. 7.41 Injection for de Quervain's tenosynovitis.

Transverse friction massage for de Quervain's tenosynovitis

Alternatively, deep transverse friction massage may be applied. Place the thumb into flexion and ulnar deviation at the wrist, to put the tendons on the stretch (Fig. 7.42). Direct the transverse friction massage down on to the tendons using two fingers side by side and sweep transversely across the fibres. Apply 10 min of deep friction massage after the numbing effect is achieved. As a chronic lesion, several sessions will be required. Relative rest is advised where functional movements may continue, but no overuse or stretching until painfree on resisted testing. A splint to support the thumb in the resting position may be helpful.

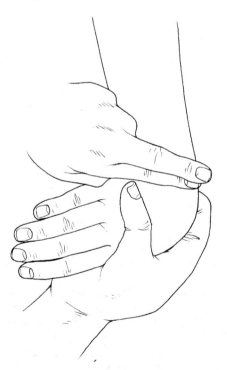

Fig. 7.42 Transverse friction massage for de Quervain's tenosynovitis.

As de Quervain's stenosing tenosynovitis is a chronic lesion, it may form part of a syndrome involving occupational overuse and it may be necessary to include a full examination of the cervical spine and upper limb, including neural tension. All components of the condition should be treated appropriately.

Lanzetta and Foucher (1994) reported an associated Wartenberg's radial neuritis in approximately 15% of patients with de Quervain's tenosynovitis. Wartenberg's syndrome is entrapment of the sensory branch of the radial nerve between the tendons of brachioradialis and extensor carpi radialis longus as the tendons converge and diverge during pronation and supination, producing a scissoring effect on the nerve. This condition is confirmed by a positive Tinel's sign elicited over the brachioradialis tendon, proximal to the styloid process. Associated nerve involvement could be a reason for poor response to the usual management of de Quervain's.

Intersection syndrome or oarsman's wrist

The intersection point between two sets of tendons (abductor pollicis longus/extensor pollicis brevis and extensor carpi radialis longus/brevis) occurs at a point on the radius approximately 4 cm proximal to the wrist (Livengood, 1992; Klug, 1995). It is a point of potential friction between the structures as they exert tension in different directions. This could produce tenosynovitis of the tendons as they pass under the extensor retinaculum or, more commonly, inflammation of the musculotendinous junction in the lower forearm. Cyriax (1982) referred to this as myosynovitis with crepitation of the muscle bellies, a condition which occasionally also affects the tibialis anterior muscle. The condition is provoked by overuse and the patient presents with acute pain and the classical signs of inflammation, heat, redness, swelling and disturbed function. Crepitation is usually audible on movement, but objective testing is difficult due to restriction by pain.

Transverse friction massage for intersection syndrome

Treatment begins immediately with rest and ice to control pain and inflammation. Gentle friction massage is given on a daily basis and the patient should recover within a week.

Position the patient comfortably on a pillow. Identify the area of inflammation, which is obvious on the lower radial aspect of the forearm. Place a thumb along the length of the inflamed tendons and by abduction and adduction of the thumb or pronation and supination of your forearm, impart the friction massage transversely across the fibres (Fig. 7.43). Begin gently to achieve the numbing effect, then follow this up with approximately six good sweeps to produce movement of the sheath around the tendon. Relative rest is advised where functional movements may continue, but no overuse or stretching until painfree on resisted testing.

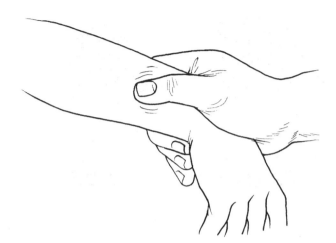

Fig. 7.43 Transverse friction massage for intersection syndrome.

Injection of tendon lesions			
Kenalog 40 mg/ml	Total steroid	Lignocaine 1%	Total volume
0.25 ml	10 mg	0.75 ml	1 ml

given as a bolus between the tendon and its sheath
given by peppering technique at the teno-osseous junction

Extensor carpi ulnaris tenosynovitis

After de Quervain's, tenosynovitis of extensor carpi ulnaris is the next most common tenosynovitis at the wrist (Klug, 1995). Tenosynovitis or tendinitis at the teno-osseous junction is usually due to repetitive overuse, sometimes occurring in the non-dominant hand of the tennis player who uses a double-handed backhand when the take back involves an extreme position of ulnar deviation (Rettig, 1994).

Direct trauma may cause subluxation of the tendon from the groove (Livengood, 1992; Rettig, 1994). The patient complains of pain and clicking on the ulnar side of the wrist. When the extended wrist is actively taken from radial to ulnar deviation, the subluxation of the tendon can be observed and this will help differentiate the condition from a triangular fibrocartilage or meniscal lesion.

Treatment applies the techniques of corticosteroid injection, either injecting between the tendon and sheath in tenosynovitis, or peppering the insertion at the base of the fifth metacarpal. Alternatively, transverse friction massage can be used, with the tendon on the stretch in tenosynovitis and against the insertion for the teno-osseous junction (Fig. 7.44).

Extensor carpi radialis longus and brevis

The lesion is usually at the teno-osseous junction where it is due to repetitive overuse, or it may be associated with a bony metacarpal

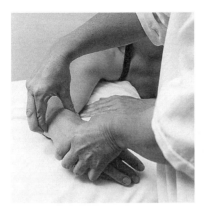

Fig. 7.44 Transverse friction massage for extensor carpi ulnaris tenosynovitis.

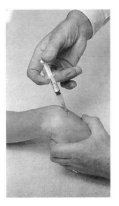

Fig. 7.45 Injection for extensor carpi radialis longus or brevis tendons at teno-osseous site.

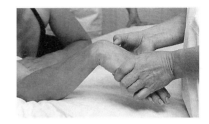

Fig. 7.46 Transverse friction massage for extensor carpi radialis longus or brevis tendons at teno-osseous site.

protuberance or boss (Rettig, 1994; Bergman, 1995). Pain is felt on resisted wrist extension and resisted radial deviation.

The principles of corticosteroid injection or transverse friction massage are applied to treat the lesion. Position the patient with the wrist in flexion to expose the base of the metacarpals and to allow the long extensor tendon to the thumb to fall out of the way. Identify the site of the lesion by palpation at the radial side of the base of the second and third metacarpals. Deliver the corticosteroid injection by a peppering technique (Fig. 7.45), or direct the transverse friction massage down on to the insertion and sweep transversely across the fibres (Fig. 7.46).

Flexor carpi ulnaris

Insertional tendinitis can occur proximal or distal to the teno-osseous junctions at the pisiform. Treatment consists of a corticosteroid injection delivered by a peppering technique into the lesion or transverse friction massage.

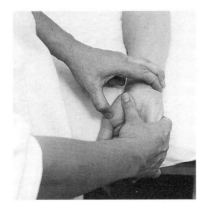

Fig. 7.47 Transverse friction massage for flexor carpi ulnaris tendinitis, proximal site.

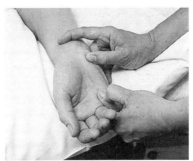

Fig. 7.48 Transverse friction massage for flexor carpi ulnaris tendinitis, distal site.

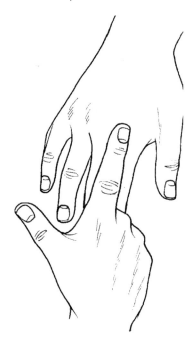

Fig. 7.49 Transverse friction massage for the dorsal interossei.

Remember the position of the ulnar nerve, lying just lateral to the tendon, to be able to avoid it if injecting.

If applying transverse friction massage at the proximal site, direct your thumb down on to pisiform (Fig. 7.47). With the patient's little finger flexed, to relax the hypothenar eminence, apply transverse friction massage to the distal site (Fig. 7.48). Sweep transversely across the fibres at either site.

Interossei

The dorsal interossei are more commonly involved, affecting musicians and tennis players, for example. The patient presents with a vague pain at the metacarpophalangeal joint or between the metacarpals, which is exacerbated by repeated gripping (Rettig, 1994). Pain will be reproduced by resisted abduction of the appropriate finger.

The treatment of choice is transverse friction massage. Palpation will determine the site, but it is often from the origin of the interosseous muscle on one metacarpal. Direct your pressure against the metacarpal and perform the sweep parallel to the shaft (Fig. 7.49).

References

Anderson, M., Tichenor, C.J. (1994) A patient with de Quervain's tenosynovitis: a case study report using an Australian approach to manual therapy. *Physical Therapy* **74**: 314–326.

Backhouse, K.M., Hutchings, R.T. (1990) *A Colour Atlas of Surface Anatomy – Clinical and Applied.* Wolfe Medical.

Bergman, A.G. (1995) Synovial lesions of the hand and wrist. *MRI Clinics of North America* **3**: 265–279.

Cailliet, R. (1990) *Soft Tissue Pain and Disability*, 2nd edn. F.A. Davis.

Chen, W.-S., Eng, H.-L. (1994) Tuberculous tenosynovitis of the wrist mimicking de Quervain's disease. *Journal of Rheumatology* **21**: 763–765.

Cyriax, J. (1982) *Textbook of Orthopaedic Medicine*, vol. 1, 8th edn. Baillière Tindall.

Cyriax, J. (1984) *Textbook of Orthopaedic Medicine*, vol. 2, 11th edn. Baillière Tindall.

Cyriax, J., Cyriax, P. (1983) *Illustrated Manual of Orthopaedic Medicine.* Butterworths.

Ditmars, D.M. (1993) Patterns of carpal tunnel syndrome. *Hand Clinics* **9**: 241–252.

Elliott, B.G. (1992a) Abductor pollicis longus – a case of mistaken identity. *Journal of Hand Surgery* **17B**: 476–478.

Elliott, B.G. (1992b) Finkelstein's test: a descriptive error that can produce a false positive. *Journal of Hand Surgery* **17B**: 481–482.

Hartley, A. (1995) *Practical Joint Assessment – Lower Quadrant*, 2nd edn. Mosby.

Hoppenfeld, S. (1976) *Physical Examination of the Spine and Extremities.* Appleton Century Crofts.

Klug, J.D. (1995) MR diagnosis of tenosynovitis about the wrist. *MRI Clinics of North America* **3**: 305–312.

Kumar, P., Clark, M. (1994) *Clinical Medicine.* Baillière Tindall.

Lanzetta, M., Foucher, G. (1994) Association of Wartenberg's syndrome and de Quervain's disease: a series of 26 cases. *Plastic and Reconstructive Surgery* **96**: 408–412.

Livengood, L. (1992) Occupational soft tissue disorders of the hand and forearm. *Wisconsin Medical Journal* 583–584.

Marini, M., Boni, S., Pingi, A. *et al.* (1994) De Quervain's disease: diagnostic imaging. *Chirurgia Degli Organi Di Movimento* **LXXIX**: 219–223.

Murphy, D., Failla, J.M., Koniuch, M.P. (1995) Steroid versus placebo injection for trigger finger. *Journal of Hand Surgery* **20A**: 628–631.

Norris, C.M. (1993) *Sports Injuries: Diagnosis and Management for Physiotherapists.* Butterworth-Heinemann.

Palastanga, N., Field, D., Soames, R. (1994) *Anatomy and Human Movement*, 2nd edn. Butterworth-Heinemann.

Rettig, A. (1994) Wrist problems in the tennis player. *Medicine and Science in Sports and Exercise* **26**: 1207–1212.

Shea, K.G., Shumsky, I.B., Shea, O.F. (1991) Shifting into wrist pain – de Quervain's disease and off-road mountain biking. *Physician and Sports Medicine* **19**: 59–63.

Smith, D.L., Wernick, R. (1994) Common nonarticular syndromes in the elbow, wrist and hand. *Postgraduate Medicine* **95**: 173–188.

Steinberg, B.D., Plancher, K.D. (1995) Clinical anatomy of the wrist and elbow. *Clinics in Sports Medicine* **14**: 299–313.

Tan, M.Y., Low, C.K., Tan, S.K. (1994) De Quervain's tenosynovitis and ganglion over first dorsal extensor retinacular compartment. *Annals Academy of Medicine* **23**: 885–886.

Vargas Busquets, M.A.V. (1994) Historical commentary: the wrist flexion test (Phalen's sign). *Journal of Hand Surgery* **19**: 521.

Weiss, A-P.C., Akelman, E., Tabatabai, M., Providence, R.I. (1994) Treatment of de Quervain's disease. *Journal of Hand Surgery* **19A**: 595–598.

Williams, P.L., Warwick, R., Dyson, M., Bannister, L.H. (1989) *Gray's Anatomy*, 37th edn. Churchill Livingstone.

Wright, T.W., del Charco, M., Wheeler, D. (1994) Incidence of ligament lesions and associated degenerative changes in the elderly wrist. *Journal of Hand Surgery* **10A**: 313–318.

8 The cervical spine

Summary

Safety is of paramount importance in the application of manual techniques to the cervical spine. As a contribution to safety this chapter begins with a summary of the key points of cervical anatomy, highlighting structures involved in the pretreatment testing procedures and the treatment techniques themselves.

Differential diagnosis and the elements of clinical examination will be discussed. Patients with a mechanical lesion, and thus suitable for the treatments subsequently described, will be identified. The contraindications to treatment will be emphasized and guidelines for safe practice will be given since both are of vital importance.

Anatomy

The spinal column is a series of motion segments each of which consists of an interbody joint and its two adjacent zygapophyseal joints, formed between the posterior arches of the vertebrae above and below. The resultant bony canal is protective but whilst the structural arrangement of the lumbar spine as a whole is suited to weight-bearing, movement and stability, the cervical spine is designed for mobility.

The cervical spine is the most mobile area of the spine (Nordin and Frankel, 1989) and its wide range and variety of movement are related to changes in the direction of vision, the positioning of the upper limbs and hands, and locomotion. It is also an area of potential danger as it gives bony protection to major blood vessels that supply the brain and the spinal cord (Taylor and Twomey, 1994).

Anatomically and functionally, the cervical spine can be divided into two segments. The *upper segment* consists of the atlas and the axis (C1 and C2). Its structure is designed for mobility, with approximately one-third of cervical flexion and extension and over half of axial rotation occurring at this level. The *lower segment* consists of the remaining cervical vertebrae (C3–7), and contributes to overall mobility.

The *atlas* (C1) is composed of two lateral masses, supporting articular facets and their joining anterior and posterior arches. The superior facets articulate with the head at the *atlanto-occipital joints* and their shape facilitates nodding movements of the head (Netter, 1987). The inferior facets articulate with the axis at the *atlantoaxial joints* where rotation is the principal movement. The *axis* (C2) supports the *dens or odontoid process* on its superior surface, the dens providing a pivot around which the atlas rotates. There is no intervertebral disc between the atlas and axis.

The internal ligaments of the upper cervical segment are particularly important to its stability (Fig. 8.1). The *tectorial membrane* is a superior extension of the posterior longitudinal ligament that covers the dens and its ligaments, acting as protection for the junction of the spinal cord and the medulla. The *transverse ligament* of the atlas is a strong horizontal band with extensions passing vertically and horizontally from its mid-point to form a ligamentous complex called the *cruciform ligament*. This, together with the *apical ligament* of the dens, is responsible for keeping the dens in close contact with the atlas. Any instability in the upper cervical segment, e.g. as occurs with rheumatoid arthritis, trauma or Down's syndrome, is an absolute contraindication to orthopaedic medicine techniques.

The lower cervical segment consists of typical cervical vertebrae C3–6 and the atypical C7 which is known as the *vertebra prominens* because of its long spinous process. A typical cervical vertebra consists of a small, broad, weight-bearing *vertebral body* (Fig. 8.2), the superior surface of which is raised on each side, rather like a bucket seat, to form *unciform processes*. The unciform processes articulate with corresponding facets on the vertebra above to form the *uncovertebral joints* or the *joints of Luschka*.

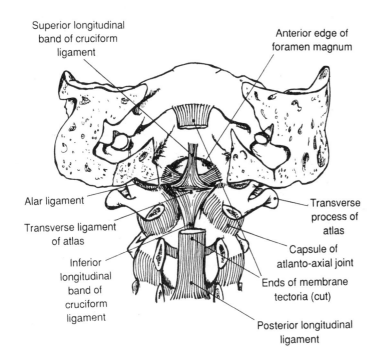

Fig. 8.1 Upper cervical internal ligaments. From Oliver and Middleditch (1991) with permission.

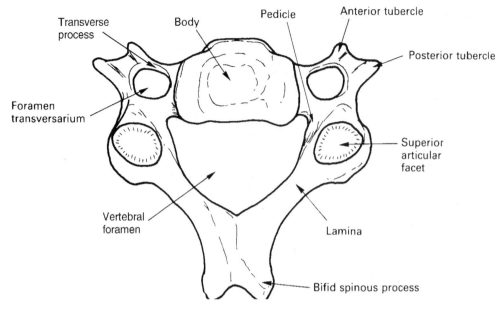

Fig. 8.2 Typical cervical vertebra.
Adapted from Palastanga *et al.* (1994) with permission.

Posteriorly lie two short *pedicles* and two long, narrow *laminae* forming the vertebral arch which, together with the vertebral body, surround a large, triangular *vertebral canal*. The laminae come together to form a bifid *spinous process*. Superior and inferior *articular processes*, at the junction of the pedicles and laminae, articulate at the synovial *zygapophyseal joints* which form an articular pillar on either side of the spine.

Short, gutter-shaped *transverse processes* slope anterolaterally to transport the emerging nerve root. The *foramen transversarium*, a distinctive feature in the transverse processes on each side of the cervical vertebrae, houses the vertebral artery.

The ligaments of the lower cervical segment assist stability and allow mobility. The *anterior longitudinal ligament* protects the anterior aspect of the intervertebral joints and, with other anterior soft tissues, limits cervical extension. The *ligamentum nuchae* is a strong, fibroelastic sheet protecting the joints posteriorly and providing an intermuscular septum. The *ligamentum flavum* is a highly elastic ligament linking adjacent laminae. In the cervical spine it allows separation of the vertebrae during flexion and assists the neck's return to the upright posture. Its elastic properties also allow it to return to its original length, so preventing buckling into the spinal canal where it can sometimes compromise the spinal cord. The *posterior longitudinal ligament* passes from the axis to the sacrum and is at its broadest in the cervical spine where it supports the posterior aspect of the intervertebral joint, preventing posterior displacement of the disc. It is taut in flexion and relaxed in extension.

The joints of the cervical spine

The joints of the lower cervical segment consist of the interbody joint anteriorly and the two zygapophyseal joints posteriorly. The interbody joint is made up of the intervertebral joint and the uncovertebral joints.

The *intervertebral joint* is a symphysis formed between the relatively avascular intervertebral disc and the adjacent vertebral bodies. The disc contributes to mobility and, as it ages, assists the uncovertebral joints in providing translatory glide to the movements of flexion and extension (see below).

The *uncovertebral joint* is formed between the unciform process and a corresponding facet on the vertebral body above (Fig. 8.3). It may be a true synovial joint or an adventitious fibrous joint which has developed through clefts in the lateral corners of the intervertebral disc. The uncovertebral joints contribute to mobility by providing a translatory gliding component to flexion and extension as well as stabilizing the spine by limiting the amount of side flexion. The gliding component produces shear which extends horizontal fissuring of the disc medially from the uncovertebral joints. This together with the degenerative process may eventually produce a bipartite disc (Taylor and Twomey, 1994).

The position of the uncovertebral joint gives bony protection to the nerve root from posterolateral disc displacement, but the joints are prone to degenerative changes with posterolateral osteophyte formation, affecting the size of the intervertebral foramen. Clinically, osteophyte formation here can threaten the nerve root or vertebral artery.

The *zygapophyseal joints* are synovial plane joints with relatively lax fibrous capsules to facilitate movement. The articular facets are angled at approximately 45° to the vertical so that side flexion and rotation of the lower cervical spine occur as a coupled movement.

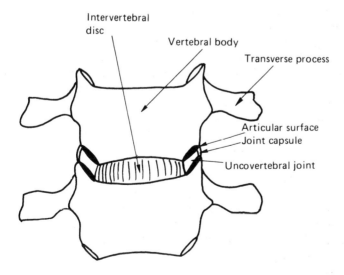

Fig. 8.3 Uncovertebral joints. From Palastanga *et al.* (1994) with permission.

This angle of inclination adds to the component of translatory glide during flexion and extension (Taylor and Twomey, 1994).

A number of intra-articular structures have been described, particularly vascular synovial folds, similar to the alar folds of the knee, as well as fat pads and meniscoid structures. All are highly innervated and can be a potential source of pain (Oliver and Middleditch, 1991; Taylor and Twomey, 1994). As synovial joints the zygapophyseal joints are prone to degenerative changes and, being placed near the exiting nerve root, they may affect the size of the intervertebral foramen.

Orthopaedic medicine treatment is based on the hypothesis of a displaced intervertebral disc, but it should be remembered that since the cervical spine is made up of individual motion segments, a lesion of one part of the segment will tend to influence the rest of that segment. Similarly, treatment directed to one part of a segment will affect the segment as a whole.

Intervertebral discs

There are six cervical discs which facilitate and restrain movement as well as transmit load from one vertebral body to the next (Fig. 8.4). Cervical discs are approximately 5 mm thick (Palastanga *et al.*, 1994) and the thinnest of all the intervertebral discs. Each forms part of the anterior wall of the intervertebral foramen and is thicker anteriorly, contributing to the cervical lordosis. The intervertebral disc consists of an annulus fibrosus, nucleus pulposus and transitional superior and inferior vertebral end-plates.

The general features of the intervertebral disc are covered in greater depth in the chapter on the lumbar spine, since much of the investigative work has been performed on lumbar discs. A brief description is given here to be able to highlight particular features of the cervical discs.

The *annulus fibrosus* is composed of type I collagen fibres arranged obliquely and parallel in concentric layers, or lamellae. Proteoglycan gel binds the fibres together to prevent buckling

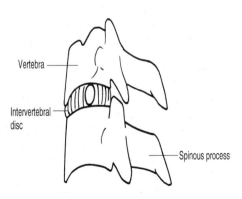

Fig. 8.4 Cervical vertebrae, interbody joint and posterior elements. Adapted from Palastanga *et al.* (1989) with permission.

Vertebra

Intervertebral disc

Spinous process

(Palastanga *et al.*, 1994). The fibres lie at an angle of approximately 65° to the vertical between adjacent vertebral bodies and run in opposite directions in adjacent lamellae. This laminated structure of the disc keeps the nucleus pulposus under pressure and facilitates mobility. There is no distinct dividing line between the annulus and the nucleus, the two blending together in a transitional region.

A small gel-like area forms the *nucleus pulposus* which is centrally placed in cervical discs and said to be the consistency of toothpaste (Bogduk and Twomey, 1991). It consists of a few irregularly placed type II collagen fibres and proteoglycan gel, which has great water-binding capacity. The nucleus is maintained under pressure by the annulus which allows it to be deformed under pressure, to be able to accommodate to movement and to transmit compressive load from one vertebra to another.

The *vertebral end-plate* offers protection by preventing the disc from bulging into the vertebral body. It acts as a semipermeable membrane which, by diffusion, facilitates the exchange of nutrients between the vertebral body and the disc.

Particular features of cervical discs

The cervical intervertebral joints and their discs should not be considered to be a miniature version of the lumbar joints and discs since they are very different. The collagen content is higher in the cervical nucleus and it exists for a relatively short period of time, being present only in children and young adults (Taylor and Twomey, 1994). There is early degeneration of cervical discs from the end of the first decade, involving horizontal fissuring of the annulus and absorption of gel-like nucleus which becomes replaced by collagen.

Cyriax (1982) stated that 'from a clinical point of view nuclear protrusions form only a small minority of cervical disc displacements'. He postulated that a true nuclear protrusion occurs only in adolescents and young adults, presenting as an acute torticollis. His hypothesis would seem to be substantiated by current knowledge of the early degeneration of the cervical nucleus, making nuclear protrusion in the cervical spine unlikely, unless precipitated by severe trauma. A central bar-like protrusion of the annulus is more likely to occur in the cervical spine (Taylor and Twomey, 1994).

Both the position of the uncovertebral joints and the large vertebral canal in the cervical spine influence disc movement. Degenerate cervical discs are more likely to displace directly posteriorly encroaching on the dura through the posterior longitudinal ligament, rather than laterally through the uncovertebral joints to affect the nerve root. Kokubun *et al.* (1996) showed herniation of the cartilaginous end-plate to be the predominant type of herniation in the cervical spine.

A protrusion may be reflected posterolaterally by the posterior longitudinal ligament to cause unilateral pressure on the dura. The triangular vertebral canal is at its largest in the cervical spine and even though the cervical cord is enlarged in this region, there is room for structures to be accommodated. Only a very large posterolateral protrusion would be able to compress the nerve root at this level, unless there is canal stenosis caused by osteophyte formation, an infolding ligamentum flavum or congenital factors. Since the extent of pain referral is thought to be related to the amount of pressure on the dural nerve root sleeve (Mooney and Robertson, 1976), brachial pain is not as commonly associated with cervical disc lesions as sciatica is with lumbar disc lesions. Dural pressure due to a cervical disc tends to produce central or unilateral scapular pain.

Cervical discs are innervated in at least the outer third and possibly the outer half of the annulus fibrosis. The nerve supply is received from branches of a posterior longitudinal plexus, derived from the cervical sinuvertebral nerves, as well as from a similar plexus formed from cervical sympathetic trunks and the vertebral nerves, and from penetrating branches from the vertebral nerve (Bogduk, 1994). Mendel *et al.* (1992) found evidence of nerve fibres and mechanoreceptors in the posterolateral region of the annulus.

The cervical disc may produce either primary disc pain or pain due to the mechanical effect of secondary compression of pain-sensitive structures with associated chemical or ischaemic effects. The mechanism of pain produced by disc displacement is covered in greater detail in Chapter 13 since, as mentioned previously with regard to anatomical studies, much of the investigative work on pain production has been performed in the lumbar region. If findings can be extrapolated to the cervical spine, herniated disc material is thought to undergo a process of degradation which contributes to disc displacement. The chemical mediators of inflammation may

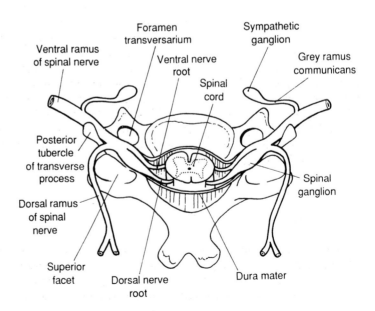

Fig. 8.5 Formation of a spinal nerve. From Oliver and Middleditch (1991) with permission.

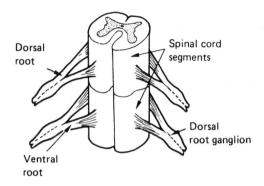

Dorsal root

Spinal cord segments

Dorsal root ganglion

Ventral root

Fig. 8.6 Horizontal direction of emerging nerve roots. From Palastanga *et al.* (1994) with permission.

play a role in the pathophysiology of cervical radiculopathy which renders the nerve root pain-sensitive (Kang *et al.*, 1995).

Cervical spinal nerves

There are eight cervical spinal nerves, each approximately 1 cm long, that, together with the dorsal root ganglion, occupy a large intervertebral foramen (Fig. 8.5). As the dorsal and ventral nerve roots exit the spinal cord they carry with them an investment of the dura mater, the dural nerve root sleeve. The *dural nerve root sleeve* is sensitive to pressure. Cervical spinal nerves emerge horizontally and therefore the nerve roots are vulnerable to pressure only from the disc at that particular level, producing signs and symptoms in one segment only (Fig. 8.6).

After it leaves the intervertebral foramen, the spinal nerve root immediately divides into ventral and dorsal rami. The *sinuvertebral nerve* is a mixed sensory and sympathetic nerve, receiving origin from the ventral ramus and the grey ramus communicans of the sympathetic system. The nerve returns through the intervertebral foramen and gives off ascending, descending and transverse branches to supply structures at, above and below the segment (Williams *et al.*, 1989; Oliver and Middleditch, 1991; Palastanga *et al.*, 1994). The structures it supplies include the dura mater, posterior longitudinal ligament and the outer part of the annulus of the intervertebral disc (Bogduk, 1994).

Vertebral artery

Anatomically the vertebral artery is divided into four sections, which include two right-angled bends, where it is vulnerable to internal and external factors which tend to compromise blood flow (Fig. 8.7) (Williams *et al.*, 1989; Oliver and Middleditch, 1991):

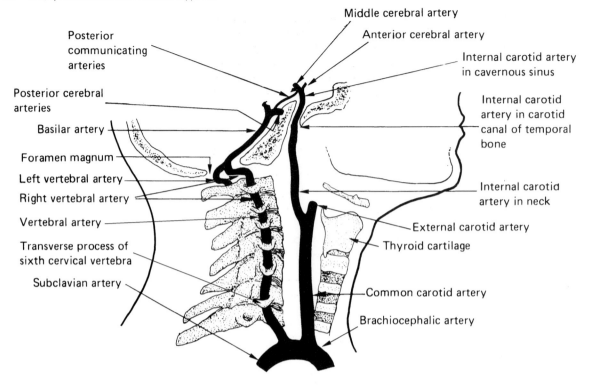

Fig. 8.7 Pathway of vertebrobasilar arteries. From Palastanga *et al.* (1994) with permission.

- Its origin from the subclavian artery.
- Its passage through each foramen transversarium except C7. In this section it gives off spinal branches which supply the spinal cord and its sheaths via the intervertebral foramen.
- The first right-angled bend, turning medially to pass behind the lateral mass of the atlas.
- The second right-angled bend, to turn vertically to enter the foramen magnum to unite with the other vertebral artery to form the basilar artery, which passes on to contribute to the circle of Willis.

Anatomical anomalies and variations exist and commonly one vertebral artery is narrower than its partner. Clinically it is important to recognize vertebrobasilar signs and symptoms since these contraindicate certain cervical manoeuvres. The artery is elastic, particularly in its first and third sections, which allow it to accommodate to movement. Degenerative changes in the artery itself, in the intervertebral canal, uncovertebral joints and zygapophyseal joints, make it vulnerable to blockage as well as possibly distorting its pathway.

Differential diagnosis at the cervical spine

An understanding of the anatomy at the cervical spine, together with a detailed history and examination of the patient, will help with the selection of patients suitable for manual treatment and contribute to safe practice. The two areas of danger in this region are the vertebral arteries and the spinal cord and certain signs and symptoms will become evident on examination which would exclude such patients from manual treatment techniques (see below).

Similarly, there are non-mechanical causes of neck pain in which manual treatment techniques are either contraindicated or not appropriate. The following section will be divided into two parts. The first covers *mechanical lesions* attributed to cervical disc pathology, which present a set of signs and symptoms that help to establish diagnosis and to rationalize treatment programmes. The second covers the *non-mechanical causes* of neck pain and associated signs and symptoms. On the whole, these patients are not appropriate for treatment with manual orthopaedic medicine treatment techniques and require suitable referral.

A central displacement produces central and bilaterally referred pain. A unilateral displacement into the vertebral canal produces unilaterally referred pain. Any structure in the canal that receives a nerve supply is a source of so-called primary somatic pain and the most likely structures to be compressed are the posterior longitudinal ligament and the dura mater. Reference of pain arising from compression of the dura mater is characteristically extrasegmental, i.e. over many segments (see Chapter 1).

The position of the uncovertebral joints offers some protection to the nerve root. However, since the disc degenerates early in the cervical spine, disc displacements tend to produce a pattern of symptoms which indicate a progression of the same condition. The symptoms are age-related with a pattern of increasing frequency and severity. Eventually the nerve root may become involved.

The anatomy of the zygapophyseal joint with its intra-articular structures makes it susceptible to possible mechanical derangement. Signs and symptoms of zygapophyseal joint derangement may mimic those of disc displacement, and treatment of the intervertebral joint will also affect these joints. Whilst acknowledging these possibilities, the approach in orthopaedic medicine is based on the hypothesis of discal pathology, since no other theory fits as well with the clinical presentation of patients. However, some would regard that conclusive proof is still wanting.

Differential diagnosis at the cervical spine

Disc displacements in the cervical spine need to be reduced to prevent them contributing further to the degenerative process. A central protrusion in particular may cause osteophyte formation through ligamentous traction which may eventually threaten the spinal cord. Cyriax (1982) was emphatic in pointing out the danger of not reducing a cervical disc protrusion for this reason. Particular attention should be paid to restoring cervical extension which would act as an indicator that reduction had been effected.

The degenerate cervical disc produces a pattern of signs and symptoms and a set of clinical models has been established to aid diagnosis and to establish treatment programmes. These are outlined later in this chapter. The history in the cervical spine is a very important factor in establishing the pattern of age-related factors. The models should be used as a general guide to the clinical diagnosis of cervical disc displacement. All show a non-capsular pattern on examination.

The following terminology will be used to describe disc displacement:

Disc protrusion

- Central disc material passes into the weakened laminate structure of the annulus, where it can produce primary disc pain since the outer annulus receives a nerve supply.

Disc prolapse

- Discal material passes through a ruptured annulus into the vertebral canal where it has a secondary effect on pain-sensitive structures: the posterior longitudinal ligament, dura mater, dural nerve root sleeve, nerve root and dorsal root ganglion. The sequela of this is sequestration of the disc.

Both forms of displacement are suitable for orthopaedic medicine manual techniques, providing no contraindications exist.

Other causes of neck pain, arm pain and associated signs and symptoms

Generally, this group of conditions does not respond to the manual techniques described in this chapter and indeed some may be absolute contraindications. There may, however, be some overlap, particularly with the degenerative conditions and the techniques may be attempted, provided contraindications have been eliminated.

Arthritis in any joint presents with the capsular pattern. Arthritis occurs in synovial joints in the cervical spine and involves the zygapophyseal and uncovertebral joints. In the cervical spine the capsular pattern is demonstrated by the cervical spine as a whole. The limited movements have the 'hard' end-feel of arthritis. The pattern of symmetrical limitation of the side flexions and rotations is distinctive when compared with the asymmetrical pattern of limitation seen in disc lesions. The early degeneration of the cervical intervertebral disc occurs concurrently with degenerative changes within the other joints. The history will indicate the type of arthritis: degenerative osteoarthrosis, inflammatory or traumatic.

Capsular pattern of the cervical spine

- Equal limitation of side flexions
- Equal limitation of rotations
- Some limitation of extension
- Usually full flexion

Degenerative osteoarthrosis involves damage to hyaline cartilage and subchondral bone with sclerosis and osteophyte formation. Cervical movements become limited in the capsular pattern. Stiffening of the neck is particularly evident on rotation when the patient may have difficulty in reversing the car. Painful symptoms occur during acute exacerbations of the condition, precipitated by trauma or overuse.

The upper cervical segments are particularly involved in the degenerative process, with marked loss of rotation. Degenerative changes in the neck are often referred to as cervical spondylosis. However, despite gross X-ray changes, there may be little in the way of symptoms.

It is possible to have a disc lesion in an older degenerative neck, i.e. non-capsular pattern, superimposed on to a capsular pattern. The disc lesion can be treated with manual techniques and the degenerative osteoarthrosis does not present a contraindication to treatment in itself.

Degenerative changes in the uncovertebral joints lead to osteophyte formation which may encroach on the nerve root or adjacent vertebral arteries, causing problems through direct compression. Degenerative changes of the synovial joints may alter or distort the path of the vertebral artery, leading to symptoms of its compromise.

Matutinal headaches may be due to ligamentous contracture around the upper two cervical joints, the atlanto-occipital and atlantoaxial joints. A condition called old man's matutinal headache exists in which the patient, an elderly male, wakes every morning with a headache which usually eases after a few hours (Cyriax, 1982). Mobilization techniques, particularly manual traction, may be appropriate for this condition.

Tinnitus and vertigo may be associated symptoms of degenerative osteoarthrosis of the cervical spine. They can respond well to the techniques, but the vertebrobasilar system must be ruled out as a cause of the symptoms.

Osteophytic root palsy produces a gradual onset of aching in the arm, usually with paraesthesia, as the osteophytes develop. The patient is usually elderly and will have objective neurological signs of weakness in the arm affecting one nerve root only. Since disc lesions presenting in this way are unusual in this age group, orthopaedic medicine techniques would be contraindicated.

Cervical myelopathy may develop in association with degenerative changes in the cervical spine. Stenosis of the central canal occurs through osteophytic formation and hypertrophy and buckling of the ligamentum flavum develops. The osteophytes, a disc protrusion or a ligamentous fold may exert pressure on the spinal cord and a gradual onset of symptoms occurs with increasing disability. Pain, dysaesthesia of the hands consisting of numbness and tingling, clumsiness and weakness of the hands, weakness and evidence of spasticity of the lower limbs may be present (Jenkins, 1979; Connell and Wiesel, 1992).

Zygapophyseal joints could conceivably produce symptoms individually and in isolation to the other joints in the segment. As synovial joints they are prone to degenerative changes along with the other joints in the segment. Aprill *et al.* (1989) suggested that distinct patterns of pain referral were associated with individual cervical zygapophyseal joints but others have refuted the existence of a facet syndrome (Schwarzer *et al.*, 1994).

Cervical or cervicogenic headache describe a pain perceived to originate in the head, but whose source is in the cervical spine (Bogduk, 1992). It consists of an aching or deep pain localized to the neck, suboccipital and frontal region, precipitated or aggravated by neck movements or sustained neck postures, especially flexion. There is limitation of passive neck movements, changes in muscle contour, texture or tone and abnormal tenderness of the neck muscles (Sjaastad, 1992; Beeton and Jull, 1994; Jull, 1994a, 1994b; Nilsson, 1995; Schoensee *et al.*, 1995). The upper three cervical segments are most commonly involved and associated symptoms may consist of nausea, visual disturbances, dizziness or light-headedness (Jull, 1994a, 1994b). There are many forms of headache and the overlapping symptoms make it difficult to isolate headache due to primary cervical dysfunction.

Polymyalgia rheumatica affects the middle and older age group – women more than men. It presents as pain and stiffness in the neck and shoulder girdle accompanied by fatigue, low-grade fever, depression and weight loss, and responds dramatically to small doses of oral corticosteroids (Hazelman, 1995).

Giant cell arteritis or temporal arteritis is a condition closely related to polymyalgia rheumatica. It is a vasculitis of unknown aetiology affecting the elderly. The patient presents with a severe temporal headache and scalp tenderness. The condition is treated urgently with high-dose steroids, to prevent blindness (Hazelman, 1995).

Rheumatoid arthritis is an inflammatory polyarthritis, affecting females more than males, with its onset usually between the ages of 40 and 50. It tends to follow a relapsing and remitting course. The synovial membrane becomes inflamed and thickened to become continuous with vascular tissue – a condition known as pannus. The pannus causes typical destructive changes of ligaments, cartilage and bone (Walker, 1995). Rheumatoid arthritis can also involve extra-articular soft tissues, e.g. Achilles tendon, plantar fascia (Kumar and Clark, 1994).

It is uncommon for rheumatoid arthritis to affect the cervical joints only, without its manifestation elsewhere, and it most commonly affects the smaller peripheral joints bilaterally. However, in patients with rheumatoid arthritis it may be silent in the cervical joints and there may be no clinical evidence of cervical spine involvement (Clark, 1994).

The mechanism of the disease in the spinal joints is the same as that seen in peripheral joints, with ligament, cartilage and bone destruction. This loss of the supporting infrastructure of the spine, particularly of the upper cervical segment, is a potential hazard for significant neurological involvement of the brainstem and cervical spinal cord. Atlantoaxial subluxation is the most common manifestation, but cranial settling (vertical intrusion of the dens) and subaxial subluxation may also occur (Clark, 1994; Zeidman and Ducker, 1994; Mathews, 1995). It is therefore an absolute contraindication to orthopaedic medicine techniques.

Traumatic arthritis is produced by significant trauma causing inflammation in the cervical synovial joints and therefore a capsular pattern. This may occur following a whiplash injury. Once the capsular pattern has settled, there may be evidence of an underlying disc lesion to which mobilization can be carefully applied, providing there is no damage to the vertebrobasilar system.

Whiplash injury occurs when a car is struck from behind, often whilst the occupants of the involved car are unaware. A hyperextension injury followed by a hyperflexion injury occurs. During the hyperextension phase the anterior structures, the intervertebral discs, anterior longitudinal ligament and anterior muscles can be damaged or torn and the posterior structures compressed. During the hyperflexion phase the dens may impact against the atlas, and the atlanto-occipital joint, posterior ligaments and zygapophyseal joints can be involved (Bogduk, 1986). Generally, a whiplash injury may produce some pain initially, but it is not until later that the ligaments stiffen and produce a secondary capsular pattern due to the trauma.

Significant bony or ligamentous damage causes immediate pain with a reluctance to move the neck. X-ray evidence of cervical instability is an absolute contraindication to orthopaedic medicine techniques. A history of recent whiplash injury is a possible risk factor of vascular accident (Kleynhans and Terrett, 1985).

Taylor and Twomey (1993) conducted an autopsy study of neck sprains and showed clefts associated with vertebral end-plate lesions in trauma victims. These were distinct from the uncovertebral clefts and central fissures associated with degeneration of cervical discs. These so-called rim lesions involved the avascular cartilage end-plates and the outer annulus and, in further experiments, showed a poor response to healing. They may be responsible for the chronic pain often associated with whiplash injuries. Posterior disc displacement through a damaged annulus and haemarthrosis of the zygapophyseal joints were also observed in the trauma victims and this is clinically significant in treating the early whiplash. The acute sprain of the joints requires pain relief and reduction of inflammation, and early mobilization may be applied providing gross bony injury and instability are not present.

Evidence exists to support early mobilization in whiplash-type injuries to avoid the chronic pain syndrome developing, with its associated psychosocial factors (Mealy *et al.*, 1986; McKinney, 1989). In the hyperacute stage, gentle techniques are applied, including Grade A mobilization, providing there is no serious pathology. The patient is given the responsibility for management of the condition, and is instructed about posture and exercise, advice to avoid excessive reliance on a collar, appropriate pillow support and adequate analgesia.

Serious, non-mechanical conditions may present with signs and symptoms similar to those of a mechanical presentation. For this reason, careful examination is necessary to eliminate serious disease which would be contraindicated for orthopaedic medicine treatment. Patients may present with local symptoms which are rarely provoked by movement or posture. On examination it may be difficult to reproduce the symptoms. Other more generalized features may also be present, such as increasing and unrelenting pain, night pain, weight loss, general malaise, fever, raised erythrocyte sedimentation rate or other symptoms, e.g. cough.

Spinal infections may include osteomyelitis or epidural abscess. The organism responsible may be *Staphylococcus aureus*, *Mycobacterium tuberculosis* or, rarely, *Brucella* (Kumar and Clark, 1994).

Malignant disease is usually extradural with bone metastases produced most commonly from primaries in the bronchus, breast, prostate, kidney or thyroid. There may be a history of a gradual onset of pain and stiffness, the pain tends to be unrelenting and night pain is usually a feature. The pain is not relieved by different postures. On examination active movements produce pain and limitation in all directions. The passive movements are prevented by the end-feel of a twang of muscle spasm and resisted movements are painful and possibly weak. All of these signs and symptoms are evidence of a gross lesion (Cyriax, 1982). Neurological examination may reveal excessive muscle weakness involving several nerve roots, possibly bilaterally, in contrast to a disc lesion that tends to involve one nerve root only (Mathews, 1995).

Primary tumours, e.g. meningioma, neurofibroma, glioma, tend to present with a gradual onset of symptoms of cord compression and pain is not usually a major feature.

Pancoast's tumour is carcinoma in the apex of the lung which may erode the ribs and involve the lower brachial plexus. There is severe pain in the shoulder and down the medial aspect of the arm, with evidence of T1 palsy. Cervical side flexion away from the painful side may be the only limited neck movement, with passive elevation of the shoulder on the symptomatic side also being painful (Cyriax, 1982). Interruption of the sympathetic ganglia can produce Horner's syndrome – constriction of the pupil and drooping of the eyelid on the side of the tumour (Kumar and Clark, 1994).

Suprascapular, long thoracic and spinal accessory neuritis usually present with pain in the scapula and upper arm for approximately 3 weeks' duration. On examination, the neck movements are full and do not reproduce the pain. There is weakness of the appropriate muscles supplied by the affected nerve. The cause may be unknown, or it may be due to trauma or follow a viral infection. Recovery is usually spontaneous over approximately 6 weeks.

- Suprascapular neuritis produces weakness of the supraspinatus and infraspinatus muscles.
- Long thoracic neuritis produces weakness of the serratus anterior muscle and winging of the scapula.
- Spinal accessory neuritis produces weakness of the sterno-cleidomastoid and trapezius muscles.

Neuralgic amyotrophy is an unusual cause of severe pain in the neck and scapular region with a bizarre pattern of muscle weakness in the infraspinatus, supraspinatus, deltoid, triceps and serratus anterior muscles. The cause of the condition is unknown, but it may follow viral infection or immunization and an allergic basis is postulated (Kumar And Clark, 1994). It usually recovers spontaneously over several weeks or months.

Thoracic outlet syndrome, reflex sympathetic dystrophy and work-related syndromes all present with upper limb signs and symptoms which are sometimes difficult to isolate into a simple diagnostic pattern, particularly if symptoms have been present for a long duration.

Thoracic outlet syndrome is a term used for compression, entrapment and/or postural alterations affecting the brachial plexus and its accompanying neurovascular structures, although debate continues about its existence (Walsh, 1994). Distal symptoms occur, usually due to compression of the lower trunk of the brachial plexus (C8, T1), but the upper and middle trunks can also be involved. The condition may be bilateral, with a burning, dull aching pain along the medial aspect of the forearm. Distal oedema may be associated with activity, sweating and heaviness, and circulatory changes may be seen in the hands. Paraesthesia occurs as the release phenomenon, coming on at night, some time after the pressure has been released.

Reflex sympathetic dystrophy describes a complex disorder of the limbs with or without obvious nerve involvement. It consists of persistent peripheral burning pain and tenderness which is termed hyperaesthesia (an abnormal response to pain) or allodynia (pain in response to stimuli which are not normally noxious). Vasomotor and sensory changes consist of sweating, colour changes and trophic skin changes together with weakness, tremor, muscle spasm and contractures (Herrick, 1995).

Work-related syndromes of the upper limb are due to repetitive occupational overuse, producing musculoskeletal symptoms, once a certain threshold of activity is exceeded. Sometimes this may present as a simple tenosynovitis or epicondylitis but much more often it presents as a catalogue of symptoms which are non-specific. Diffuse aching, stiffness, muscle or joint tiredness are present with the chronic nature of the condition perhaps leading to anxiety and depression (Bird, 1995).

The preceding conditions are usually associated with patho-neurodynamics, i.e. factors affecting the mobility and circulation of the nervous system. Each component of each condition needs to be recognized and a suitable treatment programme established. Orthopaedic medicine techniques are not usually indicated unless specific lesions are diagnosed.

Fibromyalgia presents, usually in women, as a complex of variable symptoms including widespread musculoskeletal pain of the neck, shoulders and upper limbs. Fatigue, headache, waking unrefreshed, subjective distal swelling, poor concentration, forgetfulness and weepiness have been described (Doherty, 1995). Multiple hyperalgesic tender spots and non-restorative sleep are the main diagnostic features of fibromyalgia. There are several components to management which include the use of relaxation techniques, exercise, hydrotherapy, physiotherapy, acupuncture, muscle relaxants and drugs to improve the quality of sleep. The condition is difficult to separate from endogenous depression and often responds to antidepressant medication (Huskisson, 1995, Conference note).

Drop attacks are episodes of weakness in the lower limbs, causing falling without loss of consciousness. They may be due to changes in tone in the lower limb originating in the brainstem, and appear to be related to transient ischaemic attacks (Kumar and Clark, 1994). Any instability in the upper cervical segment, i.e. congenital ligamentous laxity of the atlanto-occipital joint, deformed odontoid process, cervical spondylosis or a spondylolisthesis, can produce drop attacks (Cyriax, 1982; Hinton *et al.*, 1993). During the subjective examination the patient must be questioned about drop attacks and the result noted. Any history of drop attacks is an absolute contraindication to manual therapy.

Subluxation of the atlantoaxial joint and hypermobility of the atlanto-occipital joint are associated with Down's syndrome and may occasionally lead to compression of the spinal cord. Clinicians involved in manipulation should be aware of this risk (Pueschel *et al.*, 1992; Department of Health, 1995; Matsuda *et al.*, 1995).

Klippel–Feil syndrome is associated with a limited range of cervical movement, short neck and low hairline. Patients usually have developmental abnormalities, including congenital fusion of cervical vertebrae, which may predispose them to the risk of neurological sequelae (Pizzutillo *et al.*, 1994).

Vertebrobasilar insufficiency produces symptoms through a reduced blood flow in the vertebral arteries to the brain. Patients often relate their symptoms to particular head positions such as looking up (Toole and Tucker, 1960). Anatomical anomalies are frequently seen in the vertebral arteries and their course through the cervical foramen transversarium. Often the two arteries vary considerably in diameter (Mitchell and McKay, 1995) and extrinsic or intrinsic factors may decrease the lumen of the artery permanently or temporarily. Extrinsic factors include degenerative changes in the intervertebral, zygapophyseal and uncovertebral joints, with osteophyte formation, which may compress or alter the course of the artery. Intrinsic factors include arterial disease and thrombosis.

The position of the head and neck has been shown to affect the size of the vertebral arteries. In a cadaveric study, Brown and Tatlow (1963) looked at blood flow in the vertebral arteries in 41 subjects. Extension alone produced no occlusions. Extension and rotation produced five occlusions, involving the artery of the side opposite that to which the head was turned. The addition of traction, i.e. half body weight applied to the head, added another 27 occlusions. Twenty minutes' continuous traction in the neutral position produced a single occlusion in one cadaver and bilateral occlusion in another, whilst initial application of traction produced no occlusions.

This study is often quoted against the use of traction in conjunction with rotation manipulation. Putting it into perspective, this study was conducted on cadavers and, whilst accepting the production of occlusions, no record is made of for how long traction was maintained. The initial application of traction was said to produce no occlusions. In orthopaedic medicine, manual traction is the basis of the techniques. It is applied momentarily for the short duration of the manoeuvre, can be stopped instantly if adverse reactions are suspected or reported and is applied to assist reduction of disc displacement and principally to protect the spinal cord. The safe application of orthopaedic medicine techniques is discussed later in this chapter.

Wallenberg's syndrome or lateral medullary syndrome is probably the most recognized syndrome of brainstem infarction caused by vertebral artery pathology (Frumkin and Baloh, 1990; Kumar and Clark, 1994). The common site of injury to the vertebral artery following neck manipulation is at the level of the atlantoaxial joint. Injuries include intimal tearing, dissection or thrombus formation, intramural haematoma or vasospasm.

Dizziness and nausea are the main presenting symptoms of vertebrobasilar insufficiency. A full list of possible signs and symptoms of vertebrobasilar insufficiency are given with the description of the test later in this chapter.

Commentary on the examination

Observation

Before proceeding with the history, a general observation of the patient's *face, posture and gait* is made, noting the posture of the neck and the carriage of the head. Neck posture will give an immediate indication of the severity and possible irritability of the condition, e.g. a wry neck associated with acute pain in which the patient has developed an antalgic posture.

History (subjective examination)

The history is particularly important at the spinal joints. Selection of patients for orthopaedic medicine treatment techniques relies on a diagnosis of a displaced intervertebral disc and certain aspects of the history will assist in this diagnosis as well as highlighting patients with contraindications to treatment.

The *age, occupation, sports, hobbies and lifestyle* of the patient may give an indication of the nature of onset and its relationship to habitual postural problems associated with a particular lifestyle.

The age of the patient is important, particularly at the cervical spine, since the type of cervical disc displacement is related to age. In the young patient, child or adolescent, neck pain may be associated with an acute torticollis, considered to be a true nuclear protrusion of the disc.

Annular disc protrusions tend to occur in the middle-age group, with posterior displacement. Referred arm pain, due to a large posterolateral disc prolapse, usually occurs over the age of 35, through progressive displacement. Arm pain presenting under the age of 35 may be indicative of serious pathology and this should be noted. Degenerative changes in the intervertebral, uncovertebral and zygapophyseal joints occur in the older neck.

Occupation, sports, hobbies and lifestyle of the patient may contribute to the patient's signs and symptoms. Habitual postures can contribute to postural adjustment, altered biomechanics and muscle imbalance, for example, the head-forward posture of the visual display unit operator, the side-flexed posture of holding the telephone in the crook of the neck to leave the hands free, the flexed and rotated posture of the plumber or builder, or the head-extended posture allowing the arms to be used above the head in the painter or electrician. Athletes may assume certain postures related to their sport which may precipitate or contribute to their problem.

The *site and spread* of the symptoms give important clues to diagnosis in the cervical spine and highlight the importance of understanding the mechanisms of referred pain in a segmental or extrasegmental pattern. Pain may be localized to the neck or occur in association with symptoms felt in the scapular area, chest, upper limb or head.

Nerve root compression in the cervical spine can only occur at the levels at which the nerve root can be compressed. In the mid and lower cervical regions the roots are under threat from the intervertebral discs, uncovertebral joints and zygapophyseal joints, which form the boundaries of the intervertebral foramen. C1 and 2 nerve roots do not run in intervertebral foramina, therefore compression of these nerve roots is not the mechanism for upper cervical pain.

It is important to establish the nature of the *onset and duration* of the symptoms, not just of this current episode of pain, but of all previous episodes. Cervical disc lesions tend to be a progression of the same incident, and establishing a history of increasing and worsening episodes of pain assists diagnosis.

The onset may be sudden or gradual. It may be precipitated by a single incident such as a whiplash injury due to a motor vehicle accident or sudden unguarded movement, such as missing a footing. If traumatic in onset, the exact mechanism should be established: was it hyperflexion, hyperextension or excessive rotation? If the condition developed gradually, is it associated with habitual postures, or a change in posture, such as sleeping in a different bed?

The patient with whiplash injury, without serious bony complications, presents with pain felt at the time of the trauma which settles. Twenty-four hours later, pain and stiffness develop due to the ligamentous involvement and muscular strain. The whiplash patient who has severe pain from the time of the trauma may have more serious underlying pathology, e.g. fracture and/or dislocation.

The duration of the symptoms helps to give a prognosis of the patient's condition as well as providing an indicator for serious pathology, being always on the alert for possible contraindications to treatment. Generally, the patient who presents with a short duration of symptoms responds better to treatment. Disc pathology tends to be self-limiting and generally symptoms will resolve spontaneously. With repeated episodes, however, this tends to take longer and longer. Nerve root compression may follow a mechanism of spontaneous recovery in 3 or 4 months, providing the patient loses the central symptoms.

Recurrent symptoms may indicate a cervical disc displacement or degenerative arthrosis which tends to present with periods of exacerbation of symptoms. Inflammatory arthritis may present a similar picture, but it has usually manifested itself in other joints before involving the cervical spine.

The *symptoms and behaviour* need to be considered. The behaviour of the pain will give an indication of the irritability of the condition. Make a note of the daily pattern of the pain. If it is easier first thing in the morning and worse as the day goes on, easing up again with rest, this could indicate a compression problem or a postural problem. If it is uncomfortable and stiff in the morning and painful on certain movements, this is indicative of an active arthritis. It may be due to an acute episode of degenerative osteoarthrosis, or inflammatory arthritis such as rheumatoid arthritis or ankylosing spondylitis. Pain not at all relieved by rest, with unrelenting night pain, indicates serious pathology such as tumour or metastases.

Of what other symptoms does the patient complain? Pain on a cough, sneeze or straining, which causes an increase in the intrathecal pressure, may indicate disc compression or tumour. Paraesthesia may be related to nerve root compression. Sympathetic symptoms such as hot and cold feelings, heaviness, puffiness or circulatory symptoms may be related to nerve root compression or thoracic outlet syndrome, reflex sympathetic dystrophy or work-related upper limb disorder.

Other causes of neck pain and associated symptoms should be eliminated, such as thoracic outlet syndrome that may produce similar symptoms to upper cervical syndromes. Symptoms may include facial pain, tinnitus, auditory and visual disturbances.

From the history, specific questions must be asked to eliminate vertebrobasilar artery problems and problems of instability in the upper cervical joints, which would contraindicate treatment. Explore any complaint of dizziness, nausea, faintness, tinnitus or visual problems. Ask specific questions about drop attacks, i.e. 'Do you ever fall to the ground without losing consciousness?' Establish the presence of pins and needles and numbness and note exactly where. Consider whether the distribution of these symptoms fits with segmental referral or is more a sympathetic feature. Ask about headaches, fatigue and stress, or blurred or dull vision.

Other joint involvement will give an indication to previous problems which may or may not be related. Look for evidence of rheumatoid arthritis, usually in the smaller joints, remembering that it may be quiet in the cervical spine. Ankylosing spondylitis usually starts in the sacroiliac joint(s) and lumbar spine or hips. Note the presence of generalized degenerative osteoarthrosis. Ask about *past medical history* and consider any serious illness, operations, chemotherapy, radiotherapy or depression. It is advisable to ask about previous trauma involving the neck: a history of whiplash is considered a risk factor in vascular accidents (Kleynhans and Terret, 1985).

Check the *medications* currently taken by the patient, as anticoagulants, antidepressants or chemotherapeutic agents may present a contraindication to the treatment techniques. Ask about any pain-relieving drugs to give an indication of how much pain control is required by the patient.

Inspection

The patient should undress down to underwear, to the waist. A general inspection will reveal any **bony deformity** (Fig. 8.8 a,b). The general spinal curvatures are appreciated, assessing for any increased or decreased cervical lordosis, tilt or rotation, abnormalities in the cervicothoracic junction and upper thoracic kyphosis, scoliosis, or the presence of an antalgic posture. Abnormal fatty tissue sometimes develops over C7, in association with postural deformity at the cervicothoracic junction and this is known as a dowager's hump. Similar fatty tissue can often be seen in rugby players in the front row of the scrum. The head carriage is also noted, looking for excessive protraction or retraction.

Colour changes and swelling would not be expected in the cervical spine unless associated with a history of direct trauma.

A neuritis would give the appropriate wasting of the muscles supplied by the nerve involved and the neck, shoulder and scapular area should be assessed for obvious *muscle wasting*. Some unusual nerve pathologies produce bizarre patterns of bilateral asymmetrical wasting, e.g. neuralgic amyotrophy. In disc pathology with nerve root compression, muscle wasting may not be obvious on inspection.

State at rest

Before any movements are performed, the state at rest is established to provide a baseline for subsequent comparison.

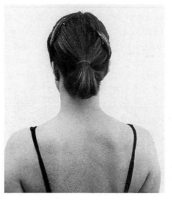
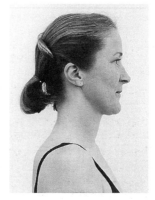

Fig. 8.8 (a, b) Inspection.   (a)   (b)

The suggested sequence for the objective examination will now be given, followed by a commentary including the reasoning in performing the movements and the significance of the possible findings.

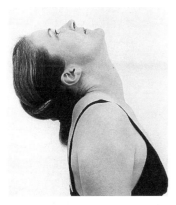

Fig. 8.9 Active extension.

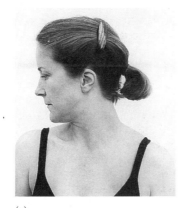

(a)

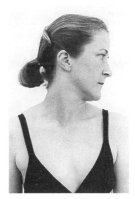

(b)

Fig. 8.10 (a, b) Active rotations.

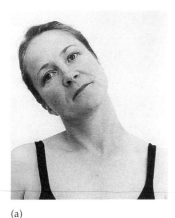

(a)

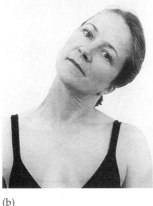

(b)

Fig. 8.11 (a, b) Active side flexions.

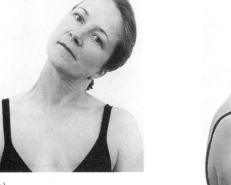

Fig. 8.12 Active flexion.

Examination by selective tension (objective examination)

Articular signs:
- Active cervical extension (Fig. 8.9)
- Active cervical right rotation (Fig. 8.10a)
- Active cervical left rotation (Fig. 8.10b)
- Active cervical right side flexion (Fig. 8.11a)
- Active cervical left side flexion (Fig. 8.11b)
- Active cervical flexion (Fig. 8.12)

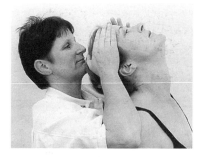

Fig. 8.13 Passive extension.

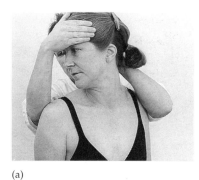

(a)

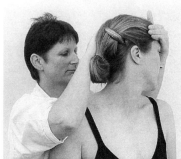

(b)

Fig. 8.14 (a, b) Passive rotations.

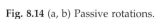

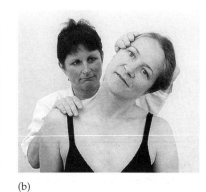

(a)

(b)

Fig. 8.15 (a, b) Passive side flexions.

- Passive cervical extension (Fig. 8.13)
- Passive cervical right rotation (Fig. 8.14a)
- Passive cervical left rotation (Fig. 8.14b)
- Passive cervical right side flexion (Fig. 8.15a)
- Passive cervical left side flexion (Fig. 8.15b)

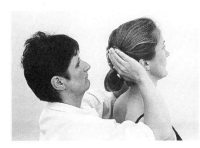

Fig. 8.16 Resisted extension.

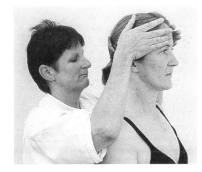

Fig. 8.17 Resisted rotations.

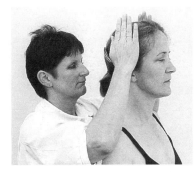

Fig. 8.18 Resisted side flexions.

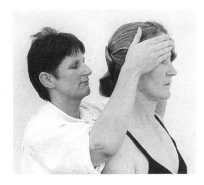

Fig. 8.19 Resisted flexion.

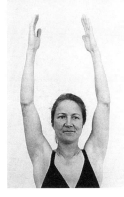

Fig. 8.20 Active shoulder elevation to eliminate the shoulder as a cause of pain.

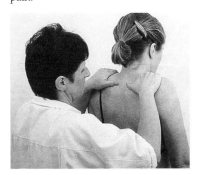

Fig. 8.21 Resisted shoulder elevation.

Resisted tests are not part of the routine examination, but may be applied here:

- Resisted cervical extension (Fig. 8.16)
- Resisted cervical rotations (Fig. 8.17)
- Resisted cervical side flexions (Fig. 8.18)
- Resisted cervical flexion (Fig. 8.19)

Elimination of the shoulder joint:

- Active shoulder elevation (fig. 8.20)

Resisted tests for objective neurological signs and alternative causes of arm pain:

- Shoulder elevation, trapezius   Spinal accessory
  (Fig. 8.21)   nerve XI C3, 4

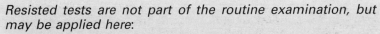

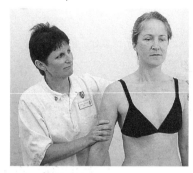

Fig. 8.22 Resisted shoulder abduction.

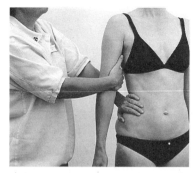

Fig. 8.23 Resisted shoulder adduction.

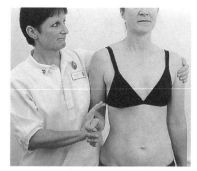

Fig. 8.24 Resisted shoulder lateral rotation.

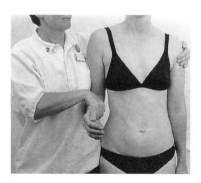

Fig. 8.25 Resisted shoulder medial rotation.

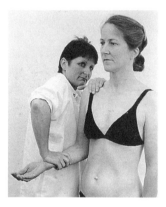

Fig. 8.26 Resisted elbow flexion.

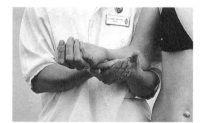

Fig. 8.27 Resisted elbow extension.

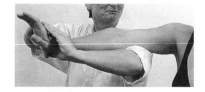

Fig. 8.28 Resisted wrist extension.

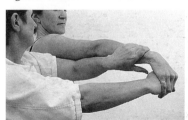

Fig. 8.29 Resisted wrist flexion.

• Shoulder abduction, supraspinatus (Fig. 8.22)	C4, *5*, 6
• Shoulder adduction, latissimus dorsi, pectoralis major, teres major and minor (Fig. 8.23)	C5, 6, *7*, 8, T1
• Shoulder lateral rotation, infraspinatus (Fig. 8.24)	C*5*, 6
• Shoulder medial rotation, subscapularis (Fig. 8.25)	C*5*, *6*
• Elbow flexion, biceps (Fig. 8.26)	C*5*, *6*
• Elbow extension, triceps (Fig. 8.27)	C6, *7*, 8
• Wrist extensors, (Fig. 8.28)	C*6*, 7, 8
• Wrist flexors, (Fig. 8.29)	C6, *7*, 8, T1

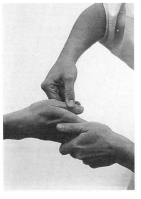

Fig. 8.30 Resisted thumb adduction.

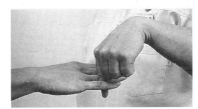

Fig. 8.31 Resisted finger adduction.

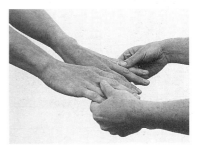

Fig. 8.32 Checking skin sensation.

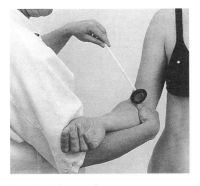

Fig. 8.33 Biceps reflex.

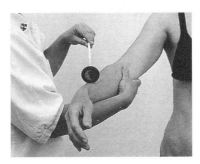

Fig. 8.34 Brachioradialis reflex.

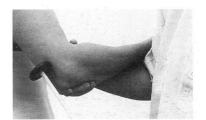

Fig. 8.35 Triceps reflex.

- Thumb adductors, adductor brevis (Fig. 8.30)   C*8*, T1
- Finger adductors, palmar interossei (Fig. 8.31)   C8, T*1*

Skin sensation (Fig. 8.32):
- Thumb and index finger: C6
- Index, middle and ring fingers: C7
- Middle, ring and little fingers: C8

Reflexes:
- Biceps (Fig. 8.33)   C*5*, 6
- Brachioradialis (Fig. 8.34)   C5, *6*, 7
- Triceps (Fig. 8.35)   C6, *7*, 8
- Babinski reflex (Fig. 8.36)

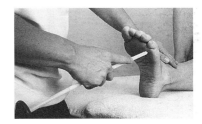

Fig. 8.36 Assessing for Babinski reflex.

The routine examination at the cervical spine includes active, passive and resisted movements. Since the spinal joints are considered to be a potential focus for 'emotional' symptoms, six active movements are conducted assessing willingness to move, range of movement and pain. The capsular or non-capsular pattern may also emerge from these active movements.

In a non-capsular pattern of the cervical spine, some movements are limited and/or painful and others are full and painfree. The presence of a non-capsular pattern indicates a possible disc displacement.

Normally movements at the cervical spine do not occur in isolation, but the examination procedure is conducted simply by assessing the individual movements. It should, however, be remembered that flexion and extension occur with a component of translatory glide whilst side flexion and rotation occur as a coupled movement.

The passive movements are assessed to determine the true limitation of range of movement and the end-feel. The pattern of limited movements should be the same as that found on active movements. Normally passive extension has a 'hard' end-feel, passive rotations an 'elastic' end-feel and passive side flexions an 'elastic' end-feel due to tissue tension. Passive flexion is not assessed because it would tend to aggravate the symptoms of disc displacement.

The resisted tests are not part of the routine examination at the cervical spine, but should be applied if there is a history of trauma, e.g. for a muscle lesion or suspected serious pathology such as fracture, metastases or pyschogenic pain. The resisted tests also assess the C1 and 2 nerve roots. Resisted flexion may produce pain in a disc lesion since it causes compression.

The shoulder joint is eliminated as a cause of pain by active elevation. If this is of full range and painfree, the shoulder can be eliminated from the examination.

Assessment for objective root signs is conducted by a series of resisted tests for the myotomes, looking for a pattern of muscle weakness which would indicate nerve root compression. Since it is also important to eliminate other causes of arm pain, the muscle groups are also assessed, looking for alternative causes of pain. This explains why the sequence appears to test the same nerve roots several times.

A quick check of skin sensation to light touch is made looking for differences. Paraesthesia commonly affects the distal end of the dermatomes and these are assessed, followed by the biceps, brachioradialis and triceps reflexes.

The Babinski reflex, the extensor plantar response, is assessed by stroking up the lateral border of the sole of the foot and across the metatarsal heads. If the response is extensor, i.e. upgoing, it is indicative of an upper motor neurone lesion. The normal response is flexor.

The objective examination sequence provides a basic assessment framework to glean important information towards the selection of patients appropriate for the treatment techniques used in

---

Capsular pattern of the cervical spine:

- **Equal limitation of side flexions**
- **Equal limitation of rotations**
- **Some limitation of extension**
- **Usually full flexion**

orthopaedic medicine. It also highlights possible contraindications and provides a guide for the specific treatments to be used.

Any other assessment procedures may be superimposed throughout the sequence or explored separately afterwards, either to elicit extra information for the purposes of the application of other treatment modalities, or to confirm findings necessitating patient referral.

Before proceeding with any of the cervical manipulation techniques it is recommended that a vertebrobasilar artery test should be performed and this is discussed in the following section.

Vertebrobasilar artery testing

In recent years the potential risk to the cerebral blood flow from cervical manipulation techniques has received much publicity in relation to incidents and accidents following cervical manipulation (Krueger and Okazaki, 1980; Weinstein and Cantu, 1991; Sinel and Smith, 1993; Rivett, 1994; Carey, 1995; Sternbach *et al.*, 1995). It must be recognized that all techniques and the testing manoeuvres themselves carry a potential risk, as indeed does turning the head in normal everyday situations, e.g. reversing the car or painting the ceiling. Intubation and resuscitation manoeuvres (Thiel, 1991) and sleeping in a position which compromises the arteries may be the reason people develop strokes whilst unconscious or in their sleep.

To put things into perspective, it has been estimated, albeit with wide variation, that one serious incident of cerebrovascular complication occurs in one to three million manipulations performed (Kunnasmaa and Thiel, 1994; Rivett, 1994). The evidence on the mechanism of injury is somewhat contradictory and it is apparent that what happens to vertebral artery flow during head and neck movements is not fully understood (Kunnasmaa and Thiel, 1994). Most evidence is related to cadaver or animal studies.

The benefit gained in pain relief and restoration of movement by an expertly applied manipulative technique should not be sacrificed in an attempt to be too cautious. However, the risk, no matter how small, does exist and techniques involving traction and rotation have received criticism for being the most hazardous (Grant, 1988).

What is often not taken into account is that there are two potential danger areas within the cervical spine – the vertebral artery and the spinal cord. In attempting to reduce disc displacement, traction is applied to assist centralization and to prevent further displacement into the vertebral canal where the prolapse can endanger the spinal cord.

Before embarking on any cervical technique the clinician is recommended to follow guidelines for safe practice as suggested below. The guidelines have been devised to minimize the risk of complication following cervical mobilization techniques. Several points need to be considered before embarking on the testing regime.

Dizziness is one of the first symptoms of vertebrobasilar insufficiency, but it is also a symptom associated with cervical dysfunction, cervicogenic headaches, benign positional vertigo and inner ear problems. The vertebrobasilar artery system supplies the vestibular nuclei in the brainstem and the labyrinth of the inner ear (Grant, 1988). A careful history will assist diagnosis. If benign postural vertigo is suspected diagnosis can be confirmed by performing Hall–Pike positional testing which, if positive, demonstrates a characteristic torsional nystagmus when the head is reclined and turned to the affected side (Lempert *et al.*, 1995).

The testing procedures may be restricted by pain which will limit the extent to which the test can be applied. The recommended test simulates, as far as possible, the position for the treatment techniques. If pain limits the range of movement achievable for the test, the test should be repeated as an increase in range of movement is achieved by other forms of mobilization.

The test itself carries a certain amount of risk. Spontaneous vascular accidents do occur and the reported average age for complications from cervical manipulation is 38, young for acquired pathology and indicating a possible congenital abnormality (Kleynhans and Terret, 1985). The test is also of limited value and does not completely eliminate a patient from risk. The test should not be considered in isolation, but in the context of the whole assessment procedure.

Cervical traction is used as a technique by itself, or in conjunction with mobilization and manipulation. It is used to decompress the cervical joints, protecting the spinal cord from further posterior displacement of the disc during the technique. Traction is always used as a first manoeuvre; it is relatively gentle and can be stopped immediately if adverse effects are noted or reported. It often achieves an increase in range and decrease in pain, making the addition of further techniques unnecessary. Manipulation is only applied when a regime of manual traction and traction with mobilization has failed to be effective. By progressing the treatment in this way, adverse vertebrobasilar artery symptoms should be picked up before a manipulation is applied.

The vertebrobasilar artery test

Position the patient in supine lying with the shoulders level with the end of the couch. Support the head comfortably. Place the head into the position of extension, side flexion and rotation (Fig. 8.37). Keep the patient talking and the eyes open whilst maintaining the position for 30 s unless symptoms are evoked before this time. Allow the patient to rest in neutral before repeating the test to the other side.

The presence of dizziness, nausea, vomiting, sweating, pallor, blurred vision, dysarthria, fainting, tinnitus and paraesthesia in the head or arm constitutes a positive test.

The main symptoms and signs of a positive vertebrobasilar artery test can be remembered using the five Ds: dizziness, diplopia, drop attacks, dysarthria and dysphagia – a useful *aide-mémoire* attributed to Coman (Grant, 1988).

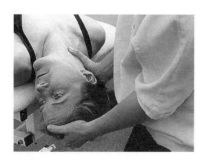

Fig. 8.37 Vertebrobasilar artery test.

If the test is found to be positive, slide the patient back on to the couch and leave them lying in supine to recover. Help the patient to sit up steadily and check by questioning and observation that the symptoms have subsided before terminating the session, or continuing with a suitable alternative treatment modality.

Following the recommended guidelines below ensures maximum safety and preparation for the unexpected. The practitioner must take all due care whilst applying the test and the treatment techniques.

Guidelines to minimize risk from cervical manipulation

Following the recommended guidelines below, ensures maximum safety and preparation for the unexpected. The practitioner must take all due care whilst applying the treatment techniques (see *Rules of Professional Conduct*, Rules 1, 2 and 4, and the *Standards of Physiotherapy Practice*, both available from the Chartered Society of Physiotherapy, 14 Bedford Road, London WC1R 4ED)

Ensure that:

A full history and examination have been completed and recorded, sufficient to establish indications and to exclude contraindications to treatment.

Specific questions have been asked relating to the following and the result recorded:

> drop attacks
> nausea, vomiting and generally feeling unwell
> dizziness or vertigo
> visual disturbances
> unsteadiness in gait or general feelings of weakness
> difficulty in speaking or swallowing
> past history of trauma
> cardiovascular disease
> anticoagulant therapy
> blood clotting disorders
> inflammatory arthritis.

From the examination, the following factors are present:

> a non capsular pattern of limited movement at the cervical spine
> a normal plantar response
> no increase in upper limb reflexes
> the recommended basilar artery test is negative, prior to cervical spine manipulation.

- If neurological signs are present, only one segment should be involved, manipulation is unlikely to succeed, but other modalities may be more effective, e.g. traction and mobilization

- Manual traction is applied as the first manoeuvre.

- You have provided sufficient information, including possible risks and advice, if manipulation is indicated, so that the patient can give informed consent. You must respect the right of the patient to refuse manipulation.

- You re-examine the patient after the application of each technique and that decisions to continue are based on the results of the previous technique.

- Any significant adverse response to treatment is reported immediately to the patient's doctor.

The following list of contraindications provides a checklist for the conditions discussed in the preceding sections of this chapter.

Absolute contraindications to cervical mobilization techniques

- Drop attacks.
- Dizziness associated with vertebrobasilar insufficiency.
- Positive vertebrobasilar artery test.
- Inflammatory arthritis – rheumatoid.
- Upper motor neuron lesion, e.g. past CVA or TIA.
- Cervical pain due to non-mechanical lesions, i.e. suspicious features, including:
  - Arm pain under age 35.
  - Pain not affected by posture and activity.
  - Side flexion away from the pain is the only painful movement.
  - Double root palsy.
  - T1 weakness.
  - Gradual onset over more than 3 months.
  - Past history of tumour of breast, prostate or bronchus.
- Anticoagulation medication and long-term steroids.
- Patients with blood-clotting disorders.

The clinical models below summarize the different presentations of disc displacement in the cervical spine and act as a guide for their diagnosis and treatment. All have a non-capsular pattern of pain and/or limitation of movement.

Cervical disc lesions – the three clinical models

1. *Cervical nuclear disc displacement – acute torticollis*

History:

- adolescent or young adult
- short central or unilateral pain
- patient wakes with severe pain.

Examination:

- antalgic posture
- non-capsular pattern
- *no* neurological signs.

The hypothesis is that a gradual displacement of nuclear material has occurred, often over night. As has already been discussed earlier in the chapter, the nucleus in the cervical spine is small and exists as true nuclear material for a relatively short time. Therefore this presentation is typical in children, adolescents and the young adult. The condition usually resolves spontaneously in 7–10 days.

Treatment consists of reassurance to both the patient and parents and progressive positioning out of the deformity may expedite reduction. Pain relieving modalities may be applied, e.g. analgesics, electrotherapy, massage and gentle mobilization.

2. *Cervical annular disc displacement*

History:

- short central or unilateral neck or scapular pain
- gradual or sudden onset
- patient may or may not recall the exact mode and time of onset.

Examination:

- non-capsular pattern
- *no* neurological signs.

The hypothesis is that since the nucleus degenerates early in the cervical spine, degenerate nuclear material may prolapse into the weakened outer annulus causing primary disc pain, or prolapsed disc material may produce secondary pain through compression of other pain sensitive structures in the vertebral canal. Pain may be extrasegmental and/or segmental in distribution. Since the vertebral canal in the cervical spine is relatively large, it may accommodate disc prolapse more readily and dural pressure may be unilateral, accounting for the unilateral neck and/or scapular pain which is typical of this presentation.

Treatment of choice is to follow the cervical mobilization routine described below, providing no contraindications to treatment exist.

3. *Cervical disc displacement – large posterolateral prolapse*

History:

- patient usually over the age of 35
- central or unilateral neck and/or scapular pain, followed by referred arm pain (the central pain ceasing or diminishing)
- sudden or gradual onset
- often part of a history of increasing, worsening episodes, therefore a progression of the above scenarios
- patient may or may not recall the exact time and mode of onset
- patient may complain of root symptoms, i.e. parasthesia felt at the distal end of the dermatome.

Examination:

- non-capsular pattern
- root signs may be present, i.e. muscle weakness, absent or reduced reflexes.

The hypothesis is that a large posterolateral prolapse of disc material has occurred, producing pain referred into the arm through compression of the dural nerve root sleeve or the nerve root itself. Pain, therefore, is segmental in distribution. If the nerve root is involved, there will be objective neurological signs. Since the nerve roots emerge horizontally in the cervical spine, only one nerve root should be involved in disc lesions. The quality of the pain helps to distinguish somatic and radicular pain (see Chapter 13).

Treatment is aimed at relieving pain. If neurological signs are present, manipulation is unlikely to succeed, but other modalities may be effective, e.g. traction and mobilization. Since the natural history of disc displacement is one of recovery, a mechanism of spontaneous recovery may occur (see Chapter 13).

Treatment of cervical disc lesions

It is recommended that a course in orthopaedic medicine is attended before the treatment techniques described later in the chapter are applied in clinical practice (see Appendix).

Treatment of cervical disc lesions depends on the nature of the pain. If the pain is subacute and the symptoms not particularly irritable, a regime of mobilization can be commenced, progressing to manipulation if necessary. If the pain is acute and the symptoms highly irritable, a gentler approach to treatment is adopted. In chronic cervical conditions, a thorough examination may reveal several components to the diagnosis, pathoneurodynamics and muscle imbalance for example, together with underlying psychological factors such as anxiety and depression. All components of the patient's condition must be addressed and the orthopaedic medicine approach and treatment techniques should form only part of the treatment programme. Their use is not intended to be exclusive.

In terms of likely response to manipulation, the ideal patient will fit into the pattern of signs and symptoms that indicate clinical model 2: a central or unilateral annular displacement of the disc.

The patient with a central or unilateral annular disc displacement into the vertebral canal has a history of sudden or gradual onset of central or unilateral neck or scapular pain. On examination there is a non-capsular pattern of limited movement and no objective neurological signs. To be ideal in terms of likely effectiveness of treatment, the symptoms should be of recent onset and have minimum reference of pain. The more peripheral the symptoms, the less successful the techniques described tend to be.

Provided there are no contraindications to treatment, a regime of cervical mobilization is commenced. Treatment techniques are chosen based on a continuous assessment approach. After every technique the patient's comparable signs are reassessed.

Following each session of treatment, advice is given about neck care, general posture, sleeping postures and pillows. Maintenance exercises are given if they are appropriate and the patient is started on a self-help programme to prevent recurrence.

Mobilization and manipulation techniques in orthopaedic medicine usually produce immediate results. One, two or three sessions of treatment would be expected. If a patient is not responding to the approach, it is abandoned and other mobilization and treatment modalities attempted.

The cervical mobilization procedure

It is important to emphasize that the treatment techniques in this section will be described carefully in a step-by-step fashion to enable their application. However, the professional judgement and existing skill of the operator will allow each technique to be adapted.

The order of the techniques as they appear here merely provides a guide towards the development of skills at each stage and it is not necessarily an order of efficacy. It is important to reassess constantly the patient's comparable signs and to decide on the next step in the light of patient response. In this way the orthopaedic medicine approach can properly be integrated into existing practice as fresh decisions are made and the underlying hypothesis is modified.

Manipulation as such, defined as a minimal-amplitude high-velocity thrust at the end of range, is only carried out if judgement deems it necessary. The mobilization procedure suggested is usually sufficient to reduce most uncomplicated cervical disc displacements, i.e. with no neurological signs or symptoms.

The enormous benefit of this cervical mobilization procedure outweighs the small risk of vertebrobasilar complications but that is not to take the risk lightly. The appropriate steps to minimize this risk, suggested in the guidelines above, should always be taken. The techniques involve traction, slight extension of the head and sometimes rotation and these are the positions which may compromise the vertebral arteries. However, it should be emphasized that the other area of danger in this region is the spinal cord, and these same positions assist centralization of the displaced disc material and aim to prevent further central displacement that could potentially endanger the cord.

It is not possible to say how many times each technique is to be attempted since the process of reassessment is the basis for each clinical decision and the circumstances vary in every clinical encounter. None the less, a balance must be found between side-stepping the question and providing a recipe for treatment. Some guidance will be given in terms of expectations, with respect to the different states and stages of the conditions presented.

Generally, the more acutely painful lesions require gentle treatment on a daily basis. For the subacute or less irritable states, if the technique is helping it is repeated; if no change occurs after a few attempts the next technique is chosen; if the patient's signs and symptoms are abolished, treatment should be stopped. Once improvement plateaus in each session, or if the progress is uncertain, the treatment is either modified to an alternative modality or ceases, with the patient being reassessed at the next session when a new status quo will have emerged.

Bridging technique

The indication for use is an acutely painful situation, either a whiplash injury or an acute torticollis. It is a method of applying gentle traction and should not produce pain.

Position the patient supine on the couch a little way down from the top edge. Sit on a chair at the head of the couch and gently adjust the patient's position so that your forearms and elbows are fully supported, with your hands resting under the patient's neck (Fig. 8.38). Make a bridge with the fingers and rest them under the occiput. Tilt the hands into radial deviation, which tips the head slightly back, and pull, flexing your forearms, to apply minimal traction. Hold the pull for a few seconds, or less if the patient is uncomfortable. Gently release and repeat as required, gradually applying more traction as the tissues relax.

Manual traction (Cyriax, 1984)

This is always the first technique to be performed for the less irritable or subacute neck. It is generally comfortable for the patient and allows both you and the patient to become used to the handling techniques. It is often not necessary to progress beyond this stage if positive results are achieved. After each technique an increase in range and/or decrease in pain is to be expected.

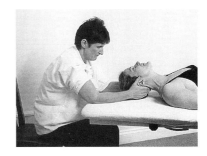

Fig. 8.38 Bridging technique.

Explain the technique and its intention to the patient. All mobilization techniques are carefully monitored by the operator for a change in symptoms. Patients are instructed to signal if they wish the manoeuvre to cease for any reason. It is important that patients appreciate that they have control over each manoeuvre – the final overpressure of the Grade C manipulation is the only exception to this – which is why feedback on discomfort should be obtained from the patient right up to the moment of its application.

Raise the couch to the level of your hips. Position the patient in supine, support their head in your hands and have the patient's shoulders level with the head of the couch. An assistant is needed to apply counterpressure at the same time as you apply the manual traction by restraining the movement of the patient's shoulders, adopting a walk-standing position at the side of the couch. If no assistant is available, restraining Cyriax 'horns' or non-slip matting may be used.

Position one of your hands to cup the occiput or support just below the occiput, allowing the head either to rest in neutral or to fall into slight extension. The other hand rests comfortably around the patient's chin, avoiding the trachea, and your forearm lies along the side of the face.

Place both feet directly under the patient's head and bend both your knees. Lean out with straight arms to apply the traction using body weight (Fig. 8.39). Perform the technique slowly, allowing the traction to establish for several seconds, then pull yourself back to the upright position and release the traction.

Sit the patient up slowly and re-examine the comparable signs, before deciding on the next manoeuvre.

Assess the patient's body weight compared with your own. If you are much heavier than the patient do not apply maximum body weight. Less body weight can be achieved by positioning the feet a little further back but the arms should still be straightened.

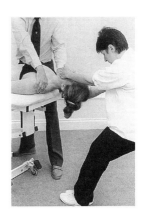

Fig. 8.39 Manual traction.

A patient with dentures should leave them *in situ* with some padding placed between the teeth to help prevent discomfort and perhaps breakage.

This technique of manual traction is essential to most other manoeuvres and it is worthwhile practising it to gain confidence and competence.

Manual traction plus rotation (Cyriax and Cyriax, 1983; Cyriax, 1984)

The painfree rotation is chosen first as this will be more comfortable for the patient. The hand holds are the same as above, with a left rotation requiring your left hand to be positioned around the chin (Fig. 8.40) and vice versa for a right rotation.

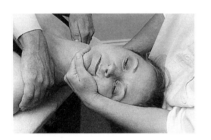

Fig. 8.40 Hand positioning for manual traction plus rotation to the left.

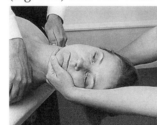

Fig. 8.41 Manual traction plus rotation, Grade A.

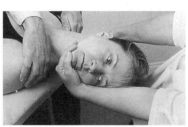

Fig. 8.42 Manual traction plus rotation, Grade B, and position at which a Grade C manipulation is applied.

Apply the traction as above. Allow it to establish for a few seconds, then rotate into the least painful rotation by side-flexing your body. Return to the mid-position and release the traction as above. Three variations of this technique can be applied, and each is a progression of the other.

- *Grade A*: mid-range rotation (Fig. 8.41).
- *Grade B*: to end of available range (Fig. 8.42). Here it is so important to understand the nature of end-feel and to be sensitive to any abnormal end-feel such as muscle spasm, which suggests the technique should be abandoned.
- *Grade C*: manipulation, the final high-velocity, minimal-amplitude thrust is applied at end of range.

If these three stages have proved unsuccessful, the procedure is now repeated using the same routine into the painful range of rotation. Under traction, this should not produce an increase in symptoms and any increase is an indication to stop. Again, progression is only made to the next step if necessary.

Antero-posterior glide under traction (Cyriax and Cyriax, 1983; Cyriax, 1984)

This technique is applied if the symptoms have centralized and the range of movement has increased, but extension remains slightly limited. The importance of fully reducing a disc displacement is based on the hypothesis that a small central bulge, if left *in situ*, will gradually cause ligamentous traction and osteophyte formation, both of which have the potential to threaten the cord in later life. Therefore extension should always be cleared.

Position the couch a little lower than for the above manoeuvres. Position the patient supine on the couch as before, with an assistant ready to apply counterpressure. Stand sideways-on to the patient with both feet parallel and close to the couch, under the patient's head. One hand cups below the occiput and the forearm supports the weight of the head whilst cradling it against your abdomen. The other hand is positioned on the chin to be able to apply both traction and retraction (Fig. 8.43). Make a bridge by spreading your index finger and thumb. Apply the web to the chin and curl the remaining fingers so that they tuck around and under the chin.

Lean out sideways as far as possible to apply traction. Once traction is established, bend your knees and apply pressure over the chin, taking the chin into maximum retraction avoiding pressure from the knuckles against the larynx. Release the pressure, allowing the chin to return to neutral, avoiding protraction. Sit the patient up and reassess. If the manoeuvre has helped it can be repeated, this time using several retractions.

Lateral glide

This manoeuvre is used to relieve post-treatment soreness and to mobilize any residual tightness in the neck.

The couch is again slightly lower than hip height, as for the position for the antero-posterior glide under traction technique. No traction is applied with this manoeuvre. The assistant stands parallel to the couch and the patient lies supine as above, but close to the assistant. The assistant grasps the patient's opposite arm with both hands and holds the patient close to prevent lateral movement of the thorax (Fig. 8.44).

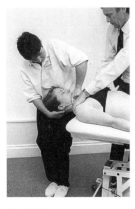
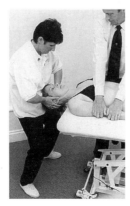

Fig. 8.43 Antero-posterior glide under traction.

Fig. 8.44 Lateral glide.

Cup the patient's head in both hands, fingers around the occiput and thumbs parallel with the mandible. Your thenar eminences should support just in front of the ears. Bend your knees and position your abdomen against the patient's head but not enough to compress it. Apply the glide by rocking from foot to foot, gradually increasing the pressure of your thenar eminences against the patient's head as the patient relaxes and more movement becomes available. To ensure that this is a rhythmical lateral gliding movement without side flexion, keep the patient's nose straight and apply gentle pressure to the chin as you move towards each side. A slight upward movement of the patient's head may occur as your weight moves from each leg.

Advanced manoeuvres

These are stronger manoeuvres and it is definitely recommended that they should not be applied without attending an orthopaedic medicine course.

> ### Traction with leverage (Cyriax and Cyriax, 1983; Cyiax, 1984)

The indication for this technique is that stronger traction is required for central or bilateral symptoms.

Position the patient in supine lying with the occiput level with the end of the couch. Cup the occiput and rest the back of your hand on the couch. Apply manual traction as described previously. At the end of the technique bend your knees smartly to apply a little more traction, using your underhand as a pivot (Fig. 8.45). Maintain the traction as you straighten your knees, having applied the technique for a few seconds.

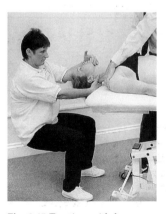

Fig. 8.45 Traction with leverage.

Manual traction plus rotation

This is the same technique as the rotation technique described previously, but it applies a different hand hold with the neck starting in a degree of rotation, which gives a stronger rotation overall.

Rotate the patient's head before applying the technique. Cup your hand, pronate your forearm and place it comfortably on the side of the patient's face with the hand on the chin, such that the fingers face the direction of the rotation you are aiming towards (Fig. 8.46). Stand with your feet rotated a little in that same direction. Conduct the rest of the technique as described previously.

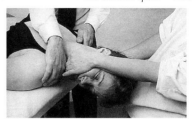

Fig. 8.46 Manual traction plus rotation. The alternative hand position produces stronger rotation.

Manual traction plus side flexion (Cyriax and Cyriax, 1983; Cyriax, 1984)

If the rotations have not cleared the symptoms, a side-flexion technique can be applied.

Always start by side-flexing the patient away from the painful side.

Position the patient as for manual traction. An assistant stands on the side to which the neck will be side-flexed and moves the patient a little closer so that the patient's shoulder fits into the corner of the couch. The assistant then reaches over to place a hand over the patient's opposite shoulder to fix it by holding on to the top edge of the couch, so resisting the side flexion movement.

If you will be moving towards the right, place your right foot against the side of the couch, or against the assistant's extended left foot. Lean out sideways to give traction, taking your left leg off the floor (Fig. 8.47). After a short pause to allow the traction to take effect, swing your body backwards, pivoting on your right foot and applying side flexion to the patient's neck. Maintaining control, apply a smart thrust at the end of range and maintain traction as you swing your body back to the straight pull position, when you can steadily put your left foot to the floor and release the traction.

As you practise this technique you will find that the momentum of the movement will help achieve a smooth transition through the various stages.

Reverse the assistant's position and the instructions if side flexion towards the left side is indicated.

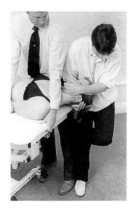

Fig. 8.47 Manual traction plus side flexion.

Cervical traction

Cyriax did not advocate the use of cervical traction to the same extent as lumbar and was of the opinion that it was used 'far too often' (Cyriax, 1982). He acknowledged that the principal indication for cervical traction was the presence of a nuclear disc displacement, particularly with brachial pain and neurological signs. Yates (1972) suggested that it also had a place in the treatment of degenerative spondylosis of the cervical spine.

Hickling (1972) described the application of sustained cervical traction in either sitting (cervical suspension) or lying and various studies have been published to explore the merits or disadvantages of each. Cervical suspension, the application of vertical traction with the patient sitting, appeared to be the choice of Cyriax, although from the authors' experience whilst training at St Thomas' Hospital, where Cyriax's ideas underpinned treatment techniques, traction in inclined supine lying (long traction) was used more frequently. Colachis and Strohm (1965) quoted the paper of Gartland which mentioned Krusen's list of advantages of cervical suspension over long or horizontal traction:

- Convenience of application.
- Elimination of friction.
- Accuracy of measurement.
- Facilitation of manipulation.

Stoddard (1954) was critical of cervical suspension since he observed that his patients found it difficult to relax in this position. He also believed that sustained traction impaired blood flow and favoured intermittent traction. Deets *et al.* (1977) mention that Maitland had the opposite view and preferred traction in sitting since his patients found it more comfortable. They also report that Crue found that greater foraminal separation was observed in the supine position than in sitting.

The findings of Colachis and Strohm (1965) in a study of 10 normal medical students found that the separation of the cervical vertebrae under traction increased with the angle of flexion to the horizontal of the rope applying the pull. They found that the poundage applied had a comparatively greater effect on the joint separation and the maximum of 30 lb (14 kg) used in their investigation had the greatest effect. Judovitch (1952) studied radiographs of the cervical spine under different poundages of traction and found that 25 lb (11 kg) of vertical traction straightened the cervical lordosis, whilst at 45 lb (20.5 kg) a mean stretch of 5 mm was achieved in the cervical spine.

Deets *et al.* (1977) cite a further study of Colachis and Strohm which demonstrated that the greatest elongation of the posterior portion of the disc was observed with the angle of rope pull at 35° to the horizontal.

Hickling (1972) recounted Cyriax's suggestion that cervical suspension should be just sufficient to lift the patient's buttocks from the chair, implying that forces of near body weight were being applied. However, this was for a short duration of 1–5 min. In lying, average treatments ranged from 15 to 25 lb (7–11 kg), according to the size and overall response of the patient. The traction was applied horizontally or in slight flexion at an unspecified angle but with consideration for patient comfort and preference.

Readers must weigh up for themselves the pros and cons of applying traction in the sitting versus supine position. The characteristics of the individual patients encountered will form part of the decision-making process.

Another factor in the application of cervical traction is the length of time for which it should be applied. Colachis and Strohm (1965) noted that no further increase of intervertebral separation occurred after 7 s of sustained traction and Judovitch (1952) stated that the time of application should be decreased as greater forces were applied. Hickling (1972) suggested that traction of 15–25 lb (7–11 kg) should be continued for between 15 and 25 min. This recommendation is based on empirical findings and more work needs to be done to establish the optimum duration of treatment.

Contraindications to cervical traction

These are largely the same as for cervical manipulation:

- Traction should not be applied in the presence of inflammatory joint disease such as rheumatoid arthritis, ankylosing spondylitis and psoriatic arthritis, often indicated by the report of long-term steroid therapy. The pain is likely to become worse and there is a danger of atlantoaxial subluxation which would endanger the spinal cord (Yates, 1972).
- The hyperacute or irritable neck is likely to be made worse by traction.
- Drop attacks or signs of vertebrobasilar artery insufficiency are an absolute contraindication to cervical traction.
- Upper motor neuron lesions, such as strokes or transient ischaemic attacks, are not suitable as circulatory abnormalities are implied.
- Anticoagulants or blood-clotting disorders are contraindicated since microtrauma might occur to the capillaries and a prolonged bleeding time could lead to the formation of extradural haematoma.

Care should be taken in applying traction to the elderly and they must be thoroughly questioned for the presence of any contraindications.

Most traction beds or mobile traction equipment of modern design have the facility to apply cervical and lumbar traction.

A cervical harness is required to rest under the occiput and chin, with straps or cord passing to a spreader bar above the head. There are several types of harness which these days are made of washable materials, which also have the advantage of being pliable to give comfortable support. The simplest uses two padded rectangles which mould to the head as the traction is applied but others are made of more substantial materials and have adjustable clasps to accommodate the differing shapes of patients.

The straps to the spreader bar should be long enough to give safe clearance above the head. A rope passes from the central point of the spreader bar via a pulley or pulleys to a fixing cleat in manually applied units, or directly into the housing of the automatic device.

Technique

Explain the technique carefully to the patient, mentioning possible after-effects such as stiffness or temporary increase in discomfort, and ask for consent to proceed.

If applying traction in the sitting position, use a firm chair with comfortable back support. Patients often like to have their arms resting on two or three pillows on their lap to support the arms and to encourage relaxation.

Put the cervical harness in place under the jaw and occiput, providing extra padding if necessary, and place tissue between the patient and the harness, for reasons of hygiene. Attach the harness to the traction unit and place on the appropriate setting, considering the patient's size and general demeanour.

Discuss the treatment time with patients, explaining that the treatment aims to be as 'long and strong' as is comfortable but they can call a halt to the treatment at any time. In practice, patients are usually comfortable with about 15 min' traction at the first treatment and even on subsequent attendances 20 min usually is the maximum required.

Give patients sight of a clock and an alarm bell or buzzer and apply the traction steadily. Keep in close contact with the patient whilst the traction is being applied, since occasionally they can become light-headed.

At the end of the treatment time release the traction slowly and observe the patients' response as you do so. Let them sit for a moment or two whilst they roll their shoulders and relax their tissues and allow them to get up when they feel ready.

If applying traction in supine ensure that the patient is comfortable with one or two pillows under the head and knees as desired. Apply the cervical harness in the same way as for sitting traction. Adjust the angle of pull and select the appropriate setting. Feedback from the patient will ensure that the traction is strong and comfortable. There is a convention that lesser weights are applied in traction in supine than in the sitting position, but for a longer time (Hickling, 1972) On this basis, weights of 5–7 kg might be applied on the first treatment for 20 min, for example, increasing to 10 kg for 25–30 min at subsequent attendances.

Traction should be applied, preferably on a daily basis, but weekends can be excluded, to allow any soft-tissue discomfort from the application of the harness to subside. Patients may not be able to attend daily due to time or financial constraints and the pressures on outpatient departments may also deny this frequency. However, it is still appropriate to try the technique as frequently as possible, since satisfactory results may still be achieved.

Improvement usually occurs after two to four treatments and the whole treatment episode may be continued over a 2- or 3-week period if necessary. If there is no change in the symptoms after four treatments the position, the weight, angle of pull or the time of application may be adjusted, but if there is still no change, the technique should be abandoned and another modality or course of action selected.

Advice on neck care and posture should be given to patients whilst they are undergoing treatment and an appropriate gentle exercise programme should be devised.

References

Aprill, C., Dwyer, A., Bogduk, N. (1989) Cervical zygapophyseal joint pain patterns II: a clinical evaluation. *Spine* **15**: 458–461.

Beeton, K., Jull, G. (1994) Effectiveness of manipulative physiotherapy in the management of cervicogenic headache: a single case study. *Physiotherapy* **80**: 417–423.

Bird, H.A. (1995) Work related syndromes. In: *Collected Reports on the Rheumatic Diseases*. Arthritis and Rheumatism Council for Research, pp. 162–164.

Bogduk, N. (1986) The anatomy and pathophysiology of whiplash. *Clinical Biomechanics* **1**: 92–101.

Bogduk, N. (1992) The anatomical basis for cervicogenic headache. *Journal of Manipulative and Physiological Therapeutics* **15**: 67–70.

Bogduk, N. (1994) Innervation and pain patterns of the cervical spine. In: *Physical Therapy of the Cervical and Thoracic Spine*, 2nd edn. (Grant, R. ed.). Churchill Livingstone, pp. 65–76.

Bogduk, N., Twomey L.T. (1991) *Clinical Anatomy of the Lumbar Spine*, 2nd edn. Churchill Livingstone.

Brown, B. St J., Tatlow, W.F.T. (1963) Radiographic studies of the vertebral arteries in cadavers – effects of position and traction on the head. *Radiology* **81**: 80–88.

Carey, P.F. (1995) Suggested protocol for the examination and treatment of the cervical spine – managing the risk. *Journal of the Canadian Chiropractic Association* **39**: 35–40.

Clark, C. (1994) Rheumatoid involvement of the cervical spine. *Spine* **19**: 2257–2258.

Colachis, S.C., Strohm, B.R. (1965) A study of tractive forces and angle of pull on vertebral interspaces in the cervical spine. *Archives of Physical Medicine and Rheumatology* **46**: 820–830.

Connell, M.D., Wiesel, S.W. (1992) Natural history and pathogenesis of cervical disc disease. *Orthopedic Clinics of North America* **23**: 369–380.

Cyriax, J. (1982) *Textbook of Orthopaedic Medicine*, vol. 1, 8th edn. Baillière Tindall.

Cyriax, J. (1984) *Textbook of Orthopaedic Medicine*, vol. 2, 11th edn. Baillière Tindall.

Cyriax, J., Cyriax, P. (1983) *Illustrated Manual of Orthopaedic Medicine*. Butterworths.

Deets, D., Hands, K.L., Hopp, S.S. (1977) Cervical traction. *Physical Therapy* **57**: 255–261.

Department of Health (1995) *Cervical Spine Instability in People with Down Syndrome*. Chief Medical Officer's Update, 7. HMSO.

Doherty, M. (1995) Fibromyalgia syndrome. In: *Collected Reports on the Rheumatic Diseases*. Arthritis and Rheumatism Council for Research, pp. 83–86.

Frumkin, L.R., Baloh, R.W. (1990) Wallenberg's syndrome following neck manipulation. *Neurology* **40**: 611–615.

Grant, R. (1988) Dizziness testing and manipulation of the cervical spine. In: *Physical Therapy of the Cervical and Thoracic Spines* (Grant, R. ed.). Churchill Livingstone, pp. 111–124.

Hazelman, B.L. (1995) Polymyalgia rheumatica and giant cell arteritis. In: *Collected Reports on the Rheumatic Diseases* (Lewin, I.G., Seymour, C.A. eds). Arthritis and Rheumatism Council for Research, pp. 97–100.

Herrick, A.L. (1995) Reflex sympathetic dystrophy. In: *Collected Reports on the Rheumatic Diseases* (Lewin, I.G., Seymour, C.A. eds). Arthritis and Rheumatism Council for Research, pp. 132–137.

Hickling, J. (1972) Spinal traction technique. *Physiotherapy* **58**: 58–63.

Hinton, M.A., Harris, M.B., King, A.G. (1993) Cervical spondylolysis. *Spine* **18**: 1369–1372.

Jenkins, D.G. (1979) Clinical features of arm and neck pain. *Physiotherapy* **65**: 102–105.

Judovitch, B. (1952) Herniated cervical disc. *American Journal of Surgery* **84**: 646–650.

Jull, G.A. (1994a) Headaches of cervical origin. In: *Physical Therapy of the Cervical and Thoracic Spine*, 2nd edn (Grant, R. ed.). Churchill Livingstone, pp. 261–285.

Jull, G. (1994b) Cervical headache – a review. In: *Grieve's Modern Manual Therapy*, 2nd edn (Boyling, J.D., Palastanga, N. eds). Churchill Livingstone, pp. 333–347.

Kang, J.D., Georgescu, H.I., McIntrye-Larkin, L. *et al.* (1995) Herniated cervical intervertebral discs spontaneously produce matrix metalloproteinases, nitric oxide, interleukin-6, and prostaglandin E2. *Spine* **20**: 2373–2378.

Kleynhans, A.M., Terrett, A.G.J. (1985) The prevention of complications from spinal manipulative therapy. In: *Aspects of Manipulative Therapy* (Glasgow, E.F., Twomey, L.T., Scull, E.R., Kleynhans, A.M. eds). pp. 161–175.

Kokubun, S., Sakurai, M., Tanaka, Y. (1996) Cartilaginous endplate in cervical disc herniation. *Spine* **21**: 190–195.

Krueger, B.R., Okazaki, H. (1980) Vertebral-basilar distribution infarction following chiropractic cervical manipulation. *Mayo Clinic Proceedings* **55**: 322–331.

Kumar, P., Clark, M. (1994) In: *Clinical Medicine*, 3rd edn. Baillière Tindall.

Kunnasmaa, K.T.T., Thiel, H.W. (1994) Vertebral artery syndrome — a review of the literature. *Journal of Orthopaedic Medicine* **16**: 17–20.

Lempert, T., Gresty, M.A., Bronstein, A.M. (1995) Benign positional vertigo – recognition and treatment. *British Medical Journal* **311**: 489–491.

McKinney, L.A. (1989) Early mobilisation and outcome in acute sprains of the neck. *British Medical Journal* **299**: 1006–1008.

Mathews, J.A. (1995) Acute neck pain – differential diagnosis and management. In: *Collected Reports on the Rheumatic Diseases*. Arthritis and Rheumatism Council for Research, pp. 142–144.

Matsuda, Y., Sano, N., Watanabe, S. *et al.* (1995) Atlanto-occipital hypermobility in subjects with Down's syndrome. *Spine* **20**: 2283–2286.

Mealy, K., Brennan, H., Fenelon, G.C.C. (1986) Early mobilisation of acute whiplash injuries. *British Medical Journal* **292**: 656–657.

Mendel, T., Wink, C.S., Zimny, M. (1992) Neural elements in human cervical intervertebral discs. *Spine* **17**: 132–135.

Mitchell, J., McKay, A. (1995) Comparison of left and right vertebral artery intracranial diameters. *Anatomical Record* **242**: 350–354.

Mooney, V., Robertson, J. (1976) The facet syndrome. *Clinical Orthopaedics and Related Research* **115**: 149–156.

Netter, F.H. (1987) Musculoskeletal system part I. In: *The Ciba Collection of Medical Illustrations*, vol. 8. Ciba-Giegy.

Nilsson, N. (1995) The prevalence of cervicogenic headache in a random population sample of 20–59 year olds. *Spine* **20**: 1884–1888.

Nordin, M., Frankel, V.H. (1989) *Basic Biomechanics of the Musculoskeletal System*, 2nd edn. Lea & Faber.

Oliver, J., Middleditch, A. (1991) *Functional Anatomy of the Spine*. Butterworth-Heinemann.

Palastanga, N., Field, D., Soames, R. (1994) *Anatomy and Human Movement*. Butterworth-Heinemann.

Pizzutillo, P.D., Woods, M., Nicholson, L., MacEwen, G.D. (1994) Risk factors in Klippel–Feil syndrome. *Spine* **19**: 2110–2116.

Pueschel, S.M., Moon, A.C., Scola, F.H. (1992) Computerised tomography in persons with Down syndrome and atlantoaxial instability. *Spine* **17**: 735–737.

Rivett, H.M. (1994) Cervical manipulation: confronting the spectre of the vertebral artery syndrome. *Journal of Orthopaedic Medicine* **16**: 12–16.

Schoensee, S.K., Jensen, G., Nicholson, G. *et al.* (1995) The effect of mobilisation on cervical headaches. *Journal of Orthopaedic and Sports Physical Therapy* **21**: 184–196.

Schwarzer, A.C., Aprill, C.N., Derby, R. *et al.* (1994) Clinical features of patients with pain stemming from the lumbar zygapophysial joints. *Spine* **19**: 1132–1137.

Sinel, M., Smith, D. (1993) Thalamic infarction secondary to cervical manipulation. *Archives of Physical Medicine and Rehabilitation* **74**: 543–546.

Sjaastad, O. (1992) Cervicogenic headache – the controversial headache. *Clinical Neurology and Neurosurgery* **94** (suppl): 147S–149S.

Sternbach, G., Cohen, M., Goldschmid, D. (1995) Vertebral artery injury presenting with signs of middle cerebral artery occlusion. *Journal of Vascular Disease* **46**: 843–846.

Stoddard, A. (1954) Traction for cervical nerve root irritation. *Physiotherapy* **40**: 48–49.

Taylor, J.R., Twomey, L.T. (1993) Acute injuries to cervical joints: an autopsy study of neck sprain. *Spine* **18**: 1115–1122.

Taylor, J.R., Twomey, L.T. (1994) Functional and applied anatomy of the cervical spine. In: *Clinics in Physical Therapy of the Cervical and Thoracic Spine*, 2nd edn (Grant, R. ed.). Churchill Livingstone, pp. 1–25.

Thiel, H.W. (1991) Gross morphology and pathoanatomy of the vertebral arteries. *Journal of Manipulative Physiological Therapeutics* **14**: 133–141.

Toole, J.F., Tucker, S.H. (1960) Influence of head position on cerebral circulation. *Archives of Neurology* **2**: 616–622.

Walker, D.J. (1995) Rheumatoid arthritis. In: *Collected Reports on the Rheumatic Diseases*. Arthritis and Rheumatism Council for Research, pp. 39–44.

Walsh, M.T. (1994) Therapist management of thoracic outlet syndrome. *Journal of Hand Therapy* **Apr/May**: 131–144.

Weinstein, S.M., Cantu, R.C. (1991) Cerebral stroke in a semi-pro football player – a case report. *Medicine and Science in Sports and Exercise* **22**: 1119–1121.

Williams, P.L., Warwick, R., Dyson, M., Bannister, L.H. (1989) *Gray's Anatomy*, 37th edn. Churchill Livingstone.

Yates, D.A.H. (1972) Indications and contra-indications for spinal traction. *Physiotherapy* **58**: 55–57.

Zeidman, S.M., Ducker, T.B. (1994) Rheumatoid arthritis: neuroanatomy, compression, and grading of deficits. *Spine* **19**: 2259–2266.

9 The thoracic spine

Summary

Thoracic pain is commonly encountered and provides a challenge in diagnosis, since referred pain from visceral problems can mimic pain of somatic origin, and vice versa. Disc lesions are a comparatively rare cause of thoracic pain, probably due to the supportive nature of this relatively stiff area brought about by the sternal and vertebral articulations of the ribs.

This chapter sets out to explain the anatomy of the thoracic spine and highlights the somatic structures which are a common cause of pain. Pain patterns are discussed and the non-mechanical causes of thoracic back pain are presented to aid diagnosis and appropriate management.

The clinical examination procedure is outlined and interpreted, the contraindications are emphasized and the treatments used in orthopaedic medicine are described, with notes on the indications for their use.

Anatomy

There are 12 thoracic vertebrae which gradually increase in size from above down, marking a transition between cervical and lumbar vertebrae. A typical thoracic vertebra is easily recognized by its costal facets, its heart-shaped superior surface and waisted vertebral body (Fig. 9.1). The *vertebral canal* in the thoracic region is round

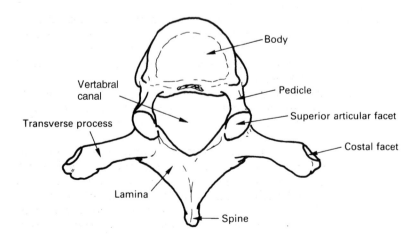

Fig. 9.1 Typical thoracic vertebra. From Palastanga *et al.* (1994) with permission.

and smaller than that found in either the cervical or lumbar spine. Short *pedicles* pass almost directly backwards and thick, broad *laminae* overlap each other from above down.

The slope of the long *spinous processes* gradually increases downwards with the fifth to eighth spinous processes overlapping each other. The eighth spinous process is the longest, whilst the 12th is shorter, horizontal and similar to the lumbar spinous processes.

Long, rounded, club-like *transverse processes* are directed posterolaterally and slightly superiorly. Except for the 11th and 12th vertebrae, oval, anterior facets lie at the tips of all transverse processes. These facets articulate with the tubercles of the corresponding ribs.

Flat *articular processes* project superiorly and inferiorly to form the thoracic zygapophyseal joints. Their direction facilitates the movement of rotation, that is coupled with side flexion, whilst also permitting a range of flexion and extension. Rotation is a particular feature of the thoracic spine and is facilitated by the direction of the articular facets and rotation or twisting of the fibres in the intervertebral discs. The shearing movement common to lumbar discs does not occur so readily in the thoracic spine (Kapandji, 1974). The orientation of the articular facets changes at T11, marking a change from the rotational segment above and the non-rotational segment of the lumbar spine below.

The thoracic *intervertebral joints* consist of the vertebral body above and below and the *intervertebral disc*. These joints are supported by anterior and posterior longitudinal ligaments, supraspinous, interspinous and intertransverse ligaments and the ligamentum flavum that connects adjacent laminae internally. Further support is gained by the costovertebral joints and ligaments which directly involve the intervertebral disc.

Nakayama *et al.* (1990), Maiman and Pintar (1992), Oppenheim *et al.* (1993), Bogduk and Valencia (1994) and Boriani *et al.* (1994) all share the opinion that disc lesions are relatively uncommon in the thoracic spine, in contrast to the claim that disc lesions account for a higher proportion of thoracic pain than is often realized (Cyriax and Cyriax, 1983). The bony anatomy, including the primary kyphotic curve, and the surrounding ligamentous structures related to the costovertebral joints may have a stabilizing effect on the intervertebral disc, making displacement less likely in this region. The rib cage also exerts a stabilizing effect by restricting movement, particularly in the upper segment where the ribs are firmly attached anteriorly and posteriorly.

Since it is apparently a less significant factor in the causes of thoracic pain, the structure and function of the disc are not covered in depth here and the reader is referred to its coverage in relation to the lumbar spine (see Chapter 13).

Twelve pairs of ribs normally attach posteriorly to the thoracic spine. The upper seven pairs are termed true ribs and attach anteriorly to the sternum. The lower five pairs consist of false and floating ribs, the false ribs attaching to the costal cartilage above.

A *typical rib* consists of a shaft and anterior and posterior ends. It is the posterior end that concerns us here. The posterior end of the rib typically has a *head, a neck and a tubercle* and articulates with the thoracic vertebrae, forming the posterior rib joints. The head of the rib is divided into two demifacets by a horizontal ridge that is attached to the disc via an intra-articular ligament. The lower facet articulates with its corresponding vertebra; the upper facet articulates with the vertebra above.

The tubercle of the rib is at the junction of the neck with the shaft and articulates with the transverse process of the corresponding vertebra. Just lateral to the tubercle the rib turns to run inferiorly forwards; this point is the *angle of the rib*.

A cervical rib may be present as an extension of the costal elements of the seventh cervical vertebra. It generally passes forwards and laterally into the posterior triangle of the neck where it is crossed by the lower trunk of the brachial plexus and the subclavian vessels. Compression of these structures may produce motor and sensory signs and symptoms.

Posterior rib joints

Two joints, the costovertebral and costotransverse joints, attach the rib firmly to the vertebral column (Fig. 9.2). These assist stabilization of the intervertebral joint whilst being relatively unstable themselves. Minor subluxations of these joints may be responsible for the mechanical pattern of signs and symptoms associated with a thoracic pain. This minor instability may also account for the ease with which subluxations occur and can be reduced in this region.

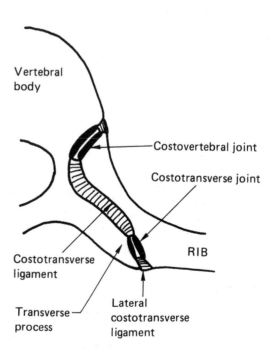

Fig. 9.2 Posterior rib joints. Costovertebral and costotransverse joints, horizontal section. From Palastanga *et al.* (1989) with permission.

The *costovertebral joint* is a synovial joint formed between the head of the rib and two adjacent vertebral bodies, except at the first, 11th and 12th ribs, where a joint is formed with a single vertebral body. The joint surfaces are covered by articular cartilage and surrounded by a fibrous capsule. The capsule is thickened anteriorly by the radiate ligament whilst the posterior aspect of the capsule blends with the nearby denticulation of the posterior longitudinal ligament. An intra-articular ligament divides the joint and attaches the transverse ridge of the rib head to the intervertebral disc.

The *costotransverse joint* joins the upper 10 ribs to the transverse processes of their corresponding vertebra. The joint is surrounded by a fibrous capsule that is reinforced posteriorly by the lateral costotransverse ligament. The joint is further stabilized by the costotransverse ligament that joins the transverse process to the neck of the rib, and the superior costotransverse ligament which connects the rib to the transverse process of the vertebra above.

Movements occur concurrently at the costovertebral and costotransverse joints and are determined by the shape and direction of the articular facets. This amounts to small rotary and gliding movements in association with the 'bucket handle' action of the ribs during respiration.

Three thin musculotendinous layers occupy the intercostal space between adjacent ribs and may become symptomatic due to strain (Fig. 9.3). The *external intercostal muscle* is the most superficial, with fibres running in an oblique direction downwards and forwards. The *internal intercostal muscle* lies beneath with fibres running in the opposite direction, and the thinnest and deepest layer is formed by the *innermost (intimi) intercostal muscle*, which is thin and possibly absent, with fibres running in the same direction as the internal intercostal muscle. The intercostal nerves and vessels run between the middle and deep intercostal layers.

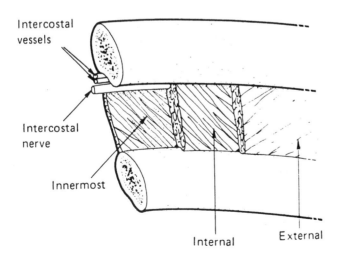

Intercostal vessels

Intercostal nerve

Innermost

Internal

External

Fig. 9.3 Layers of intercostal muscles. Adapted from Palastanga *et al.* (1994) with permission.

Differential diagnosis at the thoracic spine

Orthopaedic medicine treatment techniques for the thoracic spine are aimed at reducing a mechanical lesion, i.e. subluxation of a posterior rib joint or displacement of an intervertebral disc.

Minor subluxation of the posterior rib joints

Subluxation of one or other of the posterior rib joints is a common cause of thoracic pain. The articulating surfaces of these joints are relatively shallow and unstable, rendering them susceptible to minor subluxations. The relatively trivial incidents that provoke thoracic mechanical pain and the relative ease with which it is reduced leads us to this hypothesis. Differential diagnosis of thoracic pain is difficult because of the numerous conditions that refer pain to the area and the lesions that mimic mechanical pain.

Patients present with a sudden onset of pain; the precipitating event is usually trivial and they often feel a pop or click. More gradual onset can be associated with working in rotated postures. The pain presents a typical mechanical picture of pain aggravated by movement and posture, and eased by rest. In common with a thoracic disc lesion, a deep breath often provokes the pain, presumably because the 'bucket handle' action of the ribs during respiration translates aggravating movements to the rib joints at the spine.

On examination there is a non-capsular pattern of limited movement involving one rotation more than the other and these simple mechanical lesions usually respond rapidly to manipulation. Provided that there are no contraindications present (see below), the manipulative techniques described in this chapter can be applied. The usual postural and management advice should also be given to prevent recurrence, which is also a typical feature.

Thoracic disc lesions

It is important to reduce a thoracic disc displacement because of the potential for the displaced fragment to compromise the spinal cord. The thoracic vertebral canal is relatively small, therefore central prolapse poses the most threat.

In a review of the literature, Oppenheim *et al.* (1993) reported an estimated annual incidence of one case of thoracic disc herniation per one million population. It is primarily a condition of middle age, occurring between the third and fifth decade, and affects the lower thoracic levels more frequently. This is probably because the lower thoracic spine is free of the restriction of the rib cage, making it more mobile, and the transition to the non-rotational lumbar spine produces greater torsional stresses here. The most common level reported was T11, 12, and 75% of thoracic disc lesions occurred below T8.

Positive diagnosis of a thoracic disc lesion is difficult. There is no regular pattern to the history, signs and symptoms, as found at the cervical and lumbar spine, and it is not possible to produce a clinical model on which to base differential diagnosis. Central disc prolapse is most likely to compress the spinal cord and produce signs of myelopathy which include progressive paraparesis, increased reflexes, decreased sensation and bladder dysfunction. A postero-lateral prolapse produces segmental signs and symptoms.

The most commonly reported presentation of thoracic disc lesion is back pain and/or myelopathy. Jamieson and Ballantyne (1995) describe a rare case of prolapsed thoracic disc producing Lhermitte's sign, where neck flexion produced electric shock-like symptoms in the limbs, originally thought to be pathognomonic of multiple sclerosis. The presenting back pain can be non-specific and difficult to distinguish from visceral pain. Whitcomb *et al.* (1995) reported a case of thoracic disc prolapse mimicking chronic pancreatitis.

Small uncomplicated thoracic disc displacements may present with sudden or gradual onset of pain that may be felt posteriorly, anteriorly or radiating laterally. Pressure on the dura mater produces extrasegmental reference of pain. The pain should have a typical mechanical behaviour, i.e. aggravated by movement and posture and eased by rest. Dural symptoms of increased pain on a cough, sneeze, or deep breath may be present.

On examination, a non-capsular pattern of limited movement will be found, with one rotation being significantly more painful or limited than the other. If there are no neurological signs, and signs of cord compression are absent, the treatment techniques described in this chapter may be used. Alternatively, since lower thoracic displacements are more common, they may be treated using the techniques described for the lumbar spine.

Urgent surgical intervention is necessary for patients showing signs of spinal cord compression. Otherwise, uncomplicated thoracic disc lesions follow a path of recovery similar to that seen in cervical and lumbar disc lesions, responding to physical treatments and eventually stabilizing with time (Brown *et al.*, 1992).

Other causes of thoracic pain and associated signs and symptoms

Cervical disc lesions commonly refer pain into the thoracic region and this is particularly indicative of dural reference producing unilateral or bilateral scapular pain. The patient has a typical mechanical picture, with cervical movements increasing the pain felt in the thoracic region. Pain is not reproduced by thoracic movements. Minor chest wall pain may frequently be recognized as referred from the cervical spine, and Yeung and Hagen (1993) reported two cases of herniated C6–7 disc producing major neuropathic chest wall pain which were treated surgically.

Arthritis presents with the capsular pattern of limited movement shown in the box opposite.

Capsular pattern of the thoracic spine:

- Equal limitation of rotations
- Equal limitation of side flexions
- Some limitation of extension
- Usually full flexion

Degenerative osteoarthrosis can affect the spinal joints, causing secondary signs and symptoms. Gross degenerative changes may produce central osteophytes that may cause gradual cord compression. Anterior and lateral lipping of the vertebral body as well as wedging of mid thoracic vertebrae has been associated with degenerative osteoarthrosis of the thoracic spine (Osman *et al.*, 1994).

Inflammatory arthritis can involve the thoracic spine. Rheumatoid arthritis commonly affects the costovertebral, costotransverse and zygapophyseal joints. Reiter's disease can affect the spinal joints, although it is more frequently seen in the lower limb joints. Ankylosing spondylitis, when it involves the thoracic cage, causes a reduction in chest expansion. Thoracic pain and stiffness may be its presenting symptoms.

Serious non-mechanical conditions can affect the thoracic area and suspicions are alerted when the patient appears unwell, has a fever, night pain with or without night sweats, or reports an unexpected weight loss. The pain is not affected by movement or postures and is often unrelenting.

Malignant disease, both primary and secondary, may be a cause of pain in the thoracic spine. Bronchial carcinoma accounts for 95% of all primary tumours of the lung and may present with a cough and chest pain (Kumar and Clark, 1994). Tumours in the bronchus, breast, kidney and prostate commonly metastasize to bone. Intradural and extradural neoplasm, although relatively rare, may produce symptoms similar to nerve root irritation. Watanabe *et al.* (1992) reported a case of benign osteoblastoma in the sixth thoracic vertebra presenting with thoracodorsal pain in a 19-year-old woman, increased by coughing and shifting sleeping positions. Hodges *et al.* (1994) reports a case of intraspinal, extradural synovial cyst at the level of T4–5 in a 51-year-old woman experiencing intermittent mid thoracic and lumbar pain after lifting.

Spinal infections may include osteomyelitis or epidural abscess. The organism responsible may be *Staphylococcus aureus*, *Mycobacterium tuberculosis* or, rarely, *Brucella* (Kumar and Clark, 1994).

Bone disease can include acquired conditions or congenital abnormalities. These conditions may be asymptomatic and a chance finding on X-ray.

Scheuermann's disease is vertebral osteochondritis, most commonly seen in males in the 12–18-year age group. It usually involves the lower thoracic vertebrae, often T9. The disc may move forwards between the cartilage end-plate and the anterior longitudinal ligament, producing wedging. It may produce minor thoracic backache and a local dorsal kyphosis may be evident on spinal flexion (Corrigan and Maitland, 1989). Scheuermann's disease has been associated with Schmorl's nodes and degenerative lumbar disc disease in relatively young patients (Heithoff *et al.*, 1994).

Schmorl's nodes are protrusions of the intervertebral disc into the cancellous bone of the vertebral body. This may produce an anterior prolapse, causing separation of a small fragment of bone, seen on X-ray as a limbus vertebra (Taylor and Twomey, 1985).

Osteoporosis is a reduction in bone mass that may present a problem in postmenopausal women, who lose bone density faster than men. It is common in the sixth and seventh decades of life. Pain is not due to the condition itself, but usually to secondary wedge compression fractures of the vertebral body (Turner, 1991). The patient presents with moderate to severe episodes of thoracic back pain that gradually resolve over the course of approximately 6 weeks. Fracture produces wedging of the vertebral body on X-ray and a characteristic increase in thoracic kyphosis is seen.

Fracture may present with a history of trauma. The fracture may involve elements of the vertebra or the ribs. The position of the pain and local tenderness will give an indication to the site of possible fracture.

Visceral disease can produce local thoracic pain or pain referred to the thoracic region that mimics mechanical pain, making diagnosis difficult. In visceral conditions the patient is usually unwell, which will aid diagnosis, but this is not always so.

Angina is usually felt in the chest and can be referred into the arms. If mild, it may mimic mechanical pain. The patient experiences increased pain with exertion, e.g. climbing stairs.

Pulmonary embolism, pleurisy, pneumothorax, etc. all present with chest pain, but other distinguishing features will hopefully lead to diagnosis, which is often difficult.

Acute pancreatitis produces abdominal pain localized to the epigastrium or upper abdomen, but pain may be referred to the mid or low thoracic region.

Acute cholecystitis can cause pain in the epigastrium and right hypochondrium, but pain may also be referred to the back and shoulder.

The *testes* may refer pain to the lower thoracic area as they are supplied by nerves derived from the 10th and 11th thoracic spinal segments.

Shingles (herpes zoster) is a reawakening of the chickenpox virus infection affecting one posterior nerve root. The patient presents with a dermatomal reference of pain that may be present for some days before the typical rash appears. The rash consists of vesicles following a segmental course related to the affected nerve root.

Soft-tissue conditions can produce thoracic pain.

Muscle lesions are relatively common in the thoracic region, therefore resisted tests are included in the routine examination. Commonly the intercostal muscles are affected, particularly if there is a history of a fractured rib. Palpation determines the site of the lesion.

Tietze's syndrome is a condition affecting the costochondral or chondrosternal joints. It is usually unilateral, affecting one, two or three joints that are tender to palpation. The cause is not known, but the condition may follow a respiratory condition that involves prolonged coughing. The condition is self-limiting and may be treated with physiotherapeutic pain-relieving modalities, non-steroidal anti-inflammatory drugs or injection of corticosteroid and local anaesthetic (Kumar and Clark, 1994).

Epidemic myalgia (Bornholm disease) is due to infection by the Coxsackie B virus. The features are an upper respiratory tract illness and fever followed by pleuritic and abdominal pain and muscular tenderness. It may occur in young adults in the late summer and autumn, but resolves spontaneously within a week (Kumar and Clark, 1994).

Commentary on the examination at the thoracic spine

Observation

A general observation of the patient is made, assessing the *face, posture and gait*. Serious pathology should show in the face with the patient appearing tired and drawn. An assessment of the gait is important; the presentation of a disc displacement at the thoracic spine is relatively uncommon, but if present the serious threat to the spinal cord should be considered. Signs of myelopathy may show in the gait pattern, which if severe will be spastic in nature.

History (subjective examination)

The *age, occupation, sports, hobbies and lifestyle* of the patient will indicate possible lesions and any contributing factors to the condition that may need to be addressed to prevent recurrence. Mechanical lesions tend to be found in the middle-aged group. Osteoporosis can affect postmenopausal women. Serious conditions may present in both the very young and elderly and caution is required if these particular age groups present with symptoms, mimicking a mechanical lesion. Habitual postures may have relevance to the symptoms as will the patient's sports or hobbies.

The *site and spread* of symptoms may indicate the site of the lesion. The initial site of the symptoms may be different to the current situation and it may be helpful to know this. Mechanical lesions can produce central pain, anterior pain or both. Pain may radiate around the chest wall and this may be indicative of nerve root involvement. Progressively increasing and radiating pain is usually sinister. Symptoms may spread in an extrasegmental distribution, indicating dural involvement, or separate satellite areas of pain may be related to visceral causes. Cardiac pain characteristically radiates from the chest into one or both arms. Mechanical lesions of the posterior rib joints produce relatively local pain, but movement may provoke sharp, shooting or twinging pain.

The nature of the *onset and duration* of the symptoms will assist differentiation of mechanical lesions from more serious pathology. Minor subluxation of the posterior rib joints usually has a sudden onset, with the patient recalling the exact time of onset. The mode of onset is usually trivial and is often associated with a popping or cracking sound. The duration is generally short; patients seek help as they realize the mechanical nature of the problem, having 'felt it go'. Minor subluxation may present gradually following the adoption of an awkward posture for some time. A disc lesion may have a gradual or sudden onset. A history of trauma may indicate possible fracture. More serious pathology generally starts insidiously for no apparent reason and the duration of the symptoms may be many weeks or months. Recurrent episodes may be indicative of mechanical instability or inflammatory arthritis.

The *behaviour* of the pain is important since mechanical lesions produce a recognizable pattern of behaviour. The pain is better for rest and worse for activity. Providing the mechanical lesion does not wake the patient on turning, night pain is not a feature and the patient is usually well-rested. The provoking activities are consistent and every time the patient repeats a particular aggravating movement, the pain is produced.

The 24-h pain pattern gives an indication of severity and irritability of the condition. Inflammatory symptoms are worse at night, but if the patient does get to sleep there is stiffness on waking which may take some time to wear off. This would be generally indicative of inflammatory arthritis. If night pain is a feature, the patient will look tired and this generally indicates serious pathology.

Other *symptoms* that may indicate a mechanical lesion, particularly a minor subluxation, involve a deep breath aggravating the pain, possibly due to the 'bucket handle' action of the ribs levering the spinal rib joints. Pleurisy and pulmonary embolism, for example, may also produce pain on a deep breath, but the subsequent findings on the objective assessment will confirm whether the lesion is mechanical. Although movements are small at the posterior rib joints, the length of the ribs produces a greater proportion of movement at the anterior ends. This movement may also be painful in an intercostal muscle strain. A cough or sneeze increasing the pain could be indicative of minor subluxation or, more commonly, dural irritation.

As the vertebral canal in the thoracic spine is small, disc displacement can threaten the spinal cord and produce symptoms of myelopathy; these must be ruled out. The patient is asked about the presence of paraesthesia in the feet, weakness in the legs and difficulty in walking. A specific question must be asked about bladder and bowel function, to rule out myelopathy (Oppenheim *et al.*, 1993). If any impairment is noted, the patient should be referred for neurosurgical opinion.

Other joint involvement may give an indication of any polyarthritic condition.

Past medical history will give information concerning conditions that may be relevant to the patient's current complaint. An indication of the patient's general health will indicate any systemic illness. It may be pertinent to take the patient's temperature. The patient should be asked about any recent unexplained weight loss.

On considering *medications*, the patient should be specifically asked about anticoagulants, long-term oral steroids, chemotherapy drugs, drugs for depression and the current intake of analgesics, as a measure of pain control requirement.

Inspection

The patient should undress to underwear and an inspection is carried out in a good light. A general inspection of the posture is made assessing *bony deformity*. Note the position of the head and neck, cervical, thoracic and lumbar curves. Is there any evidence of cervical protraction or dowager's hump, excessive or local thoracic kyphosis? Note the position of the scapulae and any evidence of scoliosis, whether structural or acquired.

Colour changes or *swelling* would not be expected unless associated with a history of recent trauma. The typical appearance of shingles may be spotted or the mottled reddening (erythema ab igne) produced following prolonged application of excessive heat, giving an indication of the severity of the pain.

Muscle wasting may be seen in the scapular area associated with neuritis.

State at rest

Before any movements are performed, the state at rest is established to provide a baseline for comparison.

The suggested sequence for the objective examination will now be given, followed by a commentary including the reasoning in performing the movements and the significance of the possible findings.

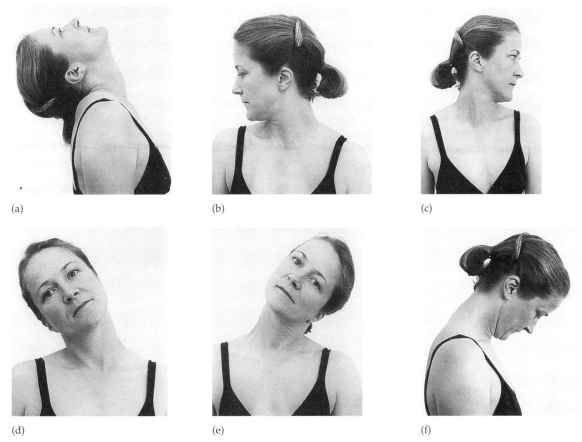

(a)

(b)

(c)

(d)

(e)

(f)

Fig. 9.4 Six active cervical movements
to eliminate the cervical spine as a
cause of pain. (a) Extension; (b, c)
rotations; (d, e) side flexions; (f) flexion.

Examination by selective tension (objective examination)

> *Eliminate the cervical spine*:
>
> - Active cervical extension (Fig. 9.4a)
> - Active right cervical rotation (Fig. 9.4b)
> - Active left cervical rotation (Fig. 9.4c)
> - Active right cervical side flexion (Fig. 9.4d)
> - Active left cervical side flexion (Fig. 9.4e)
> - Active cervical flexion (Fig. 9.4f)
>
> *Dural test*:
>
> - Scapular approximation (Fig. 9.5)

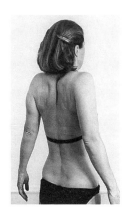

Fig. 9.5 Dural test: scapular
approximation.

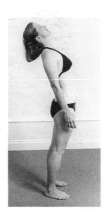

Fig. 9.6 Active extension.

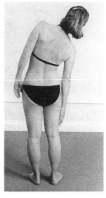
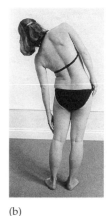

(a)   (b)

Fig. 9.7 (a, b) Active side flexions.

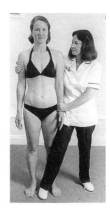

Fig. 9.8 Active flexion.

Fig. 9.9 Resisted side flexion.

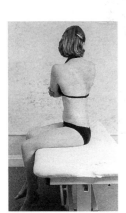

(a)

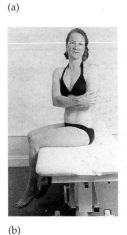

(b)

Fig. 9.10 (a, b) Active rotations.

Articular and muscle signs:

Standing:

- Active thoracic extension (Fig. 9.6)
- Active right thoracic side flexion (Fig. 9.7a)
- Active left thoracic side flexion (Fig. 9.7b)
- Active thoracic flexion (Fig. 9.8)
- Resisted thoracic side flexions (Fig 9.9)

Sitting:

- Active thoracic right rotation (Fig. 9.10a)
- Active thoracic left rotation (Fig. 9.10b)

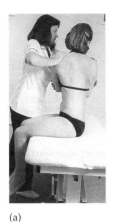
(a)

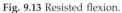
(b)

Fig. 9.11 (a, b) Passive rotations.

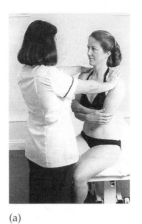
(a)

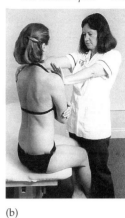
(b)

Fig. 9.12 (a, b) Resisted rotations.

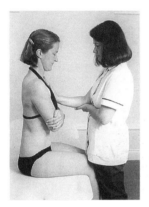

Fig. 9.13 Resisted flexion.

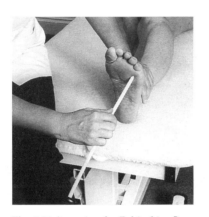

Fig. 9.14 Assessing for Babinski reflex.

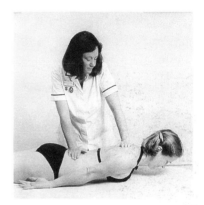

Fig. 9.15 Resisted extension.

- Passive thoracic right rotation (Fig. 9.11a)
- Passive thoracic left rotation (Fig. 9.11b)
- Resisted thoracic right rotation (Fig. 9.12a)
- Resisted thoracic left rotation (Fig. 9.12b)
- Resisted thoracic flexion (Fig. 9.13)

Supine lying:

- Babinski reflex (Fig. 9.14)

Prone lying:

- Resisted thoracic extension (Fig. 9.15)

Palpation

- Spinous processes (Fig. 9.16)

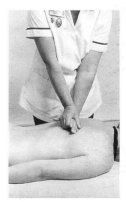

Fig. 9.16 Palpation.

The cervical spine is a possible source of pain felt in the thoracic region and it must first be eliminated. If cervical flexion is the only movement to reproduce the thoracic pain, it is considered to be a dural sign for the thoracic spine since neck flexion draws the dura upwards (Fig. 9.4f). Scapular approximation is conducted as a dural test since it pulls on the dura via the T1 and 2 nerve roots and may be positive in a disc lesion at these levels (Fig. 9.5).

In common with other regions of the spine, the thoracic spine is considered to be an 'emotional' area and the movements are assessed actively to observe willingness to perform the movements, as well as assessing the articular signs for pain and limited range of movement. The capsular or non-capsular pattern will become evident through these movements.

Resisted side flexion is assessed looking for evidence of a muscle lesion. Resisted tests may also be applied if serious pathology or psychological factors are suspected.

The patient sits to fix the pelvis whilst the rotations are assessed for pain, range of movement, end-feel and the capsular pattern. Resisted flexion may also be assessed. End-feel, which is normally elastic, is particularly pertinent to the rotations since these movements may show minimal limitation and pain in minor subluxations of the posterior rib joints. Passive overpressure can be applied to any of the other movements if appropriate.

The non-capsular pattern involves pain and or limitation of at least one of the rotations.

The patient is positioned in supine lying to apply the Babinski reflex, the extensor plantar response, by stroking up the lateral border of the sole of the foot and across the metatarsal heads. If the response is extensor, i.e. upgoing, it is indicative of an upper motor neurone lesion, the normal response is flexor.

The patient is positioned in prone lying to complete the examination. Resisted extension is applied and the spinous processes are palpated assessing pain, range of movement and end-feel (Fig. 9.15)

Treatment of thoracic lesions

Manipulation is the treatment of choice for thoracic mechanical lesions, either minor subluxation of the posterior rib joints or an uncomplicated thoracic intervertebral disc displacement. Thoracic disc lesions are relatively uncommon, but central displacement can endanger the spinal cord. The history and objective examination should reveal signs of spinal cord compression.

Indications for thoracic manipulation

- Mechanical thoracic lesion, disc displacement or minor subluxation of posterior rib joint.
- Non-capsular pattern, usually limitation and/or pain of at least one thoracic rotation.
- No neurological signs.
- No contraindications.

Capsular pattern at the thoracic spine:

- Equal limitation of rotations
- Equal limitation of side flexions
- Some limitation of extension
- Usually full flexion

Absolute contraindications to thoracic manipulation

- Signs and symptoms of spinal cord compression
- Ill patient
- Anticoagulation therapy and blood clotting disorders
- Past history of cancer
- Prolonged steroid therapy

Guidelines to minimize risk from thoracic manipulation

Following the recommended guidelines below, ensures maximum safety and preparation for the unexpected. The practitioner must take all due care whilst applying the treatment techniques (see *Rules of Professional Conduct*, Rules 1, 2 and 4, and the *Standards of Physiotherapy Practice* both available from the Chartered Society of Physiotherapy, 14 Bedford Road, London WC1R 4ED).

Ensure that:

- A full history and examination have been completed and recorded, sufficient to exclude contraindications to treatment.

- Specific questions have been asked relating to the following, and the results recorded:

  general health
  unexplained weight loss
  bilateral parasthesia in the hands and feet
  anticoagulant therapy
  long-term oral steroids
  chemotherapy drugs
  inflammatory arthritis.

- From the examination, the following factors are present:

  a non capsular pattern of pain and or limited movement at the thoracic spine
  a normal plantar response
  no neurological signs.

- You have provided sufficient information, including possible risks and advice, if manipulation is indicated, so that the patient can give informed consent. You must respect the right of the patient to refuse manipulation.

- You re-examine the patient after the application of each technique and decisions to continue are based on the results of the previous technique.

- Any significant adverse response to treatment should be reported immediately to the patient's doctor.

Thoracic manipulation techniques

As with the cervical spine, the treatment techniques in this section will be described carefully in a step-by-step fashion to enable their application. However, the professional judgement and existing skill of the operator will allow each technique to be adapted. The techniques described have been adapted from those originally described by Cyriax and Cyriax (1983) and Cyriax (1984). Clinically, minor subluxation of a posterior rib joint is a more common lesion than thoracic disc displacement, hence the techniques are not carried out under traction. As with all manipulations, the comparable signs are reassessed after each manoeuvre and a decision made about the next. If the techniques fail to produce a reduction in signs and symptoms, they can be applied under traction (Cyriax and Cyriax, 1983; Cyriax, 1984).

The position of the bed for each manoeuvre is a matter of personal choice. The extension thrust techniques are best conducted with the bed as low as possible.

It is recommended that a course in orthopaedic medicine is attended before the treatment techniques in the chapter are applied in clinical practice (see Appendix).

Straight extension thrust

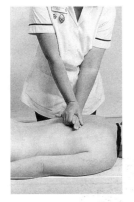

Fig. 9.17 Straight extension thrust.

Position the patient comfortably in prone lying, preferably with the head in neutral, with the face positioned in the nose hole, and the arms resting over the edge of the couch or at the patient's side. Palpate for the tender thoracic level. Apply the ulnar border of your hand, reinforced with the other hand, to the most tender spinous process (Fig. 9.17). Take up the skin slack and ask the patient to take in a small breath. Apply pressure downwards with straight arms, following the breath out. Apply a minimal-amplitude, high-velocity thrust once all the slack is taken up.

This technique is uncomfortable for the patient as the thrust is applied to the tender bony spinous process. The following manoeuvre is much more comfortable for the patient. Both techniques may have to be applied at one or two levels. It is common to find one, two or even three tender levels, in which case the most tender level is chosen first.

Extension with a rotational component

Position the patient as for the above manoeuvre and again locate the most tender spinous process. The technique can be applied in one of two ways but it may be necessary to do both.

1. Locate the painful level. Position your hands as follows on either side of the spinous process over the paraspinal muscle bulk approximately over the underlying transverse processes.

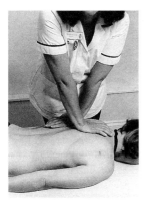

Fig. 9.18 Extension with a rotational component.

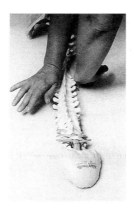

Fig. 9.19 Extension with a rotational component; hand position demonstrated on spine.

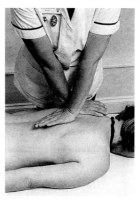

Fig. 9.20 Extension with a rotational component, alternative position.

Place the pisiform of the hand which is nearest to the patient's head, at the painful level, adjacent to the spinous process (Figs 9.18 and 9.19). Place the trapeziofirst-metacarpal joint of your other hand adjacent to the spinous process on the level above. Take up some of the slack in a rotational direction, ask the patient to take a small breath in, follow the movement down as the patient breathes out. Apply a minimal-amplitude, high-velocity thrust through straight arms once all of the slack is taken up.

2. This technique is the reverse of that described above. Place the trapeziofirst-metacarpal joint of the hand that is nearest to the patient's head adjacent to the spinous process at the painful level. Place the pisiform of your other hand on the level above (Figs 9.20 and 9.21). Repeat as described above.

Sitting rotation

Position the patient astride the end of a narrow couch to fix the pelvis, with the patient's back towards you at the end of the couch and his or her arms folded across the chest. Stand close to the patient and bend your knees. Hug the patient so that the patient's shoulder fits into the front of your axilla (Fig. 9.22). Maintain the patient as close as possible, whilst the heel of your other hand rests on the posterior thoracic spine just above the painful level (Fig. 9.23). Ask the patient to rotate actively as far as possible. Rotate a little further passively and straighten your knees to apply some traction to the patient's upper trunk (Fig. 9.24). Apply a minimal-amplitude, high-velocity thrust towards rotation once all of the slack is taken up, by smartly rotating your body and pushing through the heel of your hand.

Rotate the patient into the least painful rotation first. If that fails to improve symptoms, the technique can be repeated in the opposite direction.

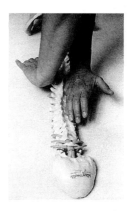

Fig. 9.21 Extension with a rotational component, alternative position; hand position demonstrated on spine.

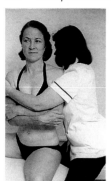

Fig. 9.22 Sitting rotation, starting position.

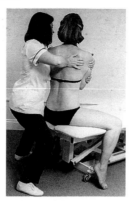

Fig. 9.23 Sitting rotation, showing hand position just above painful level.

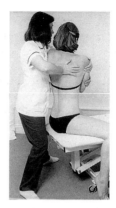

Fig. 9.24 Sitting rotation, traction applied by straightening knees, before application of the Grade C manipulation.

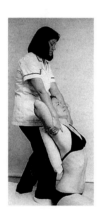

Fig. 9.25 Sitting extension thrust with a degree of traction.

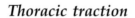

Sitting extension thrust with a degree of traction

Position the patient in sitting on the side of the couch with the patient's hands behind his or her head. Stand on the couch behind the patient and place one knee at the painful level, with a pillow or padding placed between your knee and the patient's back. Wrap your hands over and below the patient's upper arms and lean the patient back over your knee, applying traction by moving your body weight backwards on to your other leg (Fig. 9.25). Once the patient has relaxed, extend the thoracic spine by applying a small-amplitude, high-velocity upward lift of your knee against the back.

Thoracic traction

Thoracic traction is difficult to apply and is not as effective as in the cervical and lumbar joints, probably due to the comparative rigidity of the spine and to the sternal and vertebral attachments of the ribs.

The higher and lower thoracic levels form part of the cervico-thoracic and thoracolumbar transition levels respectively, and traction, or mobilization under traction, applied to the cervical and lumbar regions will affect these levels. For mid to lower thoracic levels the thoracic harness needs to be placed higher on the rib cage, which can lead to uncomfortable pressure in the axillae that is not well-tolerated by the patient.

If the history, signs and symptoms do warrant its use, it is applied on the same lines as for the lumbar spine.

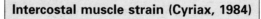

Intercostal muscle strain (Cyriax, 1984)

Generally, muscle lesions at the spinal joints are rare. However, it is not uncommon to find a lesion in the intercostal muscles. The onset of pain may follow a chest infection with prolonged coughing, overexertion or as the result of a fractured rib. Pain is felt locally and reproduced on resisted testing. Palpation reveals an area of tenderness in one intercostal space.

The lesion responds well to transverse friction massage. Position the patient in half lying and locate the tender area. Using an index or middle finger, direct the pressure up or down against the affected rib and apply transverse friction massage, according to the general principles.

References

Australian Physiotherapy Association (1988) Protocol for pre-manipulative testing of the cervical spine. *Australian Journal of Physiotherapy* **34**: 97–100.

Bogduk, N., Valencia, F. (1994) Innervations and pain patterns of the thoracic spine. In: *Clinics in Physical Therapy, Physical Therapy of the Cervical and Thoracic Spine*, 2nd edn (Grant, R. ed.). Churchill Livingstone, pp. 77–87.

Boriani, S., Biagini, R., de Lure, F. *et al.* (1994) Two-level thoracic disc herniation. *Spine* **19**: 2461–2466.

Brown, C.W., Deffer, P.A., Akmakjian, J. *et al.* (1992) The natural history of thoracic disc herniation. *Spine* **17**: S97–S102.

Corrigan, B., Maitland, G.D. (1989) *Practical Orthopaedic Medicine*. Butterworths.

Cyriax, J. (1984) *Textbook of Orthopaedic Medicine*, vol. 2, 11th edn. Baillière Tindall.

Cyriax, J., Cyriax, P. (1983) *Illustrated Manual of Orthopaedic Medicine*. Butterworths.

Heithoff, K.B., Gundry, C.R., Burton, C.V., Winter, R.B. (1994) Juvenile discogenic disease. *Spine* **19**: 335–340.

Hodges, S.D., Fronczak, S., Zindrick, M.R. *et al.* (1994) Extradural synovial thoracic cyst. *Spine* **19**: 2471–2473.

Jamieson, D.R.S., Ballantyne, J.P. (1995) Unique presentation of a prolapsed thoracic disc – Lhermitte's symptom in a golf player. *Neurology* **45**: 1219–1221.

Kapandji, I.A. (1974) *The Physiology of the Joints, Trunk and the Vertebral Column*, vol. 3. Churchill Livingstone.

Kumar, P., Clark, M. (1994) *Clinical Medicine*, 3rd edn. Baillière Tindall.

Maiman, D.J., Pintar, F.A. (1992) Anatomy and clinical biomechanics of the thoracic spine. *Clinical Neurosurgery* **38**: 296–324.

Nakayama, H., Hashimoto, H., Hase, H. *et al.* (1990) An 80 year old man with thoracic disc herniation. Spine **15**: 1234–1235.

Oppenheim, J.S., Rothman, A.S., Sachdev, V.P. (1993) Thoracic herniated discs – review of the literature and 12 cases. *Mount Sinai Journal of Medicine* **60**: 321–326.

Osman, A.A., Bassiouni, H., Koutri, R. *et al.* (1994) Ageing of the thoracic spine: distinction between wedging on osteoarthritis and fracture in osteoporosis – a cross-sectional and longitudinal study. *Bone* **15**: 437–442.

Palastanga, N., Field, D., Soames, R. (1994) *Anatomy and Human Movement*. Butterworth-Heinemann.

Taylor, J.R., Twomey, L.T. (1985) Vertebral column development and its relation to adult pathology. *Australian Journal of Physiotherapy* **31**: 83–88.

Turner, P. (1991) Osteoporotic back pain – its prevention and treatment. *Physiotherapy* **77**: 642–646.

Watanabe, M., Kihara, Y., Matsuda, Y., Shibata, T. (1992) Benign osteoblastoma in the vertebral body of the thoracic spine – a case report. *Spine* **17**: 1432–1434.

Whitcomb, D.C., Martin, S.P., Schoen, R.E., Jho, H.-D.(1995) Chronic abdominal pain caused by thoracic disc herniation. *American Journal of Gastroenterology* **90**: 835–837.

Yeung, M.C., Hagen, N.A. (1993) Cervical disc herniation presenting with chest wall pain. *Le Journal Canadien des Sciences Neurologiques* **20**: 59–61.

10 The hip

Summary

Degenerative osteoarthrosis of the hip, even before the development of X-ray changes, is frequently overlooked as a treatable condition when symptomatic relief can often be obtained by the mobilization or injection techniques described in orthopaedic medicine.

   Pain in the hip region can be incorrectly attributed to the lumbar spine, whilst the bursae in the area may not be considered, and can evade diagnosis. Groin strain and hamstring injury are familiar to the clinician, though worthy of mention to enhance effective treatment.

   This chapter describes the anatomy relevant to common lesions in the hip region, to which orthopaedic medicine principles of treatment can be applied. A commentary follows, highlighting the relevant points of the history and suggesting a methodical sequence for objective examination. Lesions are then discussed with treatment alternatives and overall management.

Anatomy

Inert structures

The *hip joint* is a synovial joint formed between the head of the femur and the acetabulum of the innominate bone. The *head of the femur* is slightly more than half a sphere and faces anteriorly, superiorly and medially to articulate with the acetabulum forming a stable ball-and-socket joint. This articulation offers great stability and provides sufficient mobility for gait. The close-packed position of the hip joint is full extension, with a degree of abduction and medial rotation (Williams *et al.*, 1989; Hartley, 1995).

   The *acetabulum* is deepened by the fibrocartilaginous acetabular labrum and all articular surfaces are covered by articular cartilage. The *fibrous capsule*, lined with synovium, surrounds most of the neck of the femur, attaching above to the acetabular rim, below to the intertrochanteric line anteriorly and 1 cm above the intertrochanteric crest posteriorly. Both the joint capsule and the articular cartilage tend to be thicker anterosuperiorly, which is the position of most stress in weight-bearing.

   Three ligaments reinforce the articular capsule and control movement. All three are taut in extension and relaxed in flexion. The *iliofemoral ligament* has strong medial and lateral bands which form a Y-shape, passing from the anterior inferior iliac spine to the intertrochanteric line. The *pubofemoral ligament* passes from the superior pubic ramus to blend distally with the capsule and the medial border of the iliofemoral ligament. The *ischiofemoral ligament* passes from the ischium and winds superiorly and laterally to the upper part of the femoral neck, blending with the capsule of the hip joint and supporting it posteriorly.

The *psoas bursa* (L2–3; Cyriax, 1982) is the largest single bursa in the body, measuring 5–7 cm in length and 2–4 cm in width in its normal collapsed state (Underwood *et al.*, 1988; Toohey *et al.*, 1990, Flanagan *et al.*, 1995; Zimmermann *et al.*, 1995). In 15% of cadaveric specimens, the psoas bursa was seen to communicate with the hip joint via an aperture between the iliofemoral and pubofemoral ligaments (Flanagan *et al.*, 1995). It may be a simple bursa or multiloculated with well-defined thin walls (Meaney *et al.*, 1992).

The psoas bursa lies beneath the musculotendinous junction of the iliopsoas muscle and the front of the capsule of the hip joint (Fig. 10.1). It cushions the iliopsoas tendon as it winds round the front of the hip joint to its posteromedial insertion on the lesser trochanter. It is related anteromedially to the femoral artery and anteriorly to the femoral nerve (Canoso, 1981). Its point of location is just distal to the mid-point of the inguinal ligament, deep to the femoral artery.

The *gluteal bursa* (L4–5; Cyriax and Cyriax, 1983) is not a single entity, but for clinical purposes is considered to be so. At least four separate bursae lie between the different planes of the gluteal

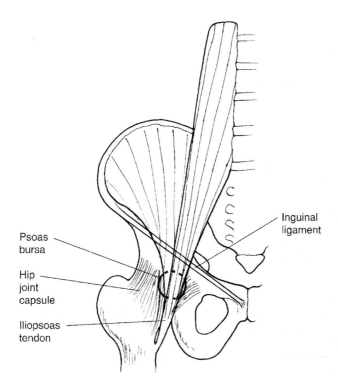

Fig. 10.1 Position of the psoas bursa.

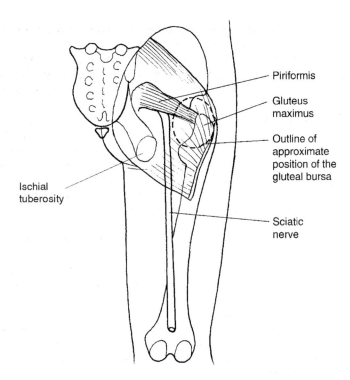

Piriformis

Gluteus maximus

Outline of approximate position of the gluteal bursa

Sciatic nerve

Ischial tuberosity

Fig. 10.2 Position of gluteal bursa.

muscles as they attach to or pass over the greater trochanter, collectively forming the gluteal bursa (Fig. 10.2).

Two bursae are associated with gluteus maximus: a large trochanteric bursa separating it from the greater trochanter, and a gluteofemoral bursa lying between it and vastus lateralis (Williams *et al.*, 1989). The trochanteric bursa of gluteus medius lies between its tendon and the anterosuperior aspect of the greater trochanter. The trochanteric bursa of gluteus minimus separates its insertion from the medial part of the greater trochanter (Williams *et al.*, 1989). One further bursa may be present, the ischial bursa, lying between the ischial tuberosity and the lower part of gluteus maximus.

Since the gluteal muscles lie in different planes, the depth and the extent of the different bursae constituting the gluteal bursa must be considered when placing a corticosteroid injection.

Contractile structures

Functionally the anterior muscles are flexors of the hip, although they may also assist other hip movements. Some pass over the knee where they also have an effect. Resisted flexion of the hip tests mainly psoas major; with the knee flexed it is also testing rectus femoris.

Psoas major (ventral rami L1–3) has its origin from the lumbar spine. It descends to pass under the centre of the inguinal ligament receiving the fibres of iliacus on its lateral side. The iliopsoas tendon crosses the front of the hip joint where it is cushioned by the underlying psoas bursa. The combined tendon winds posteriorly to insert into the lesser trochanter of the femur.

Sartorius (femoral nerve L2–3) passes from the anterior superior iliac spine to cross the thigh medially, inserting into the upper medial aspect of the tibia. It marks the lateral border of the femoral triangle.

Rectus femoris (femoral nerve L2–4) is part of the quadriceps mechanism and has its main effect at the knee. However, its origin above the hip makes it a two-joint muscle and it also acts as a powerful hip flexor, being most efficient when the knee is flexed (Kapandji, 1970). It has two heads of origin: a straight head from the anterior inferior iliac spine and a reflected head from just above the acetabular rim. It joins the rest of the quadriceps to insert into the patellar tendon.

Gluteus maximus acts principally as a hip extensor whilst the hamstrings assist hip extension, but their main effect is in flexing the knee. Since the hamstring muscles run over two joints, their efficiency in extending the hip increases if the knee is locked into extension (Kapandji, 1970). The small, deep muscles of the hip are responsible for lateral rotation.

Gluteus maximus (inferior gluteal nerve L5, S1–2) is the largest and most superficial of the gluteal muscles. It passes from behind the posterior gluteal line on the blade of the ilium to the iliotibial tract and upper femur.

Biceps femoris (sciatic nerve L5, S1–2) is the lateral hamstring with two heads of origin. A long head arises from an inferomedial facet on the ischial tuberosity (which it shares with semitendinosus) and a short head from the lateral lip of the linea aspera. Its fibres converge into a fusiform muscle belly and its tendon of insertion attaches to the head of the fibula.

Semitendinosus and semimembranosus are the medial hamstrings. *Semitendinosus* (sciatic nerve L5, S1–2) takes origin from the inferomedial facet on the ischial tuberosity. Its muscle belly ends in the middle of the thigh and its long tendon of insertion lies on semimembranosus before winding around to the medial aspect of the upper tibia. *Semimembranosus* (sciatic nerve L5, S1–2) takes origin from the superolateral facet on the ischial tuberosity and has its main insertion on to the posterior aspect of the medial tibial condyle into the tuberculum tendinis.

Piriformis (L5, S1–2) originates in the pelvis, exiting through the greater sciatic foramen to attach to the upper border of the greater trochanter.

Obturator externus (posterior branch of the obturator nerve L3–4) and *obturator internus* (nerve to obturator internus L5, S1) pass posteriorly to the hip joint and insert into the medial surface of the greater trochanter and trochanteric fossa.

Gemelli (L5, S1) pass from the ischial spine and ischial tuberosity to the medial aspect of the greater trochanter.

Quadratus femoris (nerve to quadratus femoris L5, S1) passes from the ischial tuberosity to the quadrate tubercle in the middle of the trochanteric crest.

Gluteus medius is the main hip abductor whilst medius and minimus together are responsible for maintaining the position of the opposite side of the pelvis in single-leg stance. Weakness of the hip abductors produces a positive Trendelenburg sign. Tensor fascia lata and the anterior fibres of gluteus medius and minimus also produce medial rotation and flexion because they lie anterior to the frontal plane of the hip joint. Lying posteriorly, some fibres of gluteus medius and minimus are responsible for lateral rotation and extension (Kapandji, 1970).

Gluteus medius (superior gluteal nerve L5, S1) is partially overlapped by maximus and lies in a slightly deeper plane. It originates from the blade of the ilium between posterior and anterior gluteal lines and inserts into the lateral aspect of the greater trochanter.

Gluteus minimus (superior gluteal nerve L5, S1) is the deepest gluteal muscle and arises between the anterior and inferior gluteal lines, inserting into the medial part of the anterior trochanteric surface.

Tensor fascia lata (superior gluteal nerve L4–5) arises from the anterior 5 cm of the outer lip of the iliac crest and the anterior superior iliac spine. It passes downwards and laterally to insert into the anterior border of the iliotibial tract.

The adductor muscles originate in the pelvis and pass to the medial aspect of the thigh.

Gracilis (obturator nerve L2–3) is the most superficial hip adductor. It passes from the lower half of the body of the pubis, the inferior pubic ramus and the adjacent ischial ramus, to run vertically downwards to just below the medial tibial condyle.

Pectineus (femoral nerve L2–3) passes from the pecten pubis running posterolaterally to a line joining the lesser trochanter to the linea aspera.

Adductor longus (obturator nerve L2–4) is the most superficial adductor. It passes from the body of the pubis, in the angle between the crest and the symphysis pubis, to descend posterolaterally to the middle third of the linea aspera.

Adductor brevis (obturator nerve L3) lies deep to adductor longus, passing from the lower aspect of the body of the pubis and the inferior pubic ramus to its attachment on the femur, between the lesser trochanter and the linea aspera.

Adductor magnus (upper fibres, obturator nerve; lower fibres, tibial branch of the sciatic nerve, L2–4) is the largest and deepest adductor muscle. It is considered to have two separate portions, one an adductor portion and the other a hamstring portion, each with its own separate nerve supply. It takes origin from the inferior pubic ramus, the adjacent ischial ramus and the inferolateral aspect of the ischial tuberosity. Its upper fibres pass mainly horizontally to the linea aspera of the femur and form the adductor part of the muscle. Its lower fibres pass more vertically to the adductor tubercle on the medial femoral condyle and are the hamstring part.

The movement of medial rotation at the hip is a secondary function of some of the following muscles: semimembranosus, semitendinosus, adductor magnus and longus, pectineus, gluteus medius and minimus and tensor fascia lata.

A guide to surface marking and palpation

Pelvic region

Palpate the *iliac crest*, which should be obvious in most people as no muscles attach to its superior border. The highest point of the crest lies just posterior to the mid-point and gives an approximate indication of the level of the spinous process of L4.

Palpate the *anterior superior iliac spine* which is subcutaneous and located at the anterior end of the iliac crest. It marks the lateral attachment of the inguinal ligament and the origin of the sartorius muscle.

Palpate the *posterior superior iliac spine* which is situated at the posterior end of the iliac crest. It is not as readily palpable as the anterior spine, but lies under a dimple in the upper buttock, approximately 4 cm lateral to the spinous process of S2. It gives attachment to the sacrotuberous ligament. Imagine a line drawn from the posterior superior iliac spine to the spinous process of S2; this line crosses the centre of the *sacroiliac joint* and gives an indication of the joint's position.

Consider the position of the *anterior and posterior inferior iliac spines* which lie below the superior spines and are not as readily palpable. The anterior inferior spine gives origin superiorly to the long head of rectus femoris and inferiorly to part of the iliofemoral ligament.

Locate the position of the *pubic tubercle* at the medial end of the inguinal crease, lying at the same level as the top of the greater trochanter. It marks the medial attachment of the inguinal ligament.

Palpate the bony *ischial tuberosity*, which lies in the buttock approximately 5 cm lateral to the midline just above the gluteal fold. In the sitting position, body weight is supported by the ischial tuberosities. Each is most easily palpated with the patient in side lying and the hip placed in flexion, to bring the ischial tuberosity out from under the bulk of gluteus maximus.

Lateral aspect of the thigh

In side lying palpate the *greater trochanter*, which is a large quadrangular bony prominence situated at the upper lateral shaft of the femur, approximately one hand's-breadth below the iliac crest. Grasp the greater trochanter with your thumb, index and middle fingers (Fig. 10.3), lifting the leg passively into abduction to relax the iliotibial tract. The greater trochanter will be a useful bony landmark for some of the injection techniques around the hip.

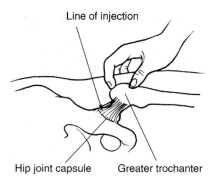

Fig. 10.3 Location of hip joint for the injection by grasping the greater trochanter.

Hip joint capsule   Greater trochanter

Anterior aspect of the thigh

Consider the position of the *femoral triangle* on the anterior thigh (Fig. 10.4). Place the leg into the FABER position – a combination of *f*lexion, *ab*duction and *e*xternal (lateral) *r*otation of the hip – to give you an idea of the borders of the triangle. The inguinal ligament forms the base of the triangle, sartorius its lateral border and adductor longus its medial border. Iliopsoas and pectineus lie in the floor of the femoral triangle.

Consider the position of the *lateral cutaneous nerve* of thigh (L2–3) as it passes under or through the inguinal ligament, just medial to the anterior superior iliac spine. It may be compressed here, causing a condition called meralgia paraesthetica, which produces paraesthesia in the nerve's distribution.

Palpate for the *femoral artery* which passes down through the middle of the triangle with the femoral vein situated medially and the femoral nerve laterally. You will locate a strong pulse just distal to the mid-point of the inguinal ligament.

Locating the femoral pulse will prove a useful landmark for the structures passing deep to it. From superficial to deep these are the iliopsoas tendon, which is en route to its insertion into the lesser trochanter, the psoas bursa, and the hip joint.

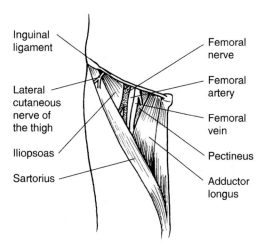

Inguinal ligament

Lateral cutaneous nerve of the thigh

Iliopsoas

Sartorius

Femoral nerve

Femoral artery

Femoral vein

Pectineus

Adductor longus

Fig. 10.4 Femoral triangle, also showing emerging lateral cutaneous nerve of thigh.

Posterior aspect of the buttock and thigh

Consider the position of the *sciatic nerve* in the buttock (Fig. 10.5). You can locate its approximate position by marking a point midway between the posterior superior iliac spine and the greater trochanter, which identifies the position of the nerve as it leaves the pelvis via the greater sciatic foramen, emerging under piriformis. Join this to another mark at a point just medial to the mid-point between the greater trochanter and the ischial tuberosity. This indicates the position of the nerve as it exits the buttock under the lower border of gluteus maximus (Williams *et al.*, 1989).

Medial aspect of the thigh

Place the leg into the FABER position to identify the thick, cord-like tendon of *adductor longus*. Palpate this tendon to appreciate its width and depth.

Commentary on the examination

Observation

A general observation is made of the patient's *face and overall posture*, but particular attention is paid to the *gait*. Since the function of the hip joint is to support body weight, lesions involving the

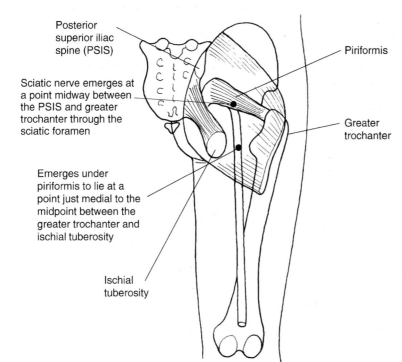

Fig. 10.5 Approximate course of the sciatic nerve in the buttock and thigh.

joint mechanics tend to cause alterations in the gait pattern. An uneven stride will indicate restricted movement, as found in arthritis, or may be due to pain on weight-bearing. Excessive lateral rotation on walking may indicate a slipped epiphysis in the young or may be present with pain or advanced capsular contracture in the elderly, indicating an arthrosis with a marked capsular pattern. A Trendelenburg gait will indicate weak abductor muscles.

Pain in the hip joint region may originate in the lumbar spine and a detailed history will help to eliminate a lesion in the area.

History (subjective examination)

The *age, occupation, sports, hobbies and lifestyle* of the patient may alert the examiner to the possible cause of the lesion.

The age of the patient is relevant to conditions at the hip. Degenerative osteoarthrosis typically presents in the middle to older age group, although it is not uncommon to find it in younger athletes, especially road runners. Muscle lesions and bursitis affect the middle age group, whilst loose bodies can present as a complication of osteoarthrosis in the older group or as osteochondritis dissecans in adolescents.

Children can develop hip problems, that if misdiagnosed can be potentially serious and an orthopaedic opinion should always be sought. Irritable hip is a non-specific diagnosis for groin pain, limited movement and a limp. Perthes disease affects boys aged 4–10 and is an osteochondritis of the femoral epiphysis. Slipped epiphysis is either sudden or gradual slipping of the superior epiphyseal plate which may produce a lateral rotation deformity. It tends to occur in overweight adolescents and is commoner in boys, who present with pain on exercise. Transient synovitis is of unknown aetiology and affects children under 10 years. Juvenile chronic arthritis usually begins in other joints, but it can also affect the hip joints.

Occupation, sports, hobbies and lifestyle will certainly indicate the aggravating factors of the condition and allow the clinician to formulate a programme of treatment and advice, tailored to the patient's individual needs.

The *site and spread* of pain may be local, indicating a superficial or less irritable lesion such as a muscle strain, or diffuse, indicating a larger lesion or gross inflammation.

Referred pain may originate from the lumbar spine. The sensory nerve supply to the hip joint is mainly through the femoral nerve L2–3, therefore the joint itself refers pain into these dermatomes depending on the size of the lesion. Part of the L2 and 3 dermatomes covers the upper buttock and a hip lesion may present as low back pain only.

Groin pain or pain referred to the knee in the child or adolescent, without obvious cause, must be considered serious and a specialist opinion sought for the possibility of the conditions mentioned above.

The *onset* of the symptoms may be gradual or sudden.

In osteoarthrosis the pain has a gradual onset, initially during weight-bearing activities, progressing to hip pain without weight-bearing, and present at rest (Cailliet, 1990). A history of previous trauma such as fracture, which alters joint biomechanics, can predispose the joint to degenerative changes.

Relatively minor trauma can fracture the pelvis in the elderly, producing severe pain of sudden onset. Loose bodies present suddenly, as do traumatic muscular lesions. Muscles around the hip joint can be easily strained, since many are two-joint muscles, and a sudden explosive contraction such as that seen in sprinting may produce overstretching (Hartley, 1995). Overuse or repetitive movements may produce chronic contractile lesions or bursitis.

The *duration* of symptoms indicates the stage of the lesion in the inflammatory process. Degenerative osteoarthrosis will present a typical history of gradually worsening episodes of pain. Bursitis tends to give a gradual onset of aching pain, therefore is often present for many months before the patient seeks treatment. A severe pain which gradually increases in intensity, and remains so, is indicative of a serious lesion. This, coupled with other findings in the history, may be indicative of the 'sign of the buttock' (see page 305).

The *symptoms and behaviour* need to be considered. The behaviour of the pain gives an indication of the nature of the lesion. For example, osteoarthrosis at the hip joint may be aggravated by activity or weight-bearing or inflamed bursae and muscle sprains are worse with use and eased by rest.

The other symptoms described by the patient may give essential clues to diagnosis. Bursae produce pain on activities which squeeze or compress them, e.g. lying on the side or sitting. Loose bodies tend to produce twinging pain and a sensation of giving way on weight-bearing. Arthritis tends to produce morning pain and stiffness due to accumulation of intracapsular swelling overnight (Hartley, 1995). Degenerative osteoarthrosis, in its early stage, often produces night pain. Unrelenting pain should be considered serious, especially if the patient is unwell with a fever, night sweats and rigors.

To determine if the pain is coming from the lumbar spine, the patient is questioned about the presence of paraesthesia and pain produced by a cough or sneeze.

An indication of *past medical history, other joint involvement* and *medications* may give a clue to diagnosis and will establish whether contraindications to treatment techniques exist. Patients should be asked about any unexpected recent weight loss, indicative of more serious lesions, such as secondary deposits which are common in the hip and pelvis (Paice, 1995).

Inspection

An inspection of the general posture, in weight-bearing, will indicate any *bony deformity* (Fig. 10.6a,b). Look for general postural asymmetry which may be relevant, the position of the buttock

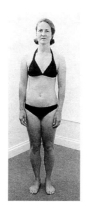

(a)

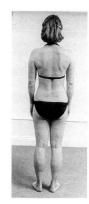

(b)

Fig. 10.6 (a, b) Inspection.

creases, posterior superior iliac spines, anterior superior iliac spines, level of the iliac crests, any leg length discrepancy and the position of the feet.

Colour changes and *swelling* are not expected at the hip because it is such a deep joint, but they may be associated with trauma, bruising and abrasions. If redness and swelling are present in the buttock area without a history of trauma, the 'sign of the buttock' (see page 305) may be suspected.

Muscle wasting may be seen in the glutei associated with a lumbar lesion, or in the quadriceps associated with degenerative osteoarthrosis of the hip or a lumbar lesion.

State at rest

Before any movements are performed, the state at rest is established to provide a baseline for subsequent comparison.

The suggested sequence for the objective examination will now be given, followed by a commentary including the reasoning in performing the movements and the significance of the possible findings.

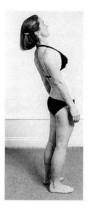

Fig. 10.7 Active extension.

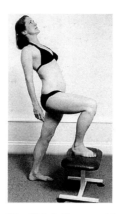

Fig. 10.8 Active extension with hip flexed to differentiate between hip and lumbar spine as the cause of pain.

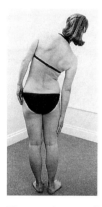

Fig. 10.9 Active right side flexion.

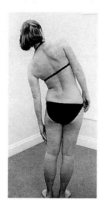

Fig. 10.10 Active left side flexion.

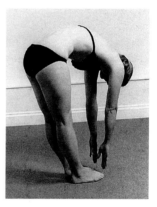

Fig. 10.11 Active flexion.

Examination by selective tension (objective examination)

Eliminate the lumbar spine:

- Active lumbar extension (Fig. 10.7)
- Extension repeated with foot on stool if necessary (Fig. 10.8)
- Active lumbar right side flexion (Fig. 10.9)
- Active lumbar left side flexion (Fig. 10.10)
- Active lumbar flexion (Fig. 10.11)

Supine lying:

- (Straight leg raise)
- Passive hip flexion (Fig. 10.12)

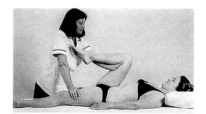

Fig. 10.12 Passive flexion.

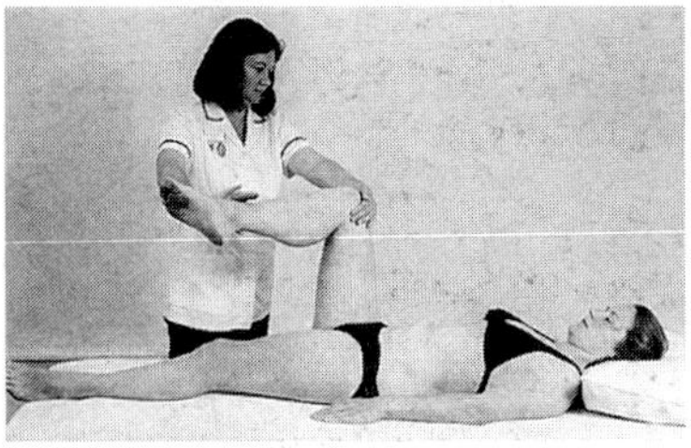

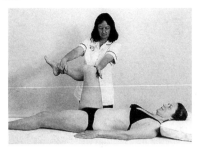

Fig. 10.13 Passive lateral rotation.

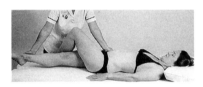

Fig. 10.14 Passive medial rotation.

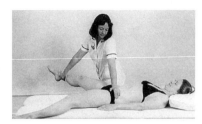

Fig. 10.15 Passive abduction.

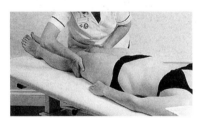

Fig. 10.16 Passive adduction.

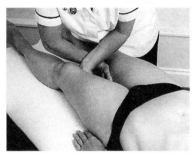

Fig. 10.17 Resisted flexion.

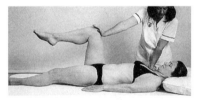

Fig. 10.18 Resisted abduction.

Fig. 10.19 Resisted adduction.

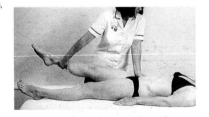

Fig. 10.20 Resisted extension.

- Passive hip lateral rotation (Fig. 10.13)
- Passive hip medial rotation for end-feel (Fig. 10.14)
- Passive hip abduction (Fig. 10.15)
- Passive hip adduction (Fig. 10.16)
- Resisted hip flexion (Fig. 10.17)
- Resisted hip abduction (Fig. 10.18)
- Resisted hip adduction (Fig. 10.19)
- Resisted hip extension (Fig. 10.20)

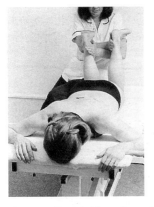

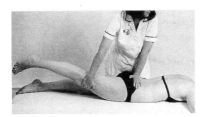

Fig. 10.21 Passive extension.

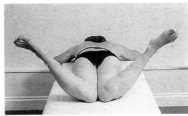

Fig. 10.22 Passive medial rotation.

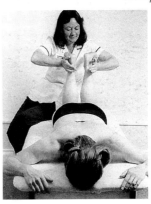

Fig. 10.23 Resisted medial rotation.

Fig. 10.24 Resisted lateral rotation.

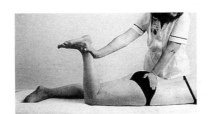

Fig. 10.25 Resisted knee flexion.

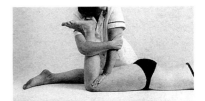

Fig. 10.26 Resisted knee extension.

Prone lying:

- Passive hip extension (Fig. 10.21)
- Passive hip medial rotation for range (Fig. 10.22)
- Resisted hip medial rotation (Fig. 10.23)
- Resisted hip lateral rotation (Fig. 10.24)
- Resisted knee flexion (Fig. 10.25)
- Resisted knee extension (Fig. 10.26)

Accessory test for the psoas bursa:

- Passive hip flexion and adduction (Fig. 10.27)

Palpation

- Once a diagnosis has been made, the structure at fault is palpated for the exact site of the lesion

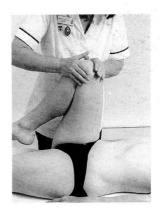

Fig. 10.27 Combined flexion and adduction to compress the psoas bursa.

The routine for the examination of the hip is conducted in the above order as it allows all tests in each position of standing, supine and prone to be completed.

The lumbar spine is first assessed by the four active movements. If active lumbar extension reproduces the pain, it should be repeated with the hip joint eliminated by placing the foot up on a stool. If extension is still painful, the lesion lies in the lumbar spine and a more thorough investigation of this must then be made.

If serious hip pathology is suspected and to clear the lumbar spine, a straight leg raise is included ('sign of the buttock' page 305). Tests for sacroiliac joint involvement may also be included at this stage, as indicated by the history, and are described in Chapter 14.

The passive hip movements test the inert structures for pain, range of movement and end-feel. Limited movement may be typical of the capsular pattern of limitation due to arthritis. Normally, passive flexion has a 'soft' end-feel whilst passive lateral rotation, medial rotation and extension have an 'elastic' end-feel. It is not possible to appreciate the end-feel of passive abduction and adduction. A bursitis or a loose body in the joint produces a non-capsular pattern of movement.

The resisted movements test the contractile structures for pain and power. At the hip, muscle lesions are commonly found in the adductors, quadriceps and hamstrings, but positive resisted tests may also be an accessory sign in bursitis. Resisted flexion tests mainly psoas, but since the knee is flexed it also tests rectus femoris. Resisted abduction tests mainly gluteus medius whilst resisted adduction tests the adductor muscles, particularly adductor longus. Resisted extension tests mainly gluteus maximus, but since the knee is extended, this also tests the hamstrings. Resisted rotations tests the medial and lateral rotators of the hip, resisted knee flexion tests the hamstring muscles and resisted knee extension tests the quadriceps muscle group.

An accessory test of combined hip flexion and adduction can be applied to compress the psoas bursa to confirm its diagnosis.

Capsular pattern of the hip joint:
• **Most limitation of medial rotation**
• **Limitation of flexion and abduction**
• **Limitation of extension**

Capsular lesions

The movements limited in the capsular pattern have a characteristically 'hard' end-feel. If, on examination, the capsular pattern exists at the hip joint then an arthritis is present. The hip can be affected by degenerative osteoarthrosis, traumatic arthritis, rheumatoid arthritis and any of the spondylarthropathies.

Arthritis at the hip is commonly primary degenerative osteoarthrosis, usually occurring in 50% of the population over the age of 60 (Kumar and Clark, 1994). It may be idiopathic or due to predisposing factors such as occupational overuse, old fractures or altered biomechanics, e.g. unequal leg length or congenital abnormality. Men and women are equally affected (Dieppe, 1995).

The pain of osteoarthrosis usually has a gradual onset and may be felt in the upper buttock, groin or referred to or beyond the knee. Pain is associated with activity in the early stages, but as the condition advances, pain is also present at rest. Joint stiffness and loss of movement such as difficulty in reaching to put on shoes and socks are also presenting factors. X-ray changes are not a good indicator of symptoms as joint pathology can be present long before symptoms present and vice versa.

After diagnosis the condition may stabilize and the prognosis can be good. However, patients referred for surgery usually have a fairly rapid deterioration and severe symptoms progress over a period of 1–2 years. It seems that osteoarthrosis progresses with periods of exacerbation and periods of remission (Dieppe, 1995).

Treatment for osteoarthrosis depends on the stage and activity of the disease. It can be divided into early, middle and late stages for the application of appropriate treatment.

Early stage osteoarthrosis of the hip

This is usually the initial phase of diagnosis of the condition. The patient complains of buttock or groin pain associated with weight-bearing activities and the pain sometimes disturbs sleep. On examination, the patient has a mild capsular pattern of limited medial rotation, flexion and perhaps abduction, with extension not yet affected. The limited movements have an abnormal 'hard' end-feel due to muscle spasm, but some elasticity remains. The principle of treatment, applied during this early stage, is to stretch the capsular adhesions using a Grade B capsular stretching technique in conjunction with heat applied to the joint. The aim of treatment is to relieve pain, allowing a greater range of painfree movement to be established.

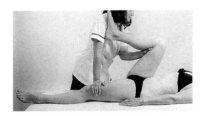

Fig. 10.28 Grade B mobilization, stretching flexion.

Grade B mobilization for early osteoarthrosis

The movements limited in the capsular pattern are stretched using Grade B mobilization. However, benefit is often gained by stretching only flexion.

To stretch flexion, position the patient in supine lying with counterpressure on the other leg to stabilize it and to ensure that maximum stretch is applied to the affected hip joint capsule (Fig. 10.28). Place one hand under the patient's lower thigh, to avoid involving the knee, and to give a little distraction, which makes the manoeuvre more comfortable. Place the patient's foot against your shoulder to assist with stretching and to help guide the movement.

To stretch extension, reverse the position described above for stretching flexion, with pressure applied to stretch extension of the affected leg (Fig. 10.29).

To stretch abduction, fix the good leg over the edge of the couch and position the affected leg in as much abduction as possible (Fig. 10.30). Increase this range of movement periodically.

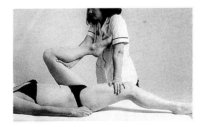

Fig. 10.29 Grade B mobilization, stretching extension.

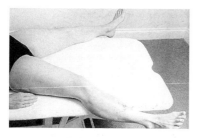

Fig. 10.30 Grade B mobilization, stretching abduction.

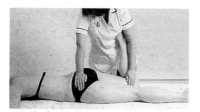

Fig. 10.31 Grade B mobilization, stretching medial rotation.

To stretch medial rotation, position the patient in prone lying with the knee flexed to 90°. Fix the opposite buttock and apply the pressure carefully to the medial aspect of the knee. Take care with this manoeuvre as it applies a strong torsion force to the neck of the femur and may also affect the knee (Fig. 10.31).

Treatment aims to provide symptomatic relief, but it relies on the patient continuing with a self-management programme.

Initially the patient is seen regularly to assess the effect of the capsular stretching and to teach the patient home management. Each treatment session of capsular stretching lasts 20–30 min and the patient should expect to feel some discomfort, as a general rule, for 2–4 h after treatment. Treatment continues until either a plateau is reached or patients are confident to continue with their own stretching exercises and management.

In this early stage of the disease the patient may experience anxiety over the diagnosis and possible prognosis. Treatment must also include education of the patient, reassurance to relieve anxiety and encouragement to empower the patient to manage the condition (Dieppe, 1995). Advice should be given about appropriate exercise, encouraging regular use and mobilization to prevent the further deterioration which immobilization would induce. A balance must be achieved between sufficient weight-bearing and rest, and avoiding prolonged overloading of the joint.

Although there is no evidence that diet changes the progressive nature of the disease, the overweight patient should be encouraged to lose weight. Obesity may increase the load on the weight-bearing surfaces, progressing the degenerative process more rapidly (Dieppe, 1995). Sticks and other walking support may be appropriate to aid daily living.

Although capsular stretching in the early stage may relieve pain and increase the range of movement, the patient may also require assistance from analgesics. Paracetomol and low-dose ibuprofen may be appropriate in the early stages of the disease (Dieppe, 1995). If non-steroidal anti-inflammatory drugs (NSAIDs) are needed to control pain, they should be prescribed for short periods of time during acute phases of the disease. The risks from NSAIDs are well-documented – gastrointestinal disturbance, renal insufficiency, and patients with osteoarthrosis fall into the older age group which is particularly susceptible to these side-effects (Dieppe, 1995; Rang *et al.*, 1995). Other forms of pain relief, such as acupuncture, may be effective (McIndoe *et al.*, 1995).

Middle stage osteoarthrosis of the hip

Here the patient's symptoms and signs indicate a progression of the disease. Pain may be present at rest as well as exacerbated by weight-bearing activities. On examination, a moderate to severe capsular pattern is found and the limited movements have a 'hard' end-feel. Capsular stretching may no longer provide benefit and the treatment of choice in the short term may be injection.

Injection of the hip joint (Cyriax and Cyriax, 1983; Cyriax, 1984)			
Adcortyl 10 mg/ml 4 ml	Total steroid 40 mg	Lignocaine 1% 1 ml	Total volume 5 ml
20G × 3½ in (0.9 × 90 mm) spinal needle			

Position the patient in side lying with the painful leg uppermost and supported in a neutral position on a pillow. Locate the greater trochanter by grasping it between thumb, index and middle fingers; the index finger should be resting on the top of the trochanter. To test you are in the correct position, move the leg passively into some abduction (Fig. 10.32), to relax the iliotibial tract, and you should feel your index finger sink in over the top of the trochanter.

The capsule of the hip joint almost completely surrounds the neck of the femur. By inserting the needle just above the index finger, i.e. above the greater trochanter, and aiming vertically downwards towards the neck of the femur, you will be intracapsular once you gently make contact with bone (Fig. 10.33). You will feel a resistance as the needle pierces first the fascia lata, then the capsule before reaching bone (Fig. 10.34). Deliver the injection as a bolus. The patient is advised to maintain a period of relative rest for approximately 2 weeks following injection.

Controversy exists concerning repeated steroid injections into weight-bearing joints and the risk of steroid arthropathy (Cameron, 1995). Therefore repeated corticosteroid injections into the hip joint are not recommended and no more than two a year should be given without monitoring the degenerative condition of the joint with X-ray investigation.

Late stage osteoarthrosis of the hip

Conservative management no longer controls the patient's pain and functional disability may now be serious. Surgery is probably indicated, but there are no agreed criteria or guidelines for electing to perform hip surgery (Dieppe, 1995). Pain, age and disability, as well as psychological factors, should all be taken into consideration by the patient and surgeon.

Injection may be given for pain relief during this stage, as described above.

Rheumatoid arthritis

This may affect the hip joint and symptomatic relief may be gained from intra-articular injection, given as described above.

Non-capsular lesions
Loose body

A loose body in the hip joint causes twinges of pain felt in the groin or radiating down the front of the leg. These twinges may be

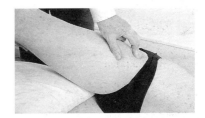

Fig. 10.32 Abducting the hip to locate the hip joint line.

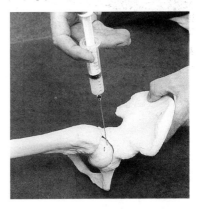

Fig. 10.33 Injection of the hip joint showing direction of approach and needle position.

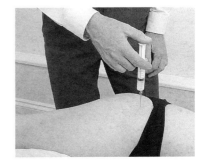

Fig. 10.34 Injection of the hip joint.

associated with a momentary sensation of giving way and an inability to weight-bear. This history suggests a loose body in the joint which periodically becomes impacted between the joint surfaces. The loose body may be associated with the rare condition osteochondritis dissecans in adolescents, but most commonly occurs secondarily to the onset of degenerative osteoarthrosis at the joint (Cyriax and Cyriax, 1983).

The diagnosis may rely solely on the history. If signs are present they consist of a non-capsular pattern, commonly with pain at the end of range of full passive hip flexion and lateral rotation. If the range of movement demonstrates limitation, a springy end-feel may be appreciated.

The principle of treatment applied is to reduce the loose body by strong traction together with Grade A mobilization. If successful, the loose body will be moved to a position within the joint where it no longer causes these typical symptoms.

Two mobilization techniques will be described (Cyriax and Cyriax, 1983; Cyriax, 1984).

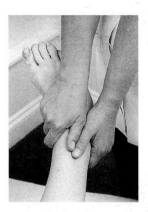

Fig. 10.35 Loose-body mobilization 1a for the hip, showing hand position for mobilization into medial rotation.

Loose-body mobilization technique 1

Position the patient in supine on the couch with an assistant applying counterpressure at the anterior superior iliac spines; padding may make it more comfortable for the patient. The assistant must start by applying pressure in an anterior–posterior direction and be prepared to change to apply cephalad pressure towards the end of the manoeuvre.

Your choice of manoeuvre with either lateral or medial rotation will depend on the physical findings during examination and the least painful rotation is attempted first: this is usually medial rotation.

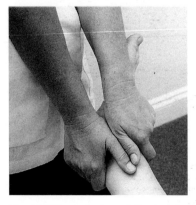

Fig. 10.36 Loose-body mobilization 1a for the hip, showing body positioning and assistant's counterpressure.

Mobilization 1a: with medial rotation
Stand on the end of the couch, with your feet close together and parallel to the edge. Face the direction of medial rotation and apply a butterfly grip with the thumbs parallel on the lateral aspect of the lower leg, taking care to avoid undue pressure around the malleoli (Fig. 10.35). The hands are wrapped comfortably around the talus and calcaneum to provide anchorage points and to pull the ankle into dorsiflexion, to prevent undue movement at the ankle joint.

Next, take your distal leg off the couch and lean out to apply traction with your elbows straight (Fig. 10.36). Maintain the traction throughout the rest of the manoeuvre, which is to rotate the patient's leg back and forth towards medial rotation whilst simultaneously stepping down off the couch, which automatically takes the hip from flexion, towards extension.

Re-examine the patient and decide on the next manoeuvre.

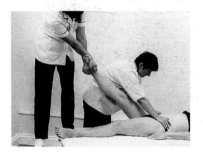

Fig. 10.37 Loose-body mobilization 1b for the hip, showing hand position for mobilization into lateral rotation.

Mobilization 1b: with lateral rotation
The manoeuvre is exactly the same as that described above, but in reverse.

Face the movement of lateral rotation and rotate the patient's leg under strong traction, back and forth towards lateral rotation (Figs 10.37 and 10.38).

> **Loose-body mobilization technique 2 (Cyriax and Cyriax, 1983; Cyriax, 1984)**

Mobilization 2a: with medial rotation
Position the patient in supine on the couch. An assistant applies counterpressure to the anterior superior iliac spines; padding may make it more comfortable for the patient (Fig. 10.39). Alternatively a seat belt can be used to maintain the patient's position on the couch.

Put your foot up on the couch, beside the patient's buttock. Flex the patient's knee so that the crook of their knee (popliteal fossa) is placed over your thigh (Fig. 10.40). Take care to avoid pressure on the gastrocnemius muscle as it is uncomfortable.

Place one hand on the lateral aspect of the patient's knee and the other on the medial aspect of the patient's ankle. Apply traction by plantarflexing your foot on the couch to lift the patient's leg (the assistant maintaining counterpressure), whilst simultaneously pushing down on the patient's ankle. Maintain this traction as you rotate the patient's leg sharply towards medial rotation, using the patient's leg as a lever.

Re-examine the patient and decide on the next manoeuvre.

Mobilization 2b: with lateral rotation
The manoeuvre is exactly the same as that described above, but reverse the hand positions to enable the patient's leg to be sharply rotated towards lateral rotation.

Bursitis

Psoas or gluteal bursitis may be a cause of pain at the hip, although they are difficult to diagnose definitively and may be overlooked. Both present a muddled clinical picture and may be misdiagnosed as a tendinitis. However, because of the close anatomical relationship of bursae to tendons, bursitis may coexist with tendinitis.

The patient commonly presents with a gradual onset of pain, often with no obvious cause. Although it is possible to induce a bursitis by direct trauma, it is usually the result of overuse activity, with the pain increased by activity and better for rest.

On examination a muddled clinical picture emerges of a non-capsular pattern with some resisted tests and some passive tests

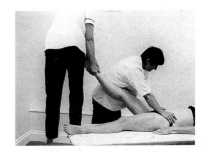
Fig. 10.38 Loose-body mobilization 1b for the hip, showing body positioning and assistant's counterpressure.

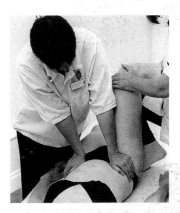
Fig. 10.39 Loose-body mobilization 2a for the hip, showing assistant's hand position.

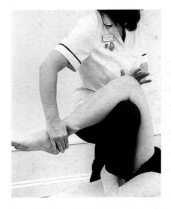
Fig. 10.40 Loose-body mobilization 2a of the hip, showing application of traction before the thrust into medial rotation.

reproducing the pain. This clinical picture may mimic that of tendinitis. Tendinitis usually produces a predictable clinical picture of pain on the appropriate resisted test and pain on passive stretching in the opposite direction. In contrast, a bursitis may produce pain when passively squeezed under a contracted muscle or tendon and thus this muddle emerges.

Psoas bursitis

Psoas bursitis commonly produces a local groin pain, but can cause pain to be referred into the L3 dermatome. It has a gradual onset of pain with the patient unable to recall the precipitating factors. It may be associated with overuse or repetitive movements and be exacerbated by hip flexion movements, e.g. bending to put on shoes and socks, rising from sitting with hips flexed, walking up stairs or hills, brisk walking, jogging or kicking (Broadhurst, 1995b). The pain may produce a shortened gait stride and, through underuse, a secondary capsulitis.

Primary effusion of the bursa is possible, but its communication with the hip joint makes it a reservoir for joint effusion. Therefore psoas bursitis is often associated with hip joint involvement, especially rheumatoid arthritis (Armstrong and Saxton, 1972; Meaney *et al.*, 1992).

On examination, a non-capsular pattern exists with a combination of passive hip flexion and adduction, squeezing the bursa and producing pain, which may be used as a comparable sign. Other signs could include pain on passive lateral rotation, passive extension and resisted flexion of the hip. However, clinically, resisted flexion is usually found to be painfree (Cyriax, 1982).

Some enlarged bursae have been reported to produce a palpable mass in the groin, causing extrinsic pressure on adjacent neurovascular structures (Underwood *et al.*, 1988; Toohey *et al.*, 1990; Meaney *et al.*, 1992). On diagnostic scanning these enlarged bursae have been shown to contain solid components consisting of various debris, e.g. cellular debris, osteocartilaginous plaques, fibrin, clot and calcium deposits (Meaney *et al.*, 1992).

Differential diagnosis should exclude other hip joint pathology and lumbar spine involvement, as well as 'Gilmore's groin'. Gilmore's groin is a disruption of the external oblique aponeurosis causing dilatation of the superficial inguinal ring, torn conjoined tendon and dehiscence between the inguinal ligament and torn conjoined tendon. It presents as a gradual onset of groin pain in athletes, particularly footballers. The pain is increased by sporting activity, on getting out of bed, especially the day after a game, and on sudden movement, e.g. sprinting or coughing. On examination there are no physical findings. Diagnosis is made by the examining doctor, inverting the scrotum and examining the superficial inguinal ring. On the symptomatic side the ring is dilated and tender and there may be a cough impulse. This condition requires surgical repair (Gilmore, 1995).

Injection of the psoas bursa (Cyriax and Cyriax, 1983; Cyriax, 1984)

Adcortyl 10 mg/ml 2 ml	Total steroid 20 mg	Procaine 0.5%* 8 ml	Total volume 10 ml

* 0.5% lignocaine can be substituted.

$20G \times 3\frac{1}{2}$ in $(0.9 \times 90$ mm) spinal needle

---

Treatment for psoas bursitis is a large-volume, low-dose local anaesthetic plus an appropriate amount of steroid.

Position the patient in supine on the couch. Locate the psoas bursa by palpating for the femoral pulse just distal to the mid-point of the inguinal ligament. This is the surface marking point for the position of the psoas bursa; mark this point. Move approximately 5 cm laterally and 5 cm distally, marking both of these points. If you draw an imaginary line to connect these three points you will form an inverted right-angled triangle. This now gives you the angle of insertion which is to follow the direction of the hypotenuse, aiming to pass deeply, in order to traverse under the neurovascular bundle in the femoral triangle, to reach the deeply located psoas bursa (Fig. 10.41).

Once the needle tip makes contact with bone it should be located in the region of the hip joint anteriorly. Withdraw it slightly into the overlying psoas bursa and inject at this point. It may be possible to inject as a bolus but, more commonly, a peppering technique is required to cover the extent of this large bursa, fanning out to cover an area approximately the size of a golf ball (Cyriax and Cyriax, 1983). The patient is advised to maintain a period of relative rest for approximately 2 weeks following injection.

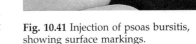

Fig. 10.41 Injection of psoas bursitis, showing surface markings.

Gluteal and trochanteric bursitis

Gluteal bursitis involves inflammation of the bursae associated with the gluteal muscles and the greater trochanter.

The cause is occasionally traumatic through direct injury (Haller *et al.*, 1989), but more commonly due to overuse through occupational or sporting activities. It may be associated with a tight iliotibial band where the bursa may be irritated by direct friction (Norris, 1993), or secondary to altered biomechanics of gait, leg length discrepancy, low back pain or sacroiliac dysfunction (Collée *et al.*, 1991; Caruso and Toney, 1994). It is common in obese, middle-aged females (Rasmussen and Fano, 1985; Allwright *et al.*, 1988; Gerber and Herrin, 1994).

The pain is usually a diffuse ache or burning pain felt in the buttock, over the lateral aspect of the hip or referred down the lateral aspect of the leg. According to Little (1979), patients who have suffered a tennis elbow associate a similar sort of pain and tenderness to that of gluteal bursitis.

Aggravating factors are walking, climbing stairs, standing for prolonged periods, crossing the legs in sitting and lying on the affected side.

On examination the typical muddled clinical picture of bursitis emerges with some or all of the following involved: a non-capsular pattern of pain on passive hip flexion, abduction and lateral rotation as the bursa is squeezed – these movements in combination may be positive (FABER test). Resisted abduction or resisted extension may produce the pain as the bursa is compressed by the contraction of adjacent muscles (Little, 1979; Cyriax and Cyriax, 1983).

Karpinski and Piggott (1985) suggested a greater trochanteric pain syndrome, to cover all symptoms of pain and tenderness felt at the greater trochanter, in association with pain on resisted abduction.

Palpation will reveal which area of the gluteal bursa is involved in the lesion. This may be above or behind the greater trochanter (gluteal bursa) or, more commonly clinically, the area over the superolateral aspect of the greater trochanter, the trochanteric bursa of gluteus maximus. Care should be taken in palpation, to compare with the unaffected side, as trigger points are commonly found in the buttock, which can be misleading.

Once diagnosis is established, the treatment of choice is an injection of low-dose, large-volume local anaesthetic with an appropriate amount of corticosteroid.

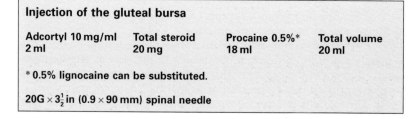

Injection of the gluteal bursa

Adcortyl 10 mg/ml 2 ml	Total steroid 20 mg	Procaine 0.5%* 18 ml	Total volume 20 ml

* 0.5% lignocaine can be substituted.

20G × 3½ in (0.9 × 90 mm) spinal needle

There are two possible approaches and it is important to recognize the depth of the lesion as the gluteal bursa lies in several different planes.

Lateral approach
Position the patient in prone or side lying and identify the position of the greater trochanter (Figs 10.42 and 10.43). Identify the full extent of the area of tenderness, usually over the superoposterior aspect of the greater trochanter, and envisage the position of the sciatic nerve in the buttock so that it can be avoided.

Insert the needle deeply into the centre of the area of tenderness. Deliver the injection using a peppering technique to cover the extent of the lesion, but also slowly withdraw the needle from deep to superficial, so that a series of droplets is deposited throughout all planes of the bursal area, fanning out to cover an area approximately the size of a tennis ball (Cyriax and Cyriax, 1983).

Vertical approach
A deep lesion of the gluteal bursa may produce symptoms on passive abduction as the bursal area is squeezed against the ilium (Cyriax and Cyriax, 1983). A deeper injection approach is possible

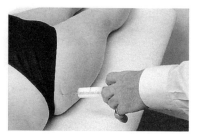

Fig. 10.42 Injection of the gluteal bursa, lateral approach in prone lying.

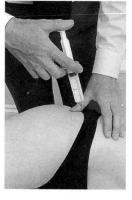

Fig. 10.43 Injection of the gluteal bursa, lateral approach in side lying.

by positioning the patient in prone with the leg supported over the edge of the couch (Fig. 10.44).

Locate the area of tenderness and insert the needle vertically until bone is reached. As the needle is withdrawn, pepper the bursal area with droplets of steroid, fanning out to ensure complete coverage from deep to superficial, again approximately the size of a tennis ball. There should be little resistance to the injection.

The patient is advised to maintain a period of relative rest for approximately 2 weeks following injection.

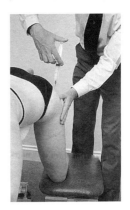

Fig. 10.44 Injection of the gluteal bursa, vertical approach.

Injection of the trochanteric bursa

Adcortyl 10 mg/ml 2 ml	Total steroid 20 mg	Lignocaine 1% 1–3 ml	Total volume 3–5 ml

$21G \times 1\frac{1}{2}$ in (0.8 × 40 mm) or $21G \times 2$ in (0.8 × 50 mm) green needle

---

Position the patient comfortably in side lying and palpate for the area of tenderness over the superolateral aspect of the greater trochanter where gluteus maximus inserts into the iliotibial tract. Deliver the injection by a peppering technique, covering the area of tenderness. The patient is advised to maintain a period of relative rest for approximately 2 weeks following injection.

Ischial bursitis

An ischial bursitis (weaver's bottom) involves the ischial bursa of gluteus maximus. It produces pain on prolonged sitting, especially on hard surfaces; the pain is relieved by standing. Pain may be reproduced near the end of range of the straight leg raise (Broadhurst, 1995a). It is a rare cause of buttock pain but the principles of treatment can be applied.

Complicated bursitis

Septic bursitis has been described, more commonly occurring in the olecranon and prepatellar bursae, where *Staphylococcus aureus* was the common organism (Hoppmann, 1993; Zimmermann *et al.*, 1995). A case of tuberculosis of the greater trochanter bursa has also been described (Rehm-Graves *et al.*, 1983). Trochanteric bursitis has been reported as a cause of hip pain associated with rheumatoid arthritis (Raman and Haslock, 1982). Pain referred from the lumbar spine may produce a similar pattern of signs and symptoms to that of gluteal bursitis and has been described as pseudotrochanteric bursitis (Traycoff, 1991). Occasionally bursitis may be complicated by calcification, making it resistant to normal conservative management (Gerber and Herrin, 1994).

Sign of the buttock

The sign of the buttock is pain produced on straight leg raise which increases on flexing the knee and hip (Cyriax and Cyriax, 1983).

An empty end-feel is appreciated as more range of movement is available, but any attempt to produce more hip flexion is abruptly stopped by voluntary muscle spasm.

A positive sign indicates a major lesion in the buttock or hip region. The history will usually reveal an unwell patient, who looks ill and may have a fever with night sweats and rigors. The pain may be unrelenting in the buttock, hip or leg. It is not eased by rest and therefore night pain is a feature.

On examination, a non-capsular pattern of movement at the hip, and often the lumbar spine, is discovered. Pain may be increased by lumbar flexion and resisted tests at the hip, but the cardinal feature of this condition is the positive sign of the buttock.

Possible causes of the sign of the buttock are neoplasm of the upper femur or ilium, fracture of the sacrum, ischiorectal abscess, sepsis, either septic bursitis or arthritis, or osteomyelitis of the upper femur (Cyriax and Cyriax, 1983). Urgent medical attention and further investigation are required.

Contractile lesions

The mode of onset of contractile lesions around the hip may be sudden through strain, gradual through overuse or traumatic through direct injury, causing muscle contusion. Lesions commonly affect the hamstrings, quadriceps and adductor longus muscles. Less common lesions of the psoas and sartorius are not described, although the principles of diagnosis and treatment would equally apply to any muscle lesion in the region.

Hamstrings

The hamstrings act to extend the hip and flex the knee and commonly present as strained, perhaps due to their relative weakness in comparison to the quadriceps (Sutton, 1984). As two-joint muscles, they are susceptible to injury, because there is a greater potential for overuse.

The onset is usually sudden, e.g. a sudden stretch or a rapid contraction against resistance such as the ballistic action of sprinting. Precipitating factors include altered posture, poor condition, inadequate warm-up and fatigue (Sutton, 1984; Worrell, 1994). The patient may report tightness or pain in the posterior thigh some time before the acute onset. Gradual onset due to overuse is possible, but chronic hamstring strain is more commonly the result of a previous acute episode which may have healed during a period of relative immobilization. Consequent tightness or shortening of the muscle belly makes it vulnerable.

On examination the patient has pain on resisted knee flexion and pain on passive straight leg raising. In most clinic situations, testing for hamstring strain is conducted statically in a non-weight-bearing position. In reality they function and are most often injured in dynamic weight-bearing situations. This is an important point to remember for full rehabilitation of any muscle lesion in the region.

Palpation reveals the site of the lesion, with muscle belly strains commonly occurring deeply in the mid-thigh region. Chonic overuse strain occurs at the origin from the ischial tuberosity. Treatment of the origin may be by deep transverse friction massage or injection.

Transverse friction massage of the origin of the hamstrings

Position the patient in prone lying with the knee supported over the edge of the bed on a stool (Fig. 10.45). This places the hip and knee into flexion and exposes the ischial tuberosity by bringing it out from under the lower border of gluteus maximus. Apply friction massage by using one thumb reinforced with the other, directed firstly up against the ischial tuberosity and then transversely across the fibres (Fig. 10.46). Start gently, then apply deep friction massage for 10 min after the numbing effect is achieved. Relative rest is advised where functional movements may continue, but no overuse or stretching until the muscle is painfree on resisted testing.

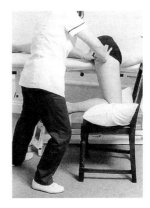

Fig. 10.45 Transverse friction massage of the origin of the hamstrings.

Injection of the origin of the hamstrings

Kenalog 40 mg/ml	Total steroid	Lignocaine 1%	Total volume
0.5 ml	20 mg	1 ml	1.5 ml

23G × 1 in (0.6 × 25 mm) blue needle (or as appropriate for the patient)

Use the position adopted for transverse friction massage of the hamstrings origin. Locate the area of tenderness over the ischial tuberosity and insert the needle perpendicular to it (Fig. 10.47). Deliver the injection by a peppering technique into the teno-osseous junction. The patient is advised to maintain a period of relative rest for approximately 2 weeks following injection.

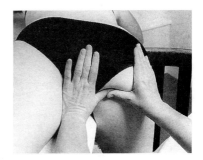

Fig. 10.46 Transverse friction massage of the origin of the hamstrings, showing hand position.

Transverse friction massage of acute muscle belly

In the first 3–5 days following injury rest, ice, compression and elevation are used to control the early inflammatory phase. Treatment is conducted on a daily basis and transverse friction massage is applied gently to maintain the muscle belly function. Position the patient in prone lying with the knee flexed, to place the muscle belly in the shortened position; this allows the muscle fibres to be moved transversely by the friction massage (Fig. 10.48). Apply the transverse friction massage gently and, once some numbing effect has been achieved, apply approximately six deeper sweeps. Follow this immediately with Grade A mobilization, encouraging an active muscle contraction within the painfree range

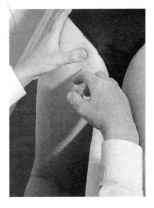

Fig. 10.47 Injection of the origin of the hamstrings.

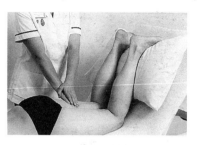

Fig. 10.48 Transverse friction massage of the hamstring muscle bellies.

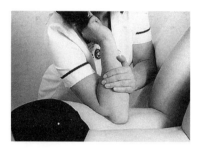

Fig. 10.49 Transverse friction massage of the hamstring muscle bellies, alternative technique (chronic).

to broaden the fibres. Teach the patient to use a normal heel–toe gait, with the aid of crutches if necessary.

After approximately 5 days the depth of friction massage and the range of Grade A mobilizations can be increased until a full range of painfree movement is achieved. Treating an acute muscle belly lesion in this way should avoid shortening of the muscle fibres and the need to apply stretching techniques.

| **Transverse friction massage of chronic muscle belly** |

Apply the transverse friction massage with the muscle belly in a relaxed position and once the numbing effect is achieved, apply deeper friction massage for 10 min (Fig. 10.49). Follow this with vigorous Grade A exercises to maintain the mobility gained.

It is important that the hamstrings are not undertreated and, to prevent recurrence of symptoms, friction massage should be continued for 1 week after cessation of symptoms. If the muscle is tight, traditional stretches can be applied once the resisted tests are painfree.

Rehabilitation following hamstring lesions

In either the acute or chronic situations, once the hamstrings have been rendered painfree by transverse friction massage and Grade A mobilizations, a full rehabilitation programme can be implemented, including stretching to lengthen the muscle if appropriate. Attention should be paid to the dynamic rather than the static function of the hamstrings. Weight-bearing activities and rehabilitation under speed are important considerations (Coole and Gieck, 1987).

Quadriceps

The mechanism of injury of the quadriceps is similar to that of the hamstrings and the principles of treatment and rehabilitation can be applied in much the same way. The patient presents with anterior thigh pain, pain on resisted knee extension and pain on resisted hip flexion (if rectus femoris is involved). As a two-joint muscle, rectus femoris is the most susceptible to injury. Palpation reveals the site of the lesion, which may be at the tendon of rectus femoris from the anterior inferior iliac spine, or in the belly of the muscle, usually mid-thigh (see Chapter 11).

| **Transverse friction massage of the origin of rectus femoris (Cyriax and Cyriax, 1983; Cyriax, 1984)** |

Position the patient in half lying to allow the hip flexors to relax. Locate the origin of rectus femoris and apply two fingers to the tendon (Fig. 10.50). Push down on to the tendon and apply transverse friction massage across the fibres. Since the lesion is usually chronic, 10 min friction massage is applied after the numbing effect is achieved. Relative rest is advised where functional movements may continue, but no overuse or stretching until the muscle is painfree on resisted testing.

Adductor longus

Adductor longus is the most common adductor muscle to be strained. It is sometimes known as a 'rider's strain' due to overuse of adductor longus in working a horse whilst riding.

The patient has groin or medial thigh pain, with pain on resisted adduction and passive abduction. The lesion is in one of two sites – either the origin from the pubis or the musculotendinous junction. Treatment of the origin is either by transverse friction massage or injection. The musculotendinous junction responds well to transverse friction massage and injection is not usually necessary.

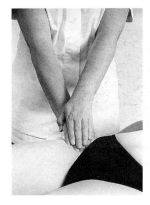

Fig. 10.50 Transverse friction massage of the origin of rectus femoris.

> ### Transverse friction massage of adductor longus

Teno-osseous site
Position the patient in supine with the leg in a degree of abduction and lateral rotation, supported on a pillow. With an index finger reinforced by the middle finger, locate the area of tenderness at the teno-osseous junction. Apply the friction massage firstly in a direction down on to the bone, then transversely across the fibres, for 10 min after numbing. This may be an embarrassing treatment for the patient and it may be more appropriate to teach patients to do the friction massage themselves.

Musculotendinous site
Position the patient as above and locate the area of tenderness at the musculotendinous junction. The friction may be imparted by a pinching manoeuvre (Fig. 10.51) (Cyriax and Cyriax, 1983; Cyriax, 1984), or by pressure directed firstly down against the tendon and then transversely across the fibres (Fig. 10.52). Apply the friction massage for 10 min after numbing.

Relative rest is advised where functional movements may continue, but no overuse or stretching until the muscle is painfree on resisted testing.

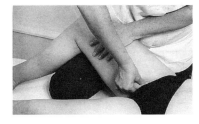

Fig. 10.51 Transverse friction massage of adductor longus, musculotendinous site.

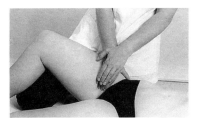

Fig. 10.52 Transverse friction massage of adductor longus, musculotendinous site, alternative hand position.

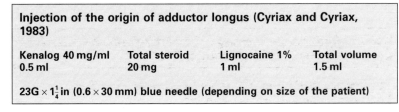

Injection of the origin of adductor longus (Cyriax and Cyriax, 1983)			
Kenalog 40 mg/ml 0.5 ml	**Total steroid** 20 mg	**Lignocaine 1%** 1 ml	**Total volume** 1.5 ml

$23G \times 1\frac{1}{4}$ in $(0.6 \times 30$ mm) blue needle (depending on size of the patient)

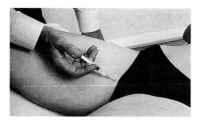

Fig. 10.53 Injection of the origin of adductor longus.

Position the patient as for the transverse friction massage (Fig. 10.53). Insert the needle into the origin of adductor longus, which is situated in the angle between the symphysis and the crest. Once in the teno-osseous junction and in contact with bone, deliver the injection by the peppering technique. The patient is advised to maintain a period of relative rest for approximately 2 weeks following injection.

References

Allwright, S.J., Cooper, R.A., Nash, P. (1988) Trochanteric bursitis: bone scan appearance. *Clinical Nuclear Medicine* **13**: 561–564.

Armstrong, P., Saxton, H. (1972) Ilio-psoas bursa. *British Journal of Rheumatology* **45**: 493–495.

Broadhurst, N. (1995a) Ischial bursitis. *Australian Family Physician* **24**: 1121.

Broadhurst, N. (1995b) Iliopsoas tendinitis and bursitis. *Australian Family Physician* **24**: 1303.

Cailliet, R. (1990) *Soft Tissue Pain and Disability*, 2nd edn. F.A. Davis.

Cameron, G. (1995) Steroid arthropathy – myth or reality? *Journal of Orthopaedic Medicine* **17**: 51–55.

Canoso, J.J. (1981) Bursae, tendons and ligaments. *Clinics in Rheumatic Diseases* **7**: 189–221.

Caruso, F.A., Toney, M.A.O. (1994) Trochanteric bursitis – a case report of plain film, scintigraphic and MRI correlation. *Clinical Nuclear Medicine* **19**: 393–395.

Collée, G., Dijkmans, B.A.C., Vandenbroucke, J.P., Cats, A. (1991) Greater trochanteric pain syndrome (trochanteric bursitis) in low back pain. *Scandinavian Journal of Rheumatology* **20**: 262–266.

Coole, W., Gieck, J.H. (1987) An analysis of hamstring strains and their rehabilitation. *Journal of Orthopaedic and Sports Physical Therapy* **9**: 77–85.

Cyriax, J. (1982) *Textbook of Orthopaedic Medicine*, vol. 1, 8th edn. Baillière Tindall.

Cyriax, J. (1984) *Textbook of Orthopaedic Medicine*, vol. 2, 11th edn. Baillière Tindall.

Cyriax, J., Cyriax, P. (1983) *Illustrated Manual of Orthopaedic Medicine*. Butterworths.

Dieppe, P. (1995) Management of hip osteoarthritis. *British Medical Journal* **311**: 853–857.

Flanagan, F.L., Sant, S., Coughlan, R.J., O'Connell, D. (1995) Symptomatic enlarged iliopsoas bursae in the presence of a normal plain hip radiograph. *British Society for Rheumatology* **34**: 365–369.

Gerber, J.M., Herrin, S.O. (1994) Conservative management of calcific trochanteric bursitis. *Journal of Manipulative and Physiological Therapeutics* **17**: 250–252.

Gilmore, O.J.A. (1995) Gilmore's groin. *Physiotherapy in Sport* **18**: 14–15.

Haller, C.C., Coleman, P.A., Estes, N.C., Grisolia, A. (1989) Traumatic trochanteric bursitis. *Kansas Medicine* **Jan**: 17–22.

Hartley, A. (1995) *Practical Joint Assessment – Lower Quadrant*, 2nd edn. Mosby.

Hoppmann, R.A. (1993) Diagnosis and management of common tendinitis and bursitis syndromes. *Journal of South Carolina Medical Association* **Nov**: 531–535.

Kapandji, I.A. (1970) *The Physiology of the Joints, Lower Limb*, vol. 2, 2nd edn. Churchill Livingstone.

Karpinski, M.R.K., Piggott, H. (1985) Greater trochanteric pain syndrome. *Journal of Bone and Joint Surgery* **67-B**: 762–763.

Kumar, P., Clark, M. (1994) *Clinical Medicine*, 3rd edn. Baillière Tindall.

Little, H. (1979) Trochanteric bursitis: a common cause of pelvic girdle pain. *Canadian Medical Association Journal* **120**: 456–458.

McIndoe, A.K., Young, K., Bone, M.E. (1995) A comparison of acupuncture with intra-articular steroid injection as analgesia for osteoarthritis of the hip. *Acupuncture in Medicine* **13**: 67–70.

Meaney, J.F., Cassar-Pullicino, V.N., Ethrington, R. *et al.* (1992) Ilio-psoas bursa enlargement. *Clinical Radiology* **45**: 161–168.

Norris, C.M. (1993) *Sports Injuries: Diagnosis and Management for Physiotherapists.* Butterworth-Heinemann.

Paice, E. (1995) Pain in the hip and knee. *British Medical Journal* **310**: 319–322.

Raman, D., Haslock, I. (1982) Trochanteric bursitis – a frequent cause of 'hip' pain in rheumatoid arthritis. *Annals of the Rheumatic Diseases* **41**: 602–603.

Rang, H.P., Dale, M.M., Ritter, J.M. (1995) *Pharmacology,* 3rd edn. Churchill Livingstone.

Rasmussen K.-J.E., Fano, N. (1985) Trochanteric bursitis: treatment by corticosteroid injection. *Scandinavian Journal of Rheumatology* **14**: 417–420.

Rehm-Graves, S., Weinstein, A.J., Calabrese, L.H. *et al.* (1983) Tuberculosis of the greater trochanter bursa. *Arthritis and Rheumatism* **26**: 77–81.

Sutton, G. (1984) Hamstrung by hamstring strains: a review of the literature. *Journal of Orthopaedics and Sports Physical Therapy* **5**: 184–195.

Toohey, A.K., LaSalle, T.L., Martinez, S., Polisson, R.P. (1990) Iliopsoas bursitis: clinical features, radiographic findings, and disease associations. *Seminars in Arthritis and Rheumatism* **20**: 41–47.

Traycoff, R.B. (1991) 'Psuedotrochanteric bursitis': the differential diagnosis of lateral hip pain. *Journal of Rheumatology* **18**: 1810–1812.

Underwood, P.L., McLeod, R.A., Ginsburg, W.W. (1988) The varied clinical manifestations of iliopsoas bursitis. *Journal of Rheumatology* **15**: 1683–1685.

Williams, P.L, Warwick, R., Dyson, M., Bannister, L.H. (1989) *Gray's Anatomy,* 37th edn. Churchill Livingstone.

Worrell, T.W. (1994) Factors associated with hamstring injuries – an approach to treatment and preventative measures. *Sports Medicine* **17**: 338–345.

Zimmermann, B., Mikolich, D.J., Ho, G. (1995) Septic bursitis. *Seminars in Arthritis and Rheumatism* **24**: 391–410.

11 The knee

Summary

Knee injuries are largely in the province of sport and developments in arthroscopic techniques have done much to facilitate diagnosis and repair. Initial diagnosis is crucial to appropriate management, particularly of the ligamentous and contractile lesions.

This chapter presents the anatomy of the knee relating to commonly encountered lesions. The commentary which follows explores the relevant points of history, aiding diagnosis, and the suggested method of objective examination adheres to the principles of selective tension. The lesions, their treatment and management are then discussed.

Anatomy

Inert structures

The lower end of the femur consists of two large femoral condyles which articulate with, and transfer weight to, corresponding surfaces on the tibial condyles at the tibiofemoral joint. The two femoral condyles are separated posteriorly and inferiorly by the intercondylar notch or fossa. The anterior aspect of the femur bears an articular surface for the patella to form the patellofemoral joint.

The lateral femoral epicondyle gives attachment to the proximal end of the *lateral (fibular) collateral ligament*. Below this lies a smooth groove which contains the tendon of popliteus in full flexion of the knee. The medial femoral condyle displays a prominent *adductor tubercle* on the medial supracondylar line and just below this the medial epicondyle gives origin to the *medial (tibial) collateral ligament*. Posteriorly the heads of gastrocnemius originate from the femoral condyles.

The tibia has an expanded upper end which posteriorly overhangs the shaft. The upper weight-bearing surface bears two shallow tibial condyles divided by the intercondylar area. Below the posterolateral tibial condyle lies an oval facet for articulation with the head of the fibula at the *superior (proximal) tibiofibular joint*. Anteriorly lies the prominent *tibial tuberosity* which gives insertion to the ligamentum patellae. *Gerdy's tubercle* lies anterolaterally and marks the insertion of the iliotibial tract (Kapandji, 1970; Burks, 1990).

The upper end of the fibula is expanded to form the head, which articulates with the tibia on its superomedial side, at the superior tibiofibular joint. The apex of the head of the fibula gives attachment to the lateral collateral ligament and the biceps femoris tendon. The common peroneal nerve winds round the neck of the fibula.

The *patella*, the largest sesamoid bone in the body, lies within the quadriceps tendon and articulates with the lower end of the femur at the *patellofemoral joint*. It is a flat triangular-shaped bone with its base uppermost and apex pointing inferiorly. It has anterior and posterior surfaces and upper, medial and lateral borders. Its anterior surface shows vertical ridges produced by fibres of the quadriceps which pass over it. This surface is separated from the skin by the subcutaneous *prepatellar bursa*.

Rectus femoris and vastus intermedius insert into the base of the patella, and the roughened posterior aspect of the apex gives attachment to the proximal end of the *ligamentum patellae*. Just proximal to this lies the infrapatellar fat pad. A subcutaneous *infrapatellar bursa* lies between the tibial tuberosity and the skin; a *deep infrapatellar bursa* lies between the ligamentum patellae and the underlying tibia.

The vastus medialis and lateralis muscles send tendinous insertions to the medial and lateral borders of the patella in the form of *quadriceps expansions*, or the *patella retinacula*. The lateral expansion receives a distinct extension from the iliotibial tract and the quadriceps expansions together are responsible for transverse stability of the patella.

The posterior articulating surface of the patella is covered with thick articular cartilage which is divided by a vertical ridge into medial and lateral articular facets for articulation with the femur, with an 'odd' facet on the medial side.

The knee joint consists of the tibiofemoral, patellofemoral and superior tibiofibular joints. The former two articulations exist within the same capsule but each has a different function:

- Tibiofemoral joint: involved in weight-bearing activities.
- Patellofemoral joint: the joint of the extensor mechanism of the knee.

The *tibiofemoral joint* is a synovial hinge joint between the convex condyles of the femur and the slightly concave articular surfaces of the tibia. Mobility is not normally compatible with stability in a joint, but the incongruent joint surfaces of the knee make it a mobile joint and the shape of the articular surfaces, the interaction of muscles, tendons and strong ligaments all contribute to stability.

Two semilunar cartilages, *the menisci*, deepen the tibial articulating surface and contribute to the congruency of the joint. The menisci facilitate load transmission, shock absorption, lubrication and stability (Bessette, 1992). The peripheral rim of each meniscus is attached to deep fibres of the capsule which secure it to the edge of the tibial condyles. These deep capsular fibres are known as the *meniscotibial* or *coronary ligaments* (*corona* Latin = around). They are strong, but lax enough to allow axial rotation to occur at the meniscotibial surface. The lateral coronary ligaments are longer than the medial to allow for the greater excursion of the lateral meniscus (Burks, 1990).

The menisci are composed of collagen fibres. The superficial collagen fibres are oriented radially and the deep fibres are circumferential (Bessette, 1992). Injury usually involves rotational strains and may result in longitudinal or transverse splitting of the fibrocartilage, or separation of the thinner inner part of the meniscus from the thicker outer portion, forming a 'bucket handle' lesion.

The *medial meniscus* is the larger of the two and is almost semicircular in shape. Its periphery has a definite attachment to the deep part of the medial collateral ligament, which forms part of the fibrous capsule of the knee joint. The *lateral meniscus* is almost circular but it is separated from the capsule of the knee joint at its periphery by the tendon of popliteus, from which it receives fibres. Posteriorly, the lateral meniscus contributes a ligamentous slip to the posterior cruciate ligament, known as the *posterior meniscofemoral ligament*.

The fibrous capsule of the knee joint is strongly supplemented by expansions from the tendons that cross it, plus ligamentous thickenings and independent ligamentous reinforcements. The medial collateral ligament, in particular, provides a strong integral reinforcement of the capsule, attaching also to the medial meniscus. The anterior capsule is reinforced by the quadriceps expansions and an extension from the iliotibial band. Independent ligaments such as the lateral collateral ligament and cruciates also have a strong stabilizing effect on the joint.

The cylindrical *fibrous capsule* is invaginated posteriorly and lined with synovial membrane. The synovium is reflected upwards anteriorly under the quadriceps, approximately three fingers' breadth, to form the *suprapatellar bursa*. The articularis genu muscle connects vastus intermedius and the upper part of the suprapatellar bursa, maintaining the bursal cavity during extension of the knee. *Plicae* (folds of synovium that protrude inwards) exist in the knee joint and may be responsible for symptoms. Two are usually recognized: the superior plica, thought to be an embryological remnant of the division between the suprapatellar bursa and the joint, and a medial plica, a vertical fold adjacent to the medial border of the patella.

Numerous bursae are associated with the knee, facilitating the function of the tendons that run more or less parallel to the bones, to exert a lengthwise pull across the joint (Palastanga *et al.*, 1994). Posteriorly a bursa sits under each head of origin of gastrocnemius. Laterally, bursae lie either side of the lateral collateral ligament, cushioning it from biceps femoris and popliteus, as well as between popliteus and the lateral femoral condyle. Medially, the *pes anserine bursa* sits between the distal medial collateral ligament and the tendons of sartorius, gracilis and semitendinosus. The semi-membranosus bursa lies between it and the medial tibial condyle and a variable number of small bursae lie deep to the medial collateral ligament.

The ligaments of the knee provide a dynamic guide during movement and act as a passive restraint to abnormal translations (Barrack and Skinner, 1990). Each ligament is oriented in a direction to produce stability and force is dissipated at the insertion by a gradual transition from ligament, to fibrocartilage, to bone (Woo *et al.*, 1990).

The *medial collateral ligament* is a strong, broad, flat band lying posteriorly over the medial joint line. Passing from the medial femoral epicondyle just distal to the adductor tubercle, it descends vertically across the joint line and runs forwards to its attachment on the medial condyle and shaft of the upper tibia. It is the primary static stabilizer of the medial side of the knee joint and is assisted by the quadriceps expansions and the tendons of sartorius, gracilis and semitendinosus, which cross over its lower part, and from which it is separated by the pes anserine bursa.

The medial collateral ligament is composed of superficial and deep layers. The superficial part of the ligament, often referred to as the tibial collateral ligament, consists of fibres which pass directly from the femur to the tibia (Staron *et al.*, 1994; Schweitzer *et al.*, 1995). These fibres are relatively strong and provide 80% of the resistance to valgus force (Schenck and Heckman, 1993). Under the superficial medial collateral ligament the capsule is thickened to form the deep medial collateral ligament or capsular ligament. This part of the ligament is relatively weaker and its fibres attach to the meniscus. Superior fibres, the *meniscofemoral ligaments*, attach the meniscus to the femur, and inferior fibres, the *coronary* or *meniscotibial ligaments*, attach the meniscus to the tibia (Burks, 1990; Staron *et al.*, 1994).

The primary stabilizing role of the medial collateral ligament is in preventing excessive valgus at the knee. Its secondary stabilizing role is in preventing lateral rotation of the tibia, anterior translation of the tibia on the femur and hyperextension of the knee. Most of the ligament is taut in full extension, but anterior and posterior parts of the superficial ligament behave differently on movement and in varying positions of the knee, displaying different strain patterns (Burks, 1990).

The *lateral collateral ligament* is a shorter, cord-like ligament separated from the capsule of the knee joint by the tendon of popliteus. It is approximately 5 cm long (Palastanga *et al.*, 1994) and roughly the size of half a pencil (Evans, 1986). It runs from the lateral femoral epicondyle to the head of the fibula where it blends with the insertion of biceps femoris. Its primary stabilizing role is to restrain varus stress (Burks, 1990), with a secondary stabilizing role in controlling posterior drawer and lateral rotation of the tibia.

The *oblique popliteal ligament* is an extension of semi-membranosus which partially blends with and strengthens the posterior capsule. The *arcuate popliteal ligament* is a Y-shaped thickening of the posterolateral capsule passing from the head of the fibular to arch over the tendon of popliteus.

The *iliotibial tract* may be considered as a dynamic stabilizer of the lateral aspect of the knee since it shows similarities in strength and direction to the medial collateral ligament.

The *cruciate ligaments* are strong intracapsular, but extrasynovial, ligaments said to be about as thick as a pencil (Evans, 1986). They are called cruciate (*crus* Latin = cross) because of the way they cross in the intercondylar fossa and are named anterior or posterior by their tibial attachments. Their primary stabilizing role is to resist anterior and posterior movement of the tibia under the femur. Their secondary stabilizing function is to act as internal collateral ligaments controlling varus, valgus and rotation (Schenck and Heckman, 1993).

The *anterior cruciate ligament* passes from the anterior tibial intercondylar area upwards, posteriorly and laterally, twisting as it goes, to attach to the posteromedial aspect of the lateral femoral condyle. Anatomically it can be divided into two parts: an anteromedial band which is lax in extension and a posterolateral band which is taut in extension; the reverse occurs in flexion. Functionally, part of the ligament has a stabilizing effect throughout the range of movement (Katz and Fingeroth, 1986; Perko *et al.*, 1992). Its primary stabilizing role resists anterior translation and medial rotation of the tibia on the femur. A secondary stabilizing role relates it to the collateral ligaments in resisting valgus, varus and hyperextension stresses (Evans, 1986). A study by Butler *et al.* (1980) showed the anterior cruciate ligament to provide 86% of the total resisting force to anterior translation, with other ligaments and capsular structures making up the remaining secondary restraint (Katz and Fingeroth, 1986).

The *posterior cruciate ligament* passes upwards, anteriorly and medially from the posterior intercondylar area to attach to the anterolateral aspect of the medial femoral condyle. The ligament is said to be twice as strong as and less oblique than the anterior cruciate ligament and its close relationship to the centre of rotation of the knee joint makes it a principal stabilizer (Palastanga *et al.*, 1994). The posterior cruciate ligament restrains posterior translation of the tibia on the femur and possibly medial rotation of the tibia, with respect to the femur (Evans, 1986).

The main function of the tibiofemoral joint is weight-bearing, therefore symptoms are usually produced on weight-bearing activities. During the gait cycle, the forces across the tibiofemoral joint amount to two to five times body weight according to position and activity. However, the forces may increase to 24 times body weight during activities such as jumping (Palastanga *et al.*, 1994).

The range of movement at the knee joint is greatest in the sagittal plane with an active range from 0° extension to 140° of flexion. Approximately 5–10° of passive extension is usually available and up to 160° of passive flexion, which is halted when the calf and hamstring muscles approximate and the heel reaches the buttock. During flexion and extension, the menisci stay with the tibia so that the movement occurs between the femoral condyles rolling and sliding over the menisci.

Active and passive axial rotation occur with the knee joint in flexion and the range available is greatest at 90° of knee flexion. Active lateral rotation amounts to approximately 45° and medial rotation of 35°, with a little more movement in each direction available passively. During axial rotation, the menisci now stay with the femur and rotation occurs between the femoral condyles and the menisci rolling and gliding over the tibial condyles. The coronary ligaments are lax enough to permit this movement.

A few degrees of automatic, involuntary rotation occurs to achieve the locked or unlocked positions of the knee. During the last 20° or so of knee extension, lateral rotation of the tibia on the femur occurs to produce the terminal screw-home or locking phase of the knee. This achieves the close-packed position of the knee joint, when it is most stable, and rotation and accessory movements are impossible to perform on the normal extended knee. The knee is unlocked by the action of popliteus medially rotating the tibia on the femur.

The locking mechanism of the knee occurs because the medial femoral condyle is slightly longer than the lateral and the shape of the tibial condyles allows the lateral femoral condyle to glide more freely and over a greater distance than the medial. The ligaments around the knee contribute to stability in extension when most fibres are under tension.

Helfet's test (Nordin and Frankel, 1989) ensures that the locking mechanism of the knee is intact. The test is performed as follows.

Position the patient in high sitting and mark the middle of the patella. Assess the position of the tibial tuberosity in respect to this midline mark and it should lie just medial to it. Extend the knee and repeat the markings. The tibial tuberosity should now lie just lateral to the midline mark, confirming that lateral rotation of the tibia has occurred.

The *patellofemoral joint* is the joint between the posterior aspect of the patella and the anterior surface of the femur. It is a joint of the extensor mechanism of the knee and therefore gives rise to symptoms on antigravity activities. The patella performs two important biomechanical functions at the knee (Nordin and Frankel, 1989):

- It produces anterior displacement of the quadriceps tendon throughout movement, assisting knee extension by increasing the lever arm of the quadriceps muscle force.
- It increases the area of contact between the patellar tendon and the femur, distributing compressive forces over a wider area.

The articular cartilage on the back of the patella is said to be the thickest in the body, at 5–6 mm thick (Evans, 1986). It is divided into areas for articulation with the medial and lateral femoral condyles in varying degrees of flexion and extension. The patella glides caudally approximately 7 cm and rotates as the knee moves from full extension to full flexion. The patella eventually sinks into the intercondylar groove in full knee flexion (Nordin and Frankel, 1989).

Patellofemoral symptoms may arise from instability, maltracking, malalignment, subluxation and dislocation, which may lead to eventual chondromalacia patellae and osteoarthrosis of the joint. There is a tendency for the patella to slip laterally, particularly as the knee moves towards full extension, and this is counteracted by:

- The high lateral border of the patellar groove on the femur.
- The active muscle pull of the oblique fibres of vastus medialis.
- The medial quadriceps expansion.

The *superior tibiofibular joint* is a synovial plane joint between the posterolateral tibia and the head of the fibula. The joint is reinforced by anterior and posterior capsular ligaments. Small accessory movements are possible at this joint which are mechanically linked to the inferior tibiofibular joint and are influenced by movements at the ankle joint.

Contractile structures

The contractile structures at the knee consist of muscles which originate from the hip region and insert at the knee, or originate at the knee and insert below the ankle. The muscles will be described in relationship to the knee and the reader is referred to the chapters on the hip and ankle for further discussion of the muscle groups.

Quadriceps femoris (femoral nerve L2–4) is composed of four muscles: rectus femoris, vastus lateralis, vastus medialis and vastus intermedius, uniting around the patella to form the *ligamentum patellae*, which passes from the apex of the patella to insert into the tibial tuberosity.

Rectus femoris originates above the hip joint and inserts into the base of the patella (upper border) with fibres continued over and on each side of the patella contributing to the ligamentum patellae.

Vastus lateralis passes from the upper anterolateral femur down to form a broad tendon which eventually tapers as it inserts into the lateral border of the patella as the lateral quadriceps expansion. Vastus lateralis contributes to the main quadriceps tendon, passing over the patella, as well as blending with fibres of the iliotibial tract to form a lateral extension and to support the anterolateral joint capsule.

Vastus medialis passes from the upper anteromedial femur downwards, to join the common quadriceps tendon and the medial border of the patella as the medial quadriceps expansion. The lower fibres, which form the medial expansion, run more horizontally and have their origin from adductor magnus, with which they share a nerve supply.

Vastus intermedius is the deepest part of the quadriceps and inserts with rectus femoris into the base of the patella.

Quadriceps femoris is the main extensor muscle of the knee joint. Vastus medialis is believed to be particularly active during the later stages of knee extension, when it exerts a stabilizing force on the patella to prevent it slipping laterally. Although quiet in standing, the muscle contracts strongly in such activities as climbing.

The *hamstrings* (sciatic nerve L5, S1–2), comprising biceps femoris, semimembranosus and semitendonosus, are responsible for flexion of the knee and medial and lateral rotation of the knee when flexed in the mid-position.

Biceps femoris inserts into the head of the fibula, splitting around the lateral collateral ligament as it does so. *Semimembranosus* has its main attachment into the posterior aspect of the medial tibial condyle, but sends slips on to blend with other structures to support the posteromedial capsule. *Semitendinosus* curves around the medial tibial condyle to the upper surface of the medial tibia together with sartorius and gracilis. These tendons blend with the medial capsule, lending it some support.

The *iliotibial tract* inserts into Gerdy's tubercle on the anterolateral aspect of the upper tibia and blends with the lateral capsule and the lateral quadriceps expansion. Tensor fascia lata, acting with gluteus maximus, tightens the tract and assists extension of the knee.

Popliteus (tibial nerve L4–5, S1) originates within the capsule of the knee joint as a tendon arising from the groove on the lateral aspect of the lateral femoral condyle. It separates the lateral collateral ligament from the fibrous capsule of the knee joint and, as it passes downwards, backwards and medially, it sends tendinous fibres to the posterior horn of the lateral meniscus. It forms a fleshy, triangular muscle belly and attaches to the posterior aspect of the tibia above the soleal line. Popliteus medially rotates the tibia on the femur, unlocking the knee joint from the close-packed position. Some consider that, through its attachment to the lateral meniscus, it pulls the meniscus backwards during rotatory movements, possibly preventing it from being trapped (Safran and Fu, 1995). Its complex attachment to the lateral meniscus, arcuate ligament, posterior capsule and femoral condyle provides an appreciable role in dynamic stability, particularly in preventing forwards displacement of the femur on the tibia (Burks, 1990; Safran and Fu, 1995).

Gastrocnemius (tibial nerve S1–2) arises by two heads from the posterior aspect of the medial and lateral femoral condyles and together with soleus and plantaris forms the triceps surae. As well as its action at the ankle, gastrocnemius is a strong flexor at the knee, but is unable to act strongly at both joints simultaneously.

A guide to surface marking and palpation

Anterior aspect (Fig. 11.1)

Locate the *patella* at the front of the knee and identify its base (upper border), apex (lower border), medial and lateral borders. With the knee extended and relaxed you should be able to shift the patella from side to side to palpate the insertion of the *quadriceps expansions (patellar retinaculum)* under the edge of each border. Tilt the base and apex to locate the *suprapatellar* and *infrapatellar tendons* respectively.

Follow the *ligamentum patellae* down to its insertion on to the tibial tuberosity, which lies approximately 5 cm below the apex of the patella in the flexed knee.

Palpate and mark in the *knee joint line* with the knee in flexion. The anterior articular surface of each femoral condyle and the anterior articular margins of the tibia should be palpable at either side of the patella. Both can be followed round on to the medial and lateral aspects, but it is not possible to palpate the joint line posteriorly since it is covered by many musculotendinous structures.

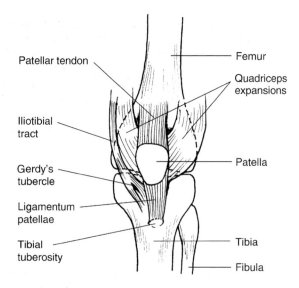

Fig. 11.1 Anterior aspect of the knee.

With the knee joint flexed, the apex of the patella marks the approximate position of the joint line. In extension, the apex of the patella lies approximately one finger's breadth above the joint line. This information may provide a useful guide if the joint is very swollen, making it difficult to palpate the joint line.

The *quadriceps muscle* forms the major anterior muscle bulk. On static contraction of this muscle, locate rectus femoris, which forms the central part of the muscle bulk. Vastus lateralis forms an obvious lateral muscle bulk, whilst vastus medialis terminates in oblique fibres which form part of the medial quadriceps expansion.

Lateral aspect (Fig. 11.2)

On the anterolateral surface of the tibia, approximately two-thirds of the way between the head of the fibula and the tibial tuberosity,

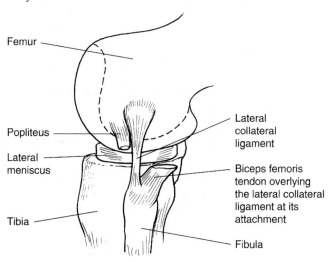

Fig. 11.2 Lateral aspect of the knee.

palpate for *Gerdy's tubercle*, which gives attachment to the *iliotibial tract*. The tract should be obvious as the quadriceps contracts.

Palpate the *head of the fibula* just below the posterior part of the lateral condyle of the tibia where it forms the proximal tibiofibular joint. The head of the fibula lies on the same plane as the tibial tuberosity. The common peroneal nerve can be rolled over the neck of the fibula.

Place the leg into the FABER position of *f*lexion, *ab*duction and *e*xternal (lateral) *r*otation, and palpate the lateral aspect of the knee joint line. You should be able to roll the cord-like *lateral collateral ligament* under your fingers.

Medial aspect (Fig. 11.3)

Palpate the medial epicondyle of the femur and locate the prominent *adductor tubercle* on the upper part of the condyle. Deep palpation is necessary and the tubercle will feel tender to palpation.

Move directly distally from the adductor tubercle until you are over the joint line and see if you can identify, by palpation, the anterior edge of the *medial collateral ligament*. This ligament is approximately 8–10 cm long (Palastanga *et al.*, 1994; Williams *et al.*, 1989) and two and a half fingers' wide as it broadens to cross the joint line. Its anterior border may be palpated in most people: this is usually in line with or just behind the central axis of the joint.

Visualize the position of the *sartorius, gracilis and semitendinosus* tendons as they cross the lower part of the medial collateral ligament to their insertion on the upper part of the medial tibia.

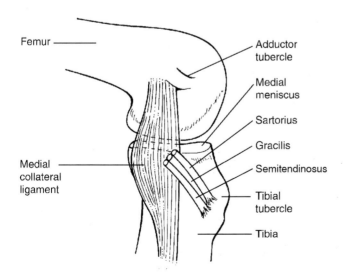

Fig. 11.3 Medial aspect of the knee.

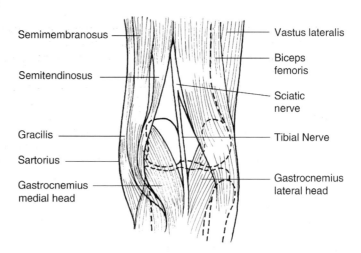

Semimembranosus

Semitendinosus

Gracilis

Sartorius

Gastrocnemius
medial head

Vastus lateralis

Biceps
femoris

Sciatic
nerve

Tibial Nerve

Gastrocnemius
lateral head

Fig. 11.4 Posterior aspect of the knee.

Posterior aspect (Fig. 11.4)

Resist knee flexion and palpate the *hamstrings*, which form the muscle bulk of the posterior thigh. The point at which the medial and lateral hamstrings separate can be identified, with biceps femoris forming the lateral wall of the popliteal fossa and semitendinosus lying on semimembranosus to form the medial wall.

Biceps femoris can be followed down to its insertion on to the head of the fibula.

On the medial side of the fossa, *semitendinosus* can be felt as an obvious tendon. Medial to it is *gracilis*, made more prominent by adding resisted medial rotation. Deeper to this is *semimembranosus*, remaining more muscular as it blends into its aponeurotic attachment.

Posteriorly, locate the two heads of *gastrocnemius* as they originate above the knee joint from the medial and lateral femoral condyles.

Commentary on the examination

Observation

A general observation is made of the patient's *face and overall posture*, but as the knee is a weight-bearing joint, particular attention is paid to the *gait* pattern. Note if an antalgic posture or gait has been adopted; a limp will be evident during gait if the patient has an abnormal stride length or is not weight-bearing evenly. Toeing-in or out, together with abnormalities of foot posture, should also be noted.

History (subjective examination)

A detailed history is required at the knee since it gives important diagnostic clues, including typical injury patterns, which may be confirmed by clinical examination. It also assists in the identification of lesions which may be better suited for specialist referral.

The *age, occupation, sports, hobbies and lifestyle* of the patient are particularly relevant.

Some conditions affect certain age groups. Knee pain in children is commonly referred from the hip and it is necessary to carry out a thorough examination of both joints. Meniscal lesions are unusual in children and increase in incidence from adolescence onwards. A gradual onset of knee pain in adolescents may be related to patellofemoral joint syndromes or Osgood–Schlatter's disease which presents as a localized pain felt over the tibial tuberosity due to traction apophysitis of the tibial tubercle.

The young adult, particularly male, may present with traumatic meniscal lesions associated with rotational injury during sporting activities. Females tend to present with instability, subluxation or episodes of dislocation of the patella.

Rheumatoid arthritis may affect the knee and onset usually occurs between the ages of 30 and 40. Degenerative osteoarthrosis affects the older age group, but may occur earlier if predisposed by previous injury or through overuse in sporting activity. It is important to remember that osteoarthrosis can affect both the patellofemoral and tibiofemoral joints. Degenerative meniscal lesions can occur in association with the degenerative ageing process of the joint.

The lifestyle of the patient will reflect whether occupational or recreational activities are a contributing factor to their condition. Sport in particular may be responsible for traumatic incidents to the relatively unstable knee, especially in positions of flexion. Progressive microtrauma may be the result of incorrect or over-training, muscle imbalances or poor joint biomechanics.

The *site* of the pain indicates whether it is local or referred. Superficial structures tend to give local pain and point tenderness, therefore lesions of the medial collateral ligament, coronary ligaments or the tendinous insertions of the muscles around the knee give reasonably accurate localization of pain. Acutely inflamed lesions or deep lesions, such as of the tibiofemoral joint, menisci or cruciate ligaments, produce a vague, more widely felt, deep pain, with the patient unable to localize the lesion accurately.

The *spread* of pain generally indicates the severity of the lesion. Whilst referred pain is expected distally to the site of the lesion, the knee as a central limb joint may also produce some proximal pain in the thigh. Pain referred from the hip or lumbar spine can be felt at the knee and both must be eliminated as a cause of pain.

Anterior knee pain is a description of the symptoms felt by the patient, although the term is often misused as a diagnosis. It usually indicates patellofemoral joint involvement, but must not be considered to be due to it exclusively.

The anatomy at the knee makes the structures susceptible to direct and indirect trauma. The menisci and ligaments are often the sites of acute lesions, whilst the contractile structures are susceptible to overuse as well as acute trauma. The superior tibiofibular joint is mechanically linked to its inferior counterpart and influenced by mechanisms of injury at the foot and ankle.

The *onset* of the pain is extremely relevant to lesions at the knee. Trauma is a common precipitating cause and the sudden nature of the injury makes it easily recalled by the patient. A direct injury can cause muscular contusion and commonly involves the quadriceps. A direct blow to the patella, such as a fall on the flexed knee, may result in fracture, or may cause contusion of the periosteum or involvement of the prepatellar bursa. A direct blow to the anterior aspect of the upper tibia or, again, a fall on the flexed knee, can injure the posterior cruciate ligament.

In contact sports such as rugby and football, the lateral side of the knee is vulnerable to impact, which may result in excessive valgus strain affecting the medial collateral ligament. Injury may be produced by excessive forces applied to the flexed knee whilst the foot is fixed, e.g. skiing injuries. The medial collateral ligament, anterior cruciate ligament and medial meniscus may be affected. The position of the coronary ligaments involves them in rotational injuries. Major ligamentous rupture, particularly of the anterior cruciate ligament, is usually accompanied by a pop or tearing sound as the patient feels the ligament 'go' (Edwards and Villar, 1993).

Hyperextension injuries can affect any of the ligaments, since all the knee ligaments are taut in extension, but the anterior cruciate ligament and medial collateral ligament are most commonly affected. Recalling the exact onset of the injury, the forces involved and the position of the leg at the time of injury will give an idea of the likely anatomy involved in the lesion.

Muscle injuries are common around the knee, as the major muscle groups span two joints and may affect the origin, insertion or mid-belly. Strain results from eccentric contraction (attempting to contract when the muscle is on the stretch), when the muscle is unable to overcome the resistance. Explosive sprinting action affects the hamstrings and the quadriceps, and rectus femoris particularly may be affected by kicking against strong resistance. Patellar instability, subluxation or dislocation affects the medial quadriceps expansions, vastus medialis or the medial capsule.

Repetitive minor injury results in microtrauma, making the onset of the lesion difficult to recall, and the examiner will have to be aware of contributing factors such as over-training, training errors, foot posture and faulty knee joint biomechanics. Iliotibial band friction syndromes are common in long-distance runners. Infrapatellar tendinitis is common in activities associated with jumping and the bursae can be inflamed if any structures passing over them are overused.

The *duration* of the symptoms will indicate the stage in the inflammatory process reached, or the recurrent nature of the condition. Different treatment approaches depend on the acute, subacute or chronic nature of a ligamentous sprain or muscle belly strain. Overuse lesions around the knee tend to be chronic in nature and are present for some considerable time before the patient seeks treatment.

Recurrent episodes of pain and swelling may be due to instability and derangement of the joint. Patellar subluxation, meniscal lesions or partial ligamentous tears may produce pain and joint effusion after use. Degenerative osteoarthrosis may be symptom-free until overuse triggers a synovitis with increased pain and swelling.

The *symptoms and behaviour* need to be considered. The behaviour of the pain and the symptoms described by the patient are very relevant to diagnosis at the knee. Immediate pain after injury indicates a severe lesion but pain developing or increasing slowly over several hours may indicate less serious pathology. The ability to continue with the sport or activity after the onset of pain is often indicative of minor ligamentous sprain, whereas major ligament disruption and muscle tears, meniscal lesions or cruciate rupture often result in the patient being totally incapacitated.

Total rupture of a ligament may produce severe pain at the time of injury but following the initial injury pain may not be a particular feature since the structure is totally disrupted. Partial ligamentous rupture continues to produce severe pain on movement.

The quality of the pain may indicate severity, but it is important to remember the subjective nature of pain. Aggravating factors can be activity, which indicates a mechanical or muscular lesion, or rest, which indicates a ligamentous lesion with an inflammatory component.

Postures such as prolonged sitting may affect the patellofemoral joint in particular. A pseudo-locking effect often occurs when the patient first gets up to weight-bear. This is due to excessive friction from changes in the articular cartilage of the patella, but it usually resolves after several steps have been taken. Walking, squatting and using stairs aggravate patellofemoral conditions, particularly going downstairs, when the forces acting on this joint are increased to approximately three times body weight.

The tibiofemoral joint, as the weight-bearing joint, usually produces symptoms on weight-bearing activities, i.e. the stance phase of walking or running or prolonged standing. Pain produced on deep knee bends, rising from kneeling and rotational strains may indicate a meniscal lesion.

The other symptoms described by the patient give important clues to diagnosis. Swelling may be a symptom and it is important to know if it is constant or recurrent or provoked by activity. Swelling occurring within 2 h of injury is indicative of haemarthrosis; the joint may feel warm to touch and the swelling may be tense. Structures responsible for a haemarthrosis are those with a good blood supply, the anterior cruciate ligament being the commonest cause of a haemarthrosis. Amiel *et al.* (1990) quoted a study by Noyes in which over 70% of patients presenting with acute haemarthrosis of the knee had an acute tear of the anterior cruciate ligament. Rupture of the posterior cruciate usually also tears the posterior capsule and blood escapes into the calf where swelling and bruising may have been noticed by the patient.

Swelling which develops over 6–24 h is synovial in origin due to traumatic arthritis. Structures with a relatively poor blood supply tend to produce this traumatic arthritis, e.g. meniscal lesions, the deep part of the medial collateral ligament involving the capsule of the knee joint, and subluxation or dislocation of the patella.

Activity may provoke swelling in conditions such as degenerative joint disease, chronic instability or internal derangement. This may be confirmed after the objective examination which may stir up the condition. Localized swelling may indicate bursitis, e.g. prepatellar bursitis, Baker's cyst (synovial effusion into the gastrocnemius or semimembranosus bursa due to effusion in the knee joint) or meniscal cyst, which more commonly affects the lateral meniscus.

The presence of an effusion may affect the gait pattern and limit full extension. Reflex inhibition of the quadriceps muscle and an inability to lock the knee gives a feeling of insecurity on weight-bearing with the patient complaining of a sensation of 'giving way'. Giving way may also be due to a loose body or meniscal lesion, which also occurs on weight-bearing, is momentary and occurs together with a twinge of pain.

True locking of the knee is indicative of a meniscal lesion and usually occurs in conjunction with a rotary component to the injury. It has a tendency to recur. The locking may resolve spontaneously over several hours or days or it may need to be manipulatively unlocked. Locking usually occurs at 10–40° short of full extension (Hartley, 1995). A ruptured anterior cruciate ligament can cause locking as the ligamentous flap catches between the joint surfaces. True locking must be distinguished from the pseudo-locking associated with the patellofemoral joint after prolonged sitting.

Provocation of pain on the stairs is important. The patellofemoral joint characteristically produces more pain on coming downstairs, due to the greater joint reaction force, although the pain may also have been provoked whilst walking upstairs.

Clicking, snapping, or catching may be due to internal derangement. Grating and pain associated with crepitation are usually indicative of degenerative changes of the tibiofemoral joint, patellofemoral joint, or both.

To exclude symptoms arising from the lumbar spine the patient should be questioned about paraesthesia and pain provoked by coughing or sneezing.

Other joint involvement should be explored to ascertain the possibility of inflammatory joint disease. *Past medical history* should exclude serious pathology and questions about *medications* will highlight any contraindications to treatment. If degenerative osteoarthrosis is considered a factor in the diagnosis, the patient can be questioned about significant weight gain. It has been suggested that obesity is a cause of osteoarthrosis in the knee (Felson *et al.*, 1988).

Inspection

The knee should be fully extended in standing. If not, some compromise of the terminal screw home or locking mechanism exists, or an effusion with limited extension is present as part of the capsular pattern.

The knee should be inspected in both the weight-bearing and non-weight-bearing positions. In standing the normal slight valgus tibiofemoral angle should be obvious.

The whole lower limb is inspected for leg length discrepancy and obvious **bony deformity** such as genu valgum, varum, recurvatum or 'wind-swept' knees (one varus, one valgus). The posture of the feet is important. Overpronation or tight Achilles tendon may be related to the knee symptoms and a detailed biomechanical assessment is then required. Position of the pelvis and obvious spinal deformities may be important to note if relevant to symptoms.

The position, shape and size of the patellae are noted if relevant to the presenting symptoms. Patellar alignment is measured by the Q-angle: the angle between the line of the quadriceps muscle (anterior superior iliac spine to the mid-point of the patella) and the patellar tendon (mid-point of the patella to the tibial tuberosity). An angle of between 15 and 20° is considered normal for patellar alignment and tracking, and less or more than this can be considered to be a malalignment (Norris, 1993).

Colour changes may be present, especially if the condition is acute, when the joint looks red due to inflammatory changes. Direct trauma may produce bruising and acute muscle lesions may show bruising, particularly in the quadriceps and hamstring muscles. Distal colour changes may be indicative of circulatory problems.

In standing, all muscle groups are inspected for *wasting*. The quadriceps wastes rapidly due to reflex inhibition if pain and swelling are present. In patellofemoral problems wasting of the oblique fibres of vastus medialis may be obvious.

Loss of the dimple on the medial aspect of the knee will indicate the presence of *swelling*, drawn out of the suprapatellar bursa by gravity. Minor swelling may not be obvious and may only be apparent on testing in the supine position.

State at rest

Before any movements are performed, the state at rest is established to provide a baseline for subsequent comparison.

The suggested sequence for the objective examination will now be given, followed by a commentary including the reasoning in performing the movements and the significance of the possible findings.

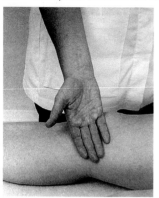

Fig. 11.5 Palpation for heat.

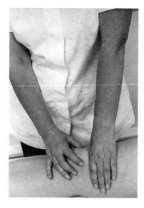

Fig. 11.6 Palpation for swelling.

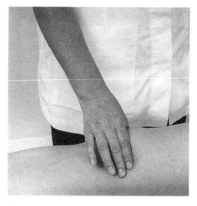

Fig. 11.7 Palpation for synovial thickening.

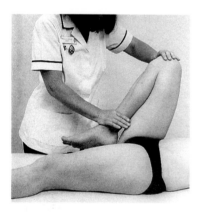

Fig. 11.8 Passive flexion.

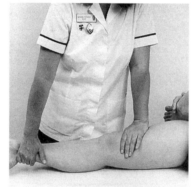

(a)

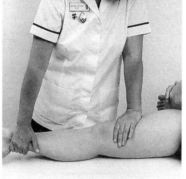

(b)

Fig. 11.9 Passive extension: (a) for range and (b) for end-feel.

Examination by selective tension (objective examination)

Supine lying:

- Palpation for heat (Fig. 11.5), swelling (Fig. 11.6) and synovial thickening (Fig. 11.7)
- Passive knee flexion (Fig. 11.8)
- Passive knee extension, once for range (Fig. 11.9a) once for end-feel (Fig. 11.9b)

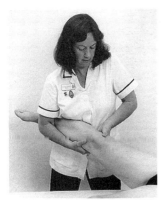

Fig. 11.10 Valgus stress.

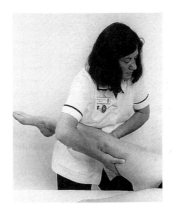

Fig. 11.11 Varus stress.

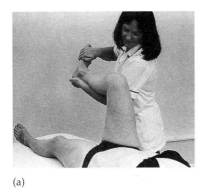

(a)

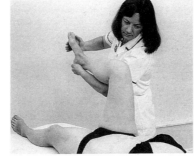

(b)

Fig. 11.12 Passive (a) lateral and (b) medial rotation.

- Passive valgus stress (Fig. 11.10)
- Passive varus stress (Fig. 11.11)
- Passive lateral rotation (Fig. 11.12a)
- Passive medial rotation (Fig. 11.12b)

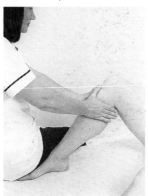

Fig. 11.13 Posterior drawer test.

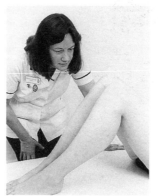

Fig. 11.14 Assessment of laxity of the posterior cruciate ligament.

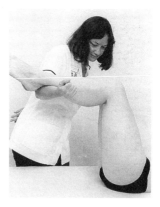

Fig. 11.15 Assessment of laxity of the posterior cruciate ligament, alternative position.

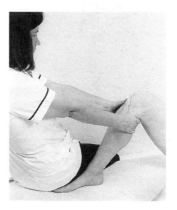

Fig. 11.16 Anterior drawer test.

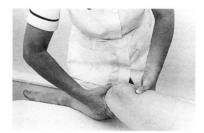

Fig. 11.17 Lachman test.

- Posterior drawer test (Figs 11.13–11.15)
- Anterior drawer test (Fig. 11.16)
- Lachman test (Fig. 11.17)

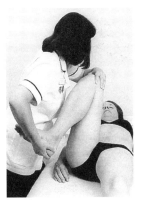

Fig. 11.18 Flexion, lateral rotation and valgus.

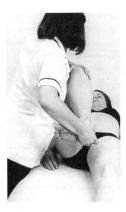

Fig. 11.19 Flexion, lateral rotation and varus.

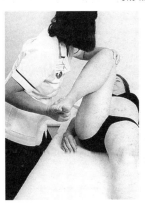

Fig. 11.20 Flexion, medial rotation and valgus.

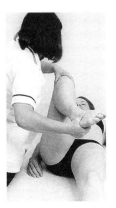

Fig. 11.21 Flexion, medial rotation and varus.

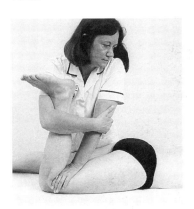

Fig. 11.22 Resisted knee extension.

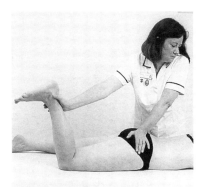

Fig. 11.23 Resisted knee flexion.

Provocation tests for the menisci:

- Flexion, lateral rotation and valgus (Fig. 11.18)
- Flexion, lateral rotation and varus (Fig. 11.19)
- Flexion, medial rotation and valgus (Fig. 11.20)
- Flexion, medial rotation and varus (Fig. 11.21)

Prone lying:

- Resisted knee extension (Fig. 11.22)
- Resisted knee flexion (Fig. 11.23)

Palpation

- Once a diagnosis has been made, the structure at fault is palpated for the exact site of the lesion

The combined history and examination are important at the knee. The symptoms described by the patient result from functional weight-bearing activities but the knee is examined clinically in a non-weight-bearing position. Lesions vary from simple contusions, muscle strains and ligament sprains to arthritis and major ligamentous rupture and instability. It is important to be able to clinically diagnose lesions at the knee, but also to appreciate the limits of clinical examination and to determine when onward referral for specialist opinion is necessary.

The acute knee should be examined as soon as possible after injury before effusion causes pain, apprehension and limited movement. Effusion makes it difficult to test accurately for ligamentous instability and to apply provocative meniscal tests. The acute knee is usually managed conservatively until the traumatic arthritis subsides. Residual instability which fails to respond to conservative management, aimed at dynamic stabilization, or internal de-rangement due to meniscal lesions can be dealt with surgically at a later date, and neither is usually considered to be an emergency.

Palpation tests are conducted for signs of activity within the joint. Temperature changes are assessed using the dorsal aspect of the same hand and comparing like with like. Inflammatory conditions will show an increase in *heat* compared with the other side. It may be necessary to repeat this test at the end of the examination to assess if an inflammatory response has been triggered by the examination, giving an indication of the irritability of the lesion.

Several tests exist for *swelling* and the choice is left to the reader on the basis of personal opinion on effectiveness and preference. A sensitive test for minor swelling involves placing the finger and thumb of one hand on either side of the patella just below the bony periphery. The web between the index finger and thumb of the other hand applies compression to the suprapatellar bursa which squeezes fluid out into the joint cavity and which is felt to part the finger and thumb of the other hand. Other tests involve wiping the fluid from one side of the joint to the other, compression of the suprapatellar bursa and the front of the joint just below the patella to assess fluctuation of fluid, or pressing down on the patella to assess for the presence of a patellar 'tap'.

Synovial thickening is assessed by palpation of the medial and lateral femoral condyles. Thickening of the synovium is normal here because of the presence of synovial plica and the medial plica is more obvious to palpation. Assessment for excessive thickening of the synovium is confirmed if the tissue feels 'boggy' to the touch.

The position of the patella should be assessed to see if it is shifted, tilted or rotated with respect to the other side. It should be emphasized here, that the orthopaedic medicine approach has limited relevance to patellofemoral lesions. Patellofemoral malalignment syndromes are not covered within this text and the reader is referred to the excellent work of Jenny McConnell.

The primary passive movements of flexion and extension are performed to assess the tibiofemoral joint. Pain, range of movement and end-feel are noted, which will indicate the presence of the capsular or non-capsular pattern. Passive flexion normally has a

Capsular pattern at the knee joint:

- **More limitation of flexion than extension**

'soft' end-feel and passive extension a 'hard' end-feel. The thigh is fixed above the knee and the foot is lifted to assess the range of hyperextension present, normally 5-10°. A further test is conducted whereby the leg is lifted into approximately 10° of flexion and dropped into extension to assess for the normal, bony 'hard' end-feel. This is sometimes known as the 'bounce home' test and an abnormally 'soft' or 'springy' end-feel indicates the end of range has not been reached due to a meniscal lesion, loose body or joint effusion. The presence of the non-capsular pattern indicates a ligamentous lesion or a loose body in the joint, or possibly a meniscal problem.

The secondary passive movements at the knee are applied to assess the ligaments. It is important to compare the two limbs since although joint motion varies considerably within the population there is very little variation between right and left in a normal subject (Daniel, 1990). The tests depend on the muscles being relaxed and the eye, feel and experience of the examiner, who is looking for an excessive range of movement compared with the asymptomatic knee, and an abnormal end-feel.

Secondary passive movements are applied to the knee in a loose packed position of slight flexion since no movement should be present with the knee in full extension. If movement can be detected in the close packed position, serious ligamentous disruption is present with accompanying damage to capsular components. Minor ligamentous laxity may be sub-clinical, therefore recognition of such symptoms from the history leads to onward referral for more detailed assessment of ligamentous laxity.

The intention here is to list the ligaments that need to be tested with the photographs providing illustrations of suggested testing methods. The methods are not proposed as the 'best' way of testing and will not be described in detail within the text. The reader is referred to the fuller descriptions of these and other methods to be found in textbooks devoted to the knee and sports injuries.

Butler *et al.*, (1980), referred to the concept of primary and secondary ligament restraints to movement in a specific direction. A ligament may act as a primary restraint in one direction and as a secondary restraint in another. Rupture of a primary restraint results in excessive movement, rupture of the secondary restraint to that movement with the primary restraint intact, does not result in increased movement. Rupture of both primary and secondary restraint produces a much greater increase in movement. For example, rupture of the anterior cruciate ligament (primary restraint) produces some increase in anterior translation, rupture of the medial collateral ligament (secondary restraint) produces no detectable increase in anterior translation and rupture of both (primary and secondary restraints) results in a much greater increase in movement.

Orthopaedic medicine treatment techniques will be directed at simple ligamentous sprains, but it is important to recognize more serious ligament disruption or intra-articular derangement due to a meniscal lesion in order to make the appropriate onward specialist referral.

Valgus and varus stresses are applied to the knee in approximately 15° of flexion and assess the primary stabilizing function of the medial and lateral collateral ligaments respectively. The range of movement available is noted and compared with the asymptomatic knee. The end-feel is assessed, which is normally firm elastic.

Axial rotation should be tested at 90° of knee flexion as the range of movement is greatest in this position. Passive lateral rotation is usually 45° and passive medial rotation is usually 35°; both test the coronary ligaments.

The posterior and anterior drawer tests are both performed with the knee at 90° of flexion. The neutral position of the resting knee must be established compared with the contralateral normal knee.

The posterior drawer test is applied first for the posterior cruciate ligament, since a deficient posterior cruciate ligament could give a false positive to anterior translation. As the tibia is pushed posteriorly, the thumbs rest over the anterior joint line to assess the 'sag-back' or step created anteriorly by the excessive posterior drawer. Isolated rupture of the posterior cruciate ligament is a rare lesion, but the posterior drawer test is a sensitive and specific test for the posterior cruciate ligament and obvious laxity is produced due to lack of resistance from the collateral ligaments and the lax posterior capsule (Palastanga *et al.*, 1994, Rubinstein *et al.*, 1994).

The anterior drawer test assesses the anterior cruciate ligament although it is considered an insensitive and poor diagnostic indicator of lesions of this ligament, especially in the acute knee (Katz and Fingeroth, 1986). The haemarthrosis and traumatic arthritis 'splint' the knee making it difficult to place the knee in 90° of flexion, and pain produces protective spasm in the hamstrings preventing anterior tibial translation. In a chronic knee, the secondary stabilizing role of an intact medial collateral ligament may prevent anterior translation at 90 degrees of knee flexion.

The Lachman test is an accurate clinical test with a high diagnostic accuracy to determine anterior cruciate laxity. It far exceeds the anterior drawer test, but is comparable to the pivot shift test (Katz and Fingeroth, 1986, Smith and Green, 1995). The Lachman test may be difficult to perform especially if the limb is large or the patient unable to relax sufficiently. Several modifications have been made to the Lachman test since it was first described by Torg *et al.* in 1976, including a 'drop leg' Lachman test described by Adler *et al.* (1995).

Similarly, the pivot-shift test (see Evans, 1986) has several methods of application. It is essentially a dynamic test to determine the degree of instability related to anterior cruciate ligament injury. However, it may also be difficult to apply in the acute knee.

Four provocation tests are applied if the history indicates a meniscal lesion. Each meniscus is put under compression and stress during combined movements of flexion, valgus, varus and both rotations.

Other traditional tests for a meniscal lesion include the 'bounce home' test of passive knee extension for end-feel, the McMurray's test which takes the leg from a position of flexion towards extension, with medial or lateral rotation of the tibia, and Apley's grind or compression test. Negative clinical testing is not conclusive evidence that a meniscal lesion does not exist. If the history is indicative, or the patient is experiencing recurrent episodes of locking and or giving way, referral should be made for specialist opinion with arthroscopy, in modern practice, the 'gold standard' for diagnosis at the knee (Curtin *et al.*, 1992).

The resisted tests are applied looking for pain and power. Resisted knee extension tests the quadriceps and resisted knee flexion the hamstrings. Having established that there is no pain on testing the muscles in the mid-position, accessory provocation tests may be included to provoke minor contractile lesions. The quadriceps and hamstrings can be tested in varying degrees of knee flexion and extension, and isotonically. The hamstring muscles may be tested in conjunction with medial or lateral rotation to isolate the lesion to the medial or lateral hamstrings (Fig. 11.24). Popliteus may be assessed by testing resisted knee flexion in conjunction with resisted medial rotation of the tibia. Although popliteal muscle lesions are unusual, its attachment to the posterior horn of the lateral meniscus may produce a positive sign on resisted testing of the muscle when there is involvement of the meniscus, as shown on the provocation tests.

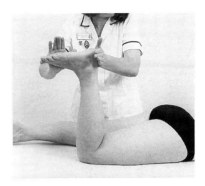

Fig. 11.24 Resisted knee flexion and medial rotation of the tibia.

Capsular lesions

The presence of the capsular pattern indicates arthritis and the history indicates the cause of the arthritis. The possibilities are an acute episode of degenerative osteoarthrosis, inflammatory arthritis such as rheumatoid arthritis or traumatic arthritis.

Traumatic arthritis is usually a secondary response to a ligamentous lesion at the knee. As a capsular ligament, damage to the medial collateral ligament produces a secondary traumatic arthritis; a ruptured cruciate ligament may also produce a haemarthrosis.

Symptomatic osteoarthrosis and inflammatory arthritis may benefit from an intra-articular injection of corticosteroid. Treatment for traumatic arthritis should be directed to the cause of the lesion, i.e. the ligamentous injury.

> **Capsular pattern at the knee**
>
> - More limitation of flexion than extension

Injection of the knee joint (Cyriax and Cyriax, 1983; Cyriax, 1984)

Adcortyl 10 mg/ml	Total steroid	Lignocaine 1%	Total volume
3 ml	30 mg	1 ml	4 ml

21G × 1½ in (0.8 × 40 mm) green needle

Position the patient comfortably in supine lying with the knee supported in extension. Glide the patella medially, pressing down on the lateral edge to lift the medial border (Fig. 11.25). Insert the

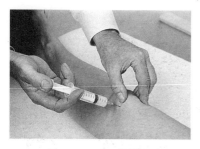

Fig. 11.25 Injection of the knee joint.

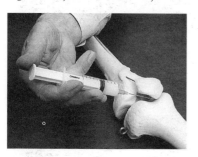

Fig. 11.26 Injection of the knee joint showing direction of approach and needle position.

needle halfway along the medial border of the patella, aiming laterally and slightly posteriorly, parallel with the articular surface of the patella (Fig. 11.26). Once the needle is intra-articular, deliver the injection as a bolus. The patient is advised to maintain a period of relative rest for approximately 2 weeks following injection.

Non-capsular lesions

Loose body

From the history, symptoms of momentary giving way on weight-bearing accompanied by twinges of pain indicate a possible loose body in the knee joint. The loose body may be a fragment of cartilage or bone associated with degenerative osteoarthrosis in the older adult, or a flap of meniscus which may momentarily give way or lock on weight-bearing.

Osteochondritis dissecans may affect the knee in adolescents, usually between the ages of 15 and 20 years. A small fragment of bone becomes demarcated from a condyle and detaches to form a loose body. Pain, swelling, locking and giving way are the symptoms and surgical intervention may be required (Paice, 1995).

On examination a non-capsular pattern is present with either limitation of flexion or extension, but not both. The end-feel is characteristically springy.

If the joint should lock, it is usually temporary and it unlocks spontaneously. A joint which requires manipulative unlocking probably requires referral for specialist opinion and possibly arthroscopy.

It may be possible to have a loose body impinged between the joint surfaces in degenerative osteoarthrosis. If the loose fragment impinges on the medial side of the joint, the patient presents with signs of an intrinsic medial collateral sprain, but in the absence of trauma. The capsular pattern of degenerative osteoarthrosis is present with a non-capsular pattern superimposed; the patient complains of increased pain on the valgus stress. The primary lesion should be treated and the secondary ligamentous sprain should therefore subside.

The treatment of choice to reduce a loose body is strong traction together with Grade A mobilization, theoretically aiming to move the loose body to another part of the joint and to restore full, painfree movement.

The strong traction is applied to the joint and a medial or lateral movement is applied simultaneously with a movement from flexion towards extension.

Loose-body mobilization technique 1

This technique may only be applied to a relatively fit patient, but it enables the technique to be applied single-handedly.

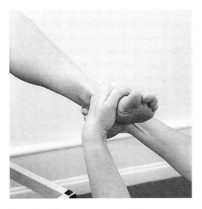

Fig. 11.27 Loose-body mobilization for the knee 1; hand position for mobilization into medial rotation.

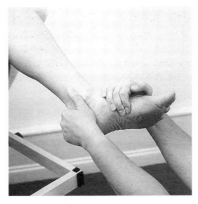

Fig. 11.28 Loose-body mobilization for the knee 1; hand position for mobilization into lateral rotation.

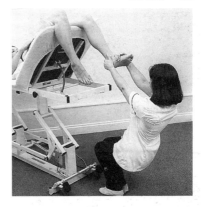

Fig. 11.29 Loose-body mobilization for the knee 1; starting position applying traction.

Position the patient in supine lying with the legs hanging over the end of the couch, the thighs supported. Arrange the couch so that it is as high as it will go and elevate the end of the bed. Run your hand down the posterior aspect of the ankle, grasping the calcaneum and pulling the ankle into dorsiflexion. Place the other hand on top of the mid-foot in order to rotate the leg into either medial or lateral rotation (Figs 11.27 and 11.28) (position your hands such that the hand on top of the foot will be pulling, not pushing, into rotation). Bend your knees and straighten your arms to apply traction (Fig. 11.29). Once traction is established, straighten your knees to extend the patient's knee, smartly rotating the leg at the same time (Figs 11.30 and 11.31).

Reassess the patient for an increase in range and a change in the end-feel. If the technique has helped, it can be repeated; if not, change your hand position to effect the opposite rotation.

The basis of this technique is traction, rotation and a movement towards extension of the knee. It can be modified to suit the patient or operator and you are encouraged to be inventive with the technique. It can be applied with the patient sitting over the edge of the bed, or a 'seat belt' may be applied to help the traction.

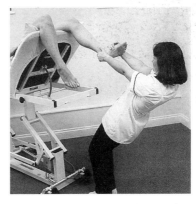

Fig. 11.30 Loose-body mobilization for the knee 1; straightening knees whilst performing the manoeuvre.

Loose-body mobilization technique 2 (Cyriax and Cyriax, 1983; Cyriax, 1984)

This technique requires an assistant. Position the patient in prone lying with the knee flexed to 90°. The assistant places two hands behind the knee joint ready to apply body weight to the thigh and therefore traction to the knee joint as the technique is applied. Stand adjacent to the patient's flexed knee, placing your foot distal to the patient, on the couch. Place the web between your index finger and thumb of one hand around the calcaneum to pull the ankle into dorsiflexion; the other hand wraps comfortably around the dorsum of the foot. Lift the patient's foot on to your flexed knee and ask the assistant to apply the traction (Fig. 11.32). Once traction is

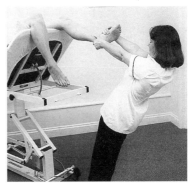

Fig. 11.31 Loose-body mobilization for the knee 1; ending the manoeuvre, avoiding full extension of the knee.

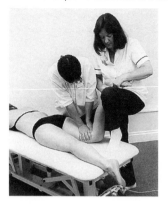

Fig. 11.32 Loose-body mobilization for the knee 2; starting position.

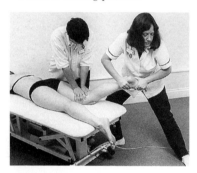

Fig. 11.33 Loose-body mobilization for the knee 2; completion of the manoeuvre.

established, remove your foot from the couch and place it to the side. Maintain the traction as you rotate the lower leg, simultaneously moving from flexion towards extension (Fig. 11.33). Reassess and repeat as necessary.

> **Loose-body mobilization technique 3 (Cyriax and Cyriax, 1983; Cyriax, 1984)**

This technique is useful if flexion is the limited movement. Position the patient comfortably in supine lying. Flex the hip on the affected side to 90° and stand adjacent to the patient. Place your forearm into the crook of the patient's flexed knee to act as a fulcrum. Take the knee into full flexion and apply a smart overpressure, releasing it immediately to achieve a brisk rocking movement of the upper tibia. Reassess the patient and repeat as necessary. This technique can be modified to include rotation, when an assistant may place a forearm into the crook of the knee to act as the fulcrum whilst you apply the flexion/rotation thrust.

Medial collateral ligament sprain

The medial collateral ligament is the ligament most vulnerable to injury at the knee, but the following treatment regime may be applied to the lateral collateral ligament if it is the site of the lesion. As the lateral collateral ligament is not associated with the fibrous joint capsule, the acute effusion common to medial collateral sprain will probably be absent.

The collateral and cruciate ligaments function together to control and stabilize the knee. The medial collateral ligament is anatomically related to the medial meniscus and functionally related to the anterior cruciate ligament. Injury may result in 'O'Donaghue's unhappy triad' affecting all three structures (Evans, 1986; Staron *et al.*, 1994). If tears of the medial meniscus and anterior cruciate ligament are confirmed by magnetic resonance imaging or arthroscopy, subtle signs of medial collateral ligament sprain should be sought, since the three conditions usually coexist (Staron *et al.*, 1994).

Rupture of the cruciate ligaments or a meniscal lesion produces an acute effusion which can be managed conservatively as for the acute phase of medial collateral ligament sprain. Once the acute phase has settled, a full assessment of the knee can be carried out, including assessment for ligamentous laxity and the provocative meniscal tests. A decision may then be taken concerning onwards referral for specialist opinion.

Ligament injuries are graded according to the amount of laxity and the end-feel (Daniel, 1990; Schenck and Heckman, 1993; Hartley, 1995). The following is applied to the medial collateral ligament:

Grade 1 injury: stretching and microfailure of some fibres of the ligament, pain, tenderness and swelling at the site of the injury, a mild capsular pattern may be present, no clinical instability noted and the end-feel is firm elastic.

Grade 2 injury: moderate–major tearing of the ligament fibres exceeding their elastic limit, pain and tenderness at the site of injury, moderate to severe swelling, movement limited in the capsular pattern, a minor degree of ligamentous laxity noted clinically, the end-feel is relatively firm elastic with a definite end point.

Grade 3 injury: macrofailure, or complete rupture of the ligament, swelling, possibly haemarthrosis and a capsular pattern of limited movement, severe pain at the time of injury, but relatively little since, definite ligamentous laxity noted and the joint may click as it returns to the neutral position, the end-feel is soft with no definite end-point.

Not all major ligamentous ruptures require surgical reconstruction and decisions are based on the lifestyle of the patient. A good functional recovery from ligamentous laxity may be achieved by strengthening the dynamic stabilizers of the knee, the hamstrings and quadriceps muscles, whilst maintaining control with appropriate braces. If haemarthrosis is present in the early acute knee, this will need to be aspirated.

From the history, medial collateral ligament sprain is possible if the knee is subjected to an excessive valgus, rotation of the flexed knee or a hyperextension stress. A combination of trauma may occur and, as already stated, the medial collateral ligament can be damaged in association with the anterior cruciate ligament and medial meniscus.

Acute medial collateral ligament sprain

Initially, the lesion is accompanied by a secondary traumatic arthritis which presents with a gross capsular pattern of limited movement. It will be impossible to apply provocative stress tests to either the ligament or menisci to assess associated damage. The history of the mechanism of the injury, the position of the leg and the forces applied will indicate medial collateral ligament sprain. The valgus test will produce pain to confirm diagnosis, but the grade of sprain will be difficult to ascertain initially since the reflex muscle spasm and effusion effectively splint the knee. Presence of haemarthrosis indicates possible anterior cruciate ligament damage and the Lachman test, at least, can be applied to this acute knee. Haemarthrosis and the presence of a positive Lachman test may indicate onward referral for specialist opinion.

The acute situation is managed conservatively with daily treatment initially, consisting of rest, ice, compression and elevation. Gentle friction massage is started as early as possible to gain some movement of the ligament over the underlying bone. This is followed by Grade A mobilization to maintain the function of the ligament.

The patient is encouraged to maintain a normal gait pattern with the aid of crutches if necessary. After approximately 3–5 days, the tensile strength of the healing ligament improves, the depth of

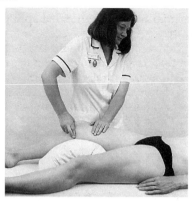

Fig. 11.34 Transverse friction massage of the acute medial collateral ligament sprain, in extension.

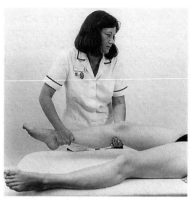

Fig. 11.35 Grade A mobilization into extension.

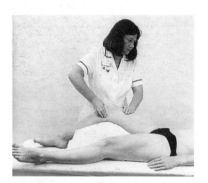

Fig. 11.36 Transverse friction massage of the acute medial collateral ligament sprain, in flexion.

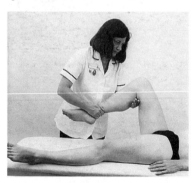

Fig. 11.37 Grade A mobilization into flexion.

friction massage is gradually increased and the range of active painfree movement becomes greater. The regime continues until a full range of painfree movement is restored, always guided by pain. Other exercises are incorporated as appropriate, aiming towards full rehabilitation of the patient.

Transverse friction massage for acute sprain of the medial collateral ligament (Cyriax and Cyriax, 1983; Cyriax, 1984)

Position the patient in half lying with enough pillows to support the knee in the maximum amount of extension that can be achieved without causing pain (Fig. 11.34). Palpate for the site of the lesion, which may be difficult to locate due to the swelling. However, the commonest site of sprain is at the joint line and this can be located by following the advice given in the surface marking and palpation section earlier in the chapter. Place two or three fingers across the site of the lesion and gently apply transverse friction massage to achieve a numbing effect. Once some numbing and depth are achieved, apply deeper friction massage for approximately six sweeps. Follow this immediately with Grade A active mobilization towards extension (Fig. 11.35).

Next, support the knee in the maximum amount of flexion that can be achieved without pain, and repeat the friction technique as above (Fig. 11.36). Follow this immediately with Grade A active exercises towards flexion (Fig. 11.37).

On a daily basis, the pain and swelling reduce and the range of movement increases. The knee should not be pushed towards extension as the medial collateral ligament is taut in extension and may become overstretched.

The usual exercises for maintenance of muscle strength should be included together with gait re-education and eventually full rehabilitation according to the patient's needs. Treating the ligament in this way maintains its mobility and function and it should not require stretching.

An uncommon complication of medial collateral ligament sprain is Stieda–Pellegrini's syndrome and this should be considered if the range of movement at the knee fails to improve (Cyriax, 1982). It is believed that, following trauma to the medial collateral ligament, calcium is deposited in the ligament, usually near the superior medial femoral condyle (Wang and Shapiro, 1995). Rest and local pain-relieving treatment together with analgesia are recommended and occasionally surgical excision if the condition fails to respond to conservative measures.

Chronic medial collateral ligament sprain

The patient has a past history of sprain to the ligament which may have largely settled without treatment. However, activity still causes pain and transient swelling around the ligament. On examination the patient may have end-range pain or limitation of movement. The valgus stress test produces the pain, as do hyperextension and passive lateral rotation – movements which tighten the ligament. Assessment should be made for instability and any associated structural damage.

The ligament has developed adhesions which interfere with function. The principle of treatment is to rupture the unwanted adhesions with a Grade C manipulation, once the ligament has been prepared by deep transverse friction massage. Following manipulative rupture, the patient is instructed to mobilize vigorously in order to maintain the movement gained through manipulation.

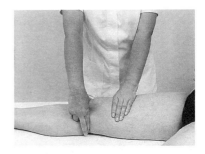

Fig. 11.38 Transverse friction massage of the chronic medial collateral ligament sprain in extension.

Transverse friction massage and Grade C manipulation for chronic sprain of the medial collateral ligament (Cyriax and Cyriax, 1983; Cyriax, 1984)

The ligament is prepared for the mobilization technique with transverse friction massage. Position the patient in half lying with the knee in maximum extension and locate the site of the lesion. Apply the friction massage with the index finger reinforced by the middle finger and the thumb placed on the opposite side of the knee for counterpressure (Fig. 11.38). Direct the pressure down on to the ligament and sweep transversely across the fibres, keeping the finger parallel to the upper border of the tibia. Treatment is maintained for approximately 10 min after the numbing effect is achieved.

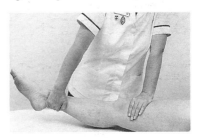

Fig. 11.39 Grade C manipulation into extension.

The Grade C manipulation follows immediately. Place one hand just above the knee to maintain the thigh on the couch. Wrap the other hand around the posterior aspect of the heel. Lean on the thigh, lifting the lower leg and, once end-range extension is achieved, a minimal-amplitude, high-velocity thrust is applied by side flexing your body (Fig. 11.39).

Next place the knee in maximum flexion (Fig. 11.40). The direction of the friction massage will have to be adjusted to run parallel to the upper tibia, remembering that the ligament moves backwards a little in flexion.

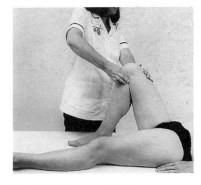

Fig. 11.40 Transverse friction massage of the chronic medial ligament sprain in flexion.

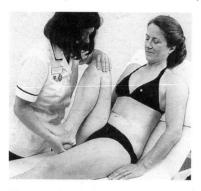

Fig. 11.41 Grade C manipulation into flexion.

The Grade C manipulation follows immediately by applying flexion with a lateral rotation stress. Place the hip and knee in maximum flexion. Cup the heel into your hand and pull the leg into lateral rotation by resting your forearm along the medial border of the foot. Maintain the lateral rotation and take the leg into maximum passive flexion. A minimal-amplitude, high-velocity thrust is applied into flexion (Fig. 11.41). The technique can be modified to apply the thrust in the direction of the lateral rotation, or to add a valgus stress if assessment of the patient shows movement to be limited in these directions.

Treatment of chronic collateral ligament sprain should be successful in two or three treatment sessions. It is important that the patient vigorously exercises the knee to maintain the mobility of the ligament.

Coronary ligaments

The patient presents with a history of rotational strain and on examination there is pain on the appropriate passive rotation. The coronary ligaments may be involved in a hyperextension injury since the menisci move forwards during extension of the tibiofemoral joint. The longer lateral coronary ligaments are less vulnerable to trauma than the shorter medial coronary ligaments and the attachment of the medial meniscus to the deep medial collateral ligament makes the medial aspect of the joint more susceptible to injury.

A sprain of the medial coronary ligaments will be discussed, but if the lesion lies in the lateral coronary ligaments, the same principles apply.

An effusion may be present depending on the severity of the lesion, but this is not as obvious as that occurring with injury to the collateral or cruciate ligaments. Medial coronary ligament sprain produces pain on passive lateral rotation of the tibia with the tibiofemoral joint at 90° of flexion. Pain may also be provoked by passive extension as the menisci move forwards on the tibia. Palpation confirms the site of the lesion, which is usually on the anteromedial joint line and the adjacent tibial plateau. It is essential that full palpation is conducted, including through the medial collateral ligament, to determine the extent of the lesion.

Transverse friction massage of the coronary ligaments

The treatment of choice is transverse friction massage. Position the patient comfortably in half lying with the knee flexed to approximately 45° and laterally rotated to expose the medial tibial plateau. Place an index finger reinforced by the middle finger on top of the medial tibial plateau at the site of the lesion. Direct the pressure down on to the ligaments and sweep transversely across the fibres (Fig. 11.42). The friction massage is given for 10 min after the numbing effect is achieved. Since the ligaments do not span the joint line, exercises or mobilization are not appropriate.

The ligaments may be injected, using the positioning as for the transverse frictions and applying the general principles with regard to dosage, using a peppering technique and advising relative rest for up to 2 weeks.

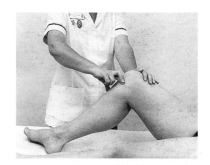

Fig. 11.42 Transverse friction massage of the medial coronary ligaments.

Bursitis

Overuse or excessive friction can affect any of the bursae around the knee. The patient presents with pain localized to the site of the lesion and there may be local swelling. The prepatellar and infrapatellar bursae are commonly involved and, if swelling is a problem, the bursa can be drained. Bursitis responds to locally applied electrotherapy or an injection of corticosteroid into the bursa. Before injecting the bursa, however, it is important to be sure that no infection is present, since septic bursitis is possible in the superficial bursae.

Pes anserinus syndrome may involve the tendons and bursa, but the condition may mimic medial collateral ligament sprain. Pain and tenderness occur 5–6 cm below the medial joint line, which is aggravated by activity and there may be slight swelling and crepitus over the bursal area. Treatment consists of locally applied anti-inflammatory modalities or by applying the principles of corticosteroid injection (Safran and Fu, 1995).

Excessive friction may cause iliotibial band syndrome involving the iliotibial tract and the underlying bursa. It particularly occurs in long-distance runners and cyclists and is often associated with tightness of the iliotibial tract (Safran and Fu, 1995). Pain is felt laterally, 2–3 cm proximal to the knee joint. Aggravating factors are downhill running and climbing stairs. Local anti-inflammatory modalities may be applied together with a change in training techniques. General principles of treatment may be applied.

Contractile lesions

Quadriceps

Direct trauma to the quadriceps muscle belly causes swelling and superficial bruising which eventually tracks down the leg. Known in sporting circles as 'dead leg', it has the potential to develop myositis ossificans traumatica, particularly if the contusion is accompanied by gross limitation of knee flexion (Norris, 1993).

Transverse friction massage to the quadriceps muscle belly

Position the patient in sitting with the knee straight. Locate the site of the lesion and, using the fingers, apply transverse friction massage

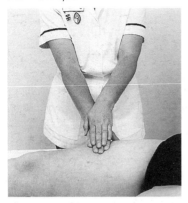

Fig. 11.43 Transverse friction massage to the quadriceps muscle belly.

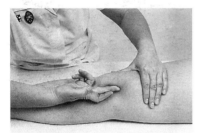

Fig. 11.44 Transverse friction massage of the quadriceps expansions, medial.

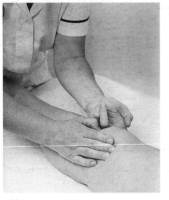

Fig. 11.45 Transverse friction massage of the quadriceps expansions, lateral.

(Fig. 11.43). After the numbing effect is achieved, apply six effective sweeps to the acute lesion and 10 min of deep friction massage for the chronic lesion, followed up by Grade A exercises.

Tendinitis of the medial and lateral quadriceps expansions (patellar retinaculum)

The patient usually presents with a gradual onset of pain felt locally at the front of the knee associated with overuse. On examination there is pain on resisted knee extension and tenderness located at the medial, lateral or both borders of the patella. Often the lesion lies at the 'corners' of the patella.

> **Transverse friction massage of the quadriceps expansions (Cyriax and Cyriax, 1983; Cyriax, 1984)**

Having established the site of the lesion, the treatment of choice is deep transverse friction massage. Position the patient comfortably with the knee supported and relaxed in extension. Push and hold the patella to one side. Use the middle finger reinforced by the index finger and rotate the forearm to direct the pressure up and under the edge of the patella (Figs 11.44 and 11.45). Sweep transversely across the fibres in a superior–inferior direction and continue treatment for 10 min after the numbing effect has been achieved. It may be necessary to treat several areas around the patella. Relative rest is advised where functional movements may continue, but no overuse or stretching until the structure is painfree on resisted testing.

Overuse lesions of the quadriceps expansions may be secondary to malalignment or abnormal tracking of the patella. Treatment may be incorporated into a regime of corrective taping and re-education of the oblique portion of vastus medialis.

Patellar tendinitis

There are two sites for patellar tendinitis:

- At the apex of the patella (infrapatellar tendon).
- At the base of the patella (suprapatellar tendon).

The most common is infrapatellar tendinitis and it may be associated with repetitive jumping actions. The repetitive overuse results in microfailure and fraying of the tendon fibres and focal degeneration (Curwin and Stanish, 1984).

The symptoms and signs are similar to those described for tendinitis of the quadriceps expansions, but the site of the lesion will be located to either the infra- or suprapatellar tendons. Treatment may be deep friction massage or corticosteroid injection followed by relative rest. Infrapatellar fat pad inflammation (Hoffa's disease) produces symptoms that mimic infrapatellar tendinitis, but pain is produced by gentle squeezing of the fat pad at either side of the patella (Curwin and Stanish, 1984).

Transverse friction massage of the infrapatellar and suprapatellar tendons (Cyriax and Cyriax, 1983; Cyriax, 1984)

Position the patient comfortably with the knee relaxed and supported in extension. Apply the web space between your index finger and thumb of one hand to the base of the patella, tilting the apex. Using the middle finger of the other hand reinforced by the index, supinate the forearm to direct the pressure up under the apex of the patella and sweep transversely across the fibres (Fig. 11.46). Ten minutes' friction massage is applied after the numbing effect is achieved. Relative rest is advised where functional movements may continue, but no overuse or stretching until the structure is painfree on resisted testing.

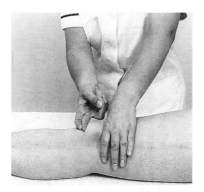

Fig. 11.46 Transverse friction massage of the infrapatellar tendon.

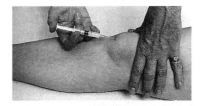

Fig. 11.47 Injection of the infrapatellar tendon.

Injection of the infrapatellar and suprapatellar tendons (Cyriax and Cyriax, 1983; Cyriax, 1984)

Kenalog 40 mg/ml	Total steroid	Lignocaine 1%	Total volume
0.5 ml	20 mg	1 ml	1.5 ml

23G × 1 in (0.6 × 25 mm) blue needle

Position the patient as described for the friction massage technique, applying pressure to the base of the patella with your stabilizing hand, to make the apex accessible (Fig. 11.47). Insert the needle just distal to the apex of the patella and advance until contact is made with bone. Deliver the injection by a peppering technique, fanning out to deposit two parallel rows of droplets of corticosteroid across the full width of the teno-osseous junction. Note that the injection is delivered into the teno-osseous junction and not the body of the tendon. The patient is advised to maintain a period of relative rest for approximately 2 weeks following injection.

For treatment of suprapatellar tendinitis, the above principles are applied (Figs 11.48 and 11.49).

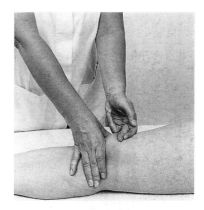

Fig. 11.48 Transverse friction massage of the suprapatellar tendon.

Tendinitis of the insertions of the hamstring muscles

The patient presents with pain localized to the posterior aspect of the knee following a history of overuse. Pain is reproduced by resisted knee flexion and the site of tenderness is located medially or laterally according to the tendons involved. Principles of treatment can be applied using either deep transverse friction massage or corticosteroid injection via a peppering technique. Relative rest is advised where functional movements may continue,

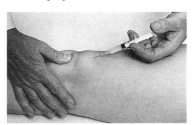

Fig. 11.49 Injection of the suprapatellar tendon.

but no overuse or stretching until the structure is painfree on resisted testing.

Lesions of the hamstrings muscle belly and the tendon of origin are discussed in Chapter 10. Lesions of gastrocnemius are discussed in Chapter 12.

References

Adler, G.G., Hoekman, R.A., Beach, D.M. (1995) Drop leg Lachman test. *American Journal of Sports Medicine* **23**: 320–323.

Amiel, D., Kuiper, S., Akeson, W.H. (1990) Cruciate ligaments. In: *Knee Ligaments: Structure, Function, Injury and Repair* (Daniel, D. *et al.*, eds). Raven Press, pp. 365–376.

Barrack, R.L., Skinner, H.B. (1990) The sensory function of knee ligaments. In: *Knee Ligaments: Structure, Function, Injury and Repair* (Daniel, D. *et al.*, eds). Raven Press, pp. 95–112.

Bessette, G.C. (1992) The meniscus. *Orthopaedics* **15**: 35–42.

Burks, R.T. (1990) Gross anatomy. In: *Knee Ligaments: Structure, Function, Injury and Repair* (Daniel, D. *et al.*, eds). Raven Press, pp. 59–75.

Butler, D.L., Noyes, F.R., Grood, E.S. (1980) Ligamentous restraints to anterior–posterior drawer in the human knee. *Journal of Bone and Joint Surgery* **62-A**: 259–270.

Curtin, W., O'Farrell, D., McGoldrick, F. *et al.* (1992) The correlation between clinical diagnosis of knee pathology and findings in arthroscopy. *Irish Journal of Medical Science* 135–136.

Curwin, S., Stanish, W.D. (1984) Jumper's knee. In: *Tendinitis – Its Etiology and Treatment*. Collamore Press.

Cyriax, J. (1982) *Textbook of Orthopaedic Medicine*, vol. 1, 8th edn. Baillière Tindall.

Cyriax, J. (1984) *Textbook of Orthopaedic Medicine*, vol. 2, 11th edn. Baillière Tindall.

Cyriax, J., Cyriax, P. (1983) *Illustrated Manual of Orthopaedic Medicine*. Butterworths.

Daniel, D.M. (1990) Diagnosis of a ligament injury. In: *Knee Ligaments: Structure, Function, Injury and Repair* (Daniel, D. *et al.*, eds). Raven Press, pp. 3–10.

Edwards, D., Villar, R. (1993) Anterior cruciate ligament injury. *The Practitioner* **237**: 113–117.

Evans, P. (1986) *The Knee Joint*. Churchill Livingstone.

Felson, D.T., Anderson, J.J., Naimark, A. *et al.* (1988) Obesity and knee osteoarthritis. *Annals of Internal Medicine* **July**: 18–24.

Hartley, A. (1995) *Practical Joint Assessment – Lower Quadrant*, 2nd edn. Mosby.

Kapandji, I.A. (1970) *The Physiology of the Joints, Lower Limb*, vol. 2, 2nd edn. Churchill Livingstone.

Katz, J.W., Fingeroth, R.J. (1986) The diagnostic accuracy of ruptures of the anterior cruciate ligament comparing the Lachman test, the anterior drawer sign, and the pivot shift test in acute and chronic knee injuries. *American Journal of Sports Medicine* **14**: 88–91.

Nordin, M., Frankel, V.H. (1989) *Basic Biomechanics of the Musculoskeletal System*, 2nd edn. Lea & Febiger.

Norris, C.M. (1993) *Sports Injuries: Diagnosis and Management for Physiotherapists*. Butterworth-Heinemann.

Paice, E. (1995) Pain in the hip and knee. *British Medical Journal* **310**: 319–322.

Palastanga, N., Field, D., Soames, R. (1994) *Anatomy and Human Movement*, 2nd edn. Butterworth-Heinemann.

Perko, M.M.J., Cross, M.J., Ruske, D., Phillip, R. (1992) Anterior cruciate ligament injuries, clues for diagnosis. *Medical Journal of Australia* **157**: 467–470.

Rubinstein, R.A., Shelbourne, K.D., McCarroll, J.R. *et al.* (1994) The accuracy of the clinical examination in the setting of posterior cruciate ligament injuries. *American Journal of Sports Medicine* **22**: 550–557.

Safran, M.R., Fu, F.H. (1995) Uncommon causes of knee pain in the athelete. *Orthopedic Clinics of North America* **26**: 547–559.

Schenck, R.C., Heckman, J.D. (1993) Injuries of the knee. *Clinical Symposia* **45**: 2–32.

Schweitzer, M.E., Tran, D., Deely, D.M., Hume, E.L. (1995) Medial collateral ligament injuries: evaluation of multiple signs, prevalence and location of associated bone bruises, and assessment with MR imaging. **March**: *Radiology* 825–829.

Smith, B.W., Green, G.A. (1995) Acute knee injuries: part I. History and physical examination. *American Family Physician* **51**: 615–621.

Staron, R.B., Haramati, N., Feldman, F. *et al.* (1994) O'Donoghue's triad: magnetic resonance imaging evidence. *International Skeletal Society* **23**: 633–636.

Wang, J.C., Shapiro, M.S. (1995) Pelligrini–Steida syndrome. *American Journal of Orthopaedics* **June**: 493–497.

Williams, P.L, Warwick, R., Dyson, M., Bannister, L.H. (1989) *Gray's Anatomy*, 37th edn. Churchill Livingstone.

Woo, S.L.-Y., Wang, C., Newton, P.O., Lyon, R.M. (1990) The response of ligaments to stress deprivation and stress enhancement. In: *Knee Ligaments: Sructure, Function, Injury and Repair* (Daniel, D. *et al.*, eds). Raven Press, pp. 337–350.

12 The ankle and foot

Summary

Sprained ankle is a commonly encountered traumatic lesion in primary care. Mismanagement leads to a chronic persistent condition and likely recurrence. Other lesions of the foot and ankle have been attributed to faulty biomechanics which may also lead to adaptive postures in the lower limb and spine, with consequent problems.

This chapter confines itself to common lesions in the ankle and foot, arising from arthritis, trauma or overuse, and begins with a presentation of the relevant anatomy and palpation techniques, to aid their identification. Points from the history are considered and a logical sequence of objective examination is given, followed by discussion of lesions and suggestions for treatment and management.

Anatomy

Inert structures

The *inferior tibiofibular joint* is the articulation between the fibular notch on the lateral aspect of the tibia and the distal end of the fibula. It is considered to be a syndesmosis because the firm union of the two bones is largely due to the interosseous membrane. Anterior and posterior ligaments reinforce the joint.

The deep part of the posterior ligament is the *inferior transverse tibiofibular ligament* which passes under the posterior ligament from the tibia, into the malleolar fossa of the fibular. It is a thickened band of yellow elastic fibres forming part of the articulating surface of the ankle joint.

The firm union of the inferior tibiofibular joint is significant to the mortise of the ankle joint and a major factor in its inherent stability. When the ankle joint is in dorsiflexion, the close-packed position, the elastic nature of the inferior tibiofibular joint ligament allows the joint to yield and separate, accommodating the wider anterior aspect of the trochlear surface of the talus. In plantarflexion the ligament recoils as the narrower posterior aspect of the talus moves into the mortise, approximating the malleoli to maintain a pinch-like grip on the talus.

Dorsiflexion and plantarflexion of the ankle will induce small accessory movements in the inferior tibiofibular joint which in turn affect the superior tibiofibular joint. Injuries of the syndesmosis usually involve forced dorsiflexion, causing widening or diastasis of the ankle mortise (Edwards and DeLee, 1984; Boytim *et al.*, 1991; Marder, 1994). However, isolated injuries are uncommon and damage usually occurs in association with other major ligamentous disruption and fracture.

The *ankle joint (talocrural joint)* is a uniaxial, synovial hinge joint between the mortise, formed by the distal ends of the tibia and fibula, and the trochlear surface and sides of the talus. It bears more weight per unit area than any other joint, and any malalignment or instability may lead to degenerative changes (Sartoris, 1994). The joint surfaces are covered with hyaline cartilage and surrounded by a fibrous capsule which attaches to the margins of the articulating surfaces. The capsule is lined with synovium and reinforced by strong collateral ligaments.

The collateral ligaments are roughly triangular in their attachments, radiating downwards from the malleoli to a wide base. Each has anterior and posterior components which link with the talus, and a central component that links with the calcaneum.

Movement at the ankle joint occurs about a transverse axis in a sagittal plane and amounts to approximately 20° of dorsiflexion and 35° of plantarflexion, allowing the foot to adjust to the surface on which it is placed. Dorsiflexion achieves the close-packed position of the ankle joint and no movement of the talus in the mortise should be possible in this position. In full plantarflexion, the loose-packed position, a small amount of side-to-side movement of the talus should be possible.

The *medial collateral (deltoid) ligament* forms a strong triangular band passing from the anterior and posterior borders of the medial malleolus and its apex. Radiating out, it forms a continuous line of attachment from the navicular in front, along the sustentaculum tali, to the talus behind. It has deep and superficial fibres. The deep fibres consist of anterior tibiotalar and posterior tibiotalar components; the superficial fibres consist of tibionavicular and tibiocalcaneal components.

As the medial collateral ligament offers such strong support to the medial aspect of the ankle joint, traumatic injuries more commonly cause fracture and disruption of the syndesmosis rather than ligamentous injury. Most strain on the ligament occurs with a plantarflexion/eversion stress. Biomechanical problems in the foot can, however, lead to an overuse lesion of gradual onset of the medial collateral ligament and treatment of this should be directed to the cause.

The *lateral collateral ligament* consists of three separate bands which leave the ligament deficient in its support of the lateral aspect of the ankle joint. Consequently inversion and forced plantarflexion injuries commonly affect the lateral collateral ligament (Liu and Jason, 1994).

The components of the lateral collateral ligament are as follows (Fig. 12.1):

- The *anterior talofibular ligament* is an integral part of the capsule of the ankle joint. It arises from the anterior border and

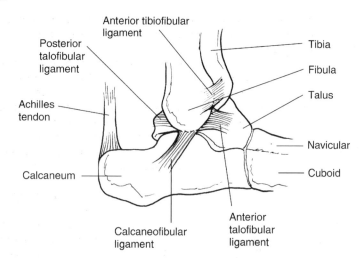

Fig. 12.1 Lateral collateral ligament of the ankle.

tip of the lateral malleolus and passes deeply and anteromedially across the ankle joint to the neck of the talus. It is a wide, flattened band approximately the width of the patient's index finger. In the neutral position, the ligament runs almost parallel to the transverse axis of the foot, whilst in plantarflexion it runs more parallel to the vertical axis of the leg (Kannus and Renstrom, 1991). It is the most vulnerable of the three components to plantarflexion injury.

- The *calcaneofibular ligament* is a narrow cord, separate from the capsule of the ankle joint. It arises from the apex of the lateral malleolus and passes obliquely inferoposteriorly, under the peroneal tendons, to attach to the calcaneum just behind the peroneal tubercle. Here it is closely related to the overlying peroneal sheath containing the tendons of peroneus longus and brevis (Marder, 1994). This component of the ligament crosses both the ankle and subtalar joints and is vulnerable to a varus stress applied in dorsiflexion.
- The *posterior talofibular ligament* is a strong, thick band arising from the posterior border of the lateral malleolus and passing horizontally and posteromedially to the posterior aspect of the talus. Clinically, it is rare to find involvement of this ligamentous component.

The anterior talofibular ligament and calcaneofibular ligament work synergistically and as one ligament relaxes, the other tenses. The anterior talofibular ligament has the weakest tensile strength (Boruta *et al.*, 1990).

The foot consists of 26 bones and 57 joints which enable it to act as a rigid structure for weight-bearing, e.g. pointing in ballet, or to be converted into a flexible structure for mobility, e.g. gait activities (Nordin and Frankel, 1989). The foot supports body weight and controls posture by maintaining the centre of gravity. It assists propulsion and lift, as well as restraining gait activities and acting as a shock absorber. To provide this variety of function, arches have developed together with the joints, ligaments and muscles, all contributing to functional activities. The main joints and ligaments of the arches, of clinical concern in orthopaedic medicine, will be described briefly here.

The *subtalar (talocalacaneal) joint* is a synovial joint between the talus and underlying calcaneum, which works in conjunction with the ankle and midtarsal joints to form a functional component. These joints together allow the foot to adapt to the surface of stance and to act as a shock absorber. They allow adjustment of the arches of the foot and, in conjunction with muscle activity, provide spring and propulsion to gait. During walking, the subtalar joint adapts to the side-to-side slope of the ground, accompanied by secondary rotation of the tibia (Evans, 1990).

Movements at the subtalar joint are complex due to the shape of the articulating facets, which allow a degree of play to occur simultaneously in three planes. The calcaneum 'pitches', 'turns' and 'rolls' (Kapandji, 1985) under the talus enabling these accessory movements to contribute to the functional movements of inversion and eversion. The movements at the subtalar joint can be expressed simply as supination, which achieves a varus position of the calcaneum, and pronation, which achieves a valgus position of the calcaneum.

The *talus* provides attachment for ligaments and many tendons pass over it, although it does not itself give insertion to any contractile unit.

The *sinus tarsi* is a tunnel formed by the sulcus tali and the calcaneal sulcus together, and is occupied by the interosseous ligament. This divides the subtalar joint into two compartments – an important point to recognize when injecting the subtalar joint.

The *midtarsal (transverse tarsal) joints* consist of the *calcaneocuboid joint*, laterally, and the *talocalcaneonavicular joint*, medially. These joints adapt the posture of the foot, keeping the sole of the foot in contact with the ground, whatever the slope of the surface or the position of the leg. Together they act as a shock absorber as well as providing elasticity and spring to gait.

The *calcaneocuboid joint* is supported by the *calcaneocuboid ligament* which is a capsular ligament that runs along the dorsolateral aspect of the joint. This ligament is sometimes involved in an inversion sprain of the ankle.

Accessory movements of dorsiflexion, plantarflexion, abduction, adduction, pronation and supination occur at the midtarsal joints, contributing to the functional, composite movements of inversion and eversion.

Eversion turns the sole of the foot laterally and consists of pronation and abduction at the midtarsal joints, pronation at the subtalar joint and dorsiflexion at the ankle joint. Inversion turns the sole of the foot medially and consists of supination and adduction at the midtarsal joints, supination at the subtalar joint and plantarflexion at the ankle. The muscles responsible for eversion and inversion all insert distal to the midtarsal joints.

A series of arches, ligaments and muscles satisfies the requirements of the foot to be able to provide both strength and mobility.

- The *medial and lateral longitudinal arches* are supported posteriorly by the calcaneum and anteriorly by the metatarsal heads. The talus forms the summit of the arch. The medial longitudinal arch is the larger of the two and has a dynamic role for gait. It consists of the calcaneum, talus, navicular, the cuneiforms and three medial metatarsals. It absorbs and transmits weight back through the calcaneum and forward to the metatarsal heads, whilst providing elasticity for propulsion. The lateral longitudinal arch has a static role for weight-bearing. It is lower than the medial, making contact with the ground throughout its length to support load in standing. The main supporting mechanism for the longitudinal arches is the plantar fascia. Acting as a cable between the heel and the toes, it locks the joints of the foot and prevents the arches from collapsing during weight-bearing.
- The *transverse arch* is formed by the distal row of tarsal bones and the bases of the metatarsals, and acts to support and transmit body weight. As body weight is applied, the metatarsal bones separate and flatten slightly.

The arches of the foot depend on ligamentous and muscular support. The important ligaments are the long and short plantar ligaments, plantar aponeurosis and the spring ligament (plantar calcaneonavicular ligament). The intrinsic muscles of the foot maintain the arches, together with some of the long muscles of the leg. Tibialis anterior supports the medial arch, whilst peroneus longus supports the lateral arch.

The *spring (plantar calcaneonavicular) ligament* is a broad band connecting the sustentaculum tali to the navicular. It supports the talus, which rests in the centre of the ligament, stabilizing the medial longitudinal arch. Laxity or rupture of the spring ligament results in a flattening of the medial longitudinal arch (Rule *et al.*, 1993).

The *plantar fascia* arises from the medial calcaneal tuberosity and consists of longitudinally arranged fibres which pass into the forefoot, widening and thinning before dividing to extend into the toes (Karr, 1994). It is a strong connecting cable passing between the pillars of the longitudinal arch, where it acts as a supporting platform for weight-bearing. It has very little ability to lengthen, but under loading gives slightly to act as a shock absorber. The intrinsic foot muscles and the ligaments aid the plantar fascia in supporting the longitudinal arches.

Contractile structures

As tendons cross the ankle joint, they change their direction from running vertically to horizontally. Several retinacula prevent the tendons from bowstringing under activity, whilst synovial sheaths protect the tendons as they pass under the retinacula.

All anterior muscles of the lower leg are supplied by the deep peroneal nerve and their principal function is dorsiflexion of the ankle and extension of the toes.

Tibialis anterior (L4–5) takes origin from the upper two-thirds of the lateral tibial shaft and adjacent interosseous membrane. It becomes tendinous in its lower third, passing across the anteromedial aspect of the ankle joint to insert into the medial aspect of the medial cuneiform and the base of the first metatarsal. Its function is to dorsiflex the ankle, during the swing-through phase of gait, and invert the foot. It raises the medial longitudinal arch and works in conjunction with other muscles to counteract gravity and to control foot placement. This tendon runs a relatively straight course and is not a common cause of pain. However, hill running or irritation from tight-fitting boots, for example, may cause lesions of tibialis anterior (Frey and Shereff, 1988; Chandnani and Bradley, 1994).

Extensor hallucis longus (L5, S1) takes origin from the middle of the anteromedial border of the fibula and passes downwards and medially to a tendon which inserts into the base of the distal phalanx of the hallux. Functionally it dorsiflexes the ankle and extends the hallux to enable the big toe and foot to clear the ground during the swing-through phase.

Extensor digitorum longus (L5, S1) takes origin from the upper two-thirds of the anterior aspect of the fibula and passes downwards under the extensor retinacula, dividing into four tendons which insert into the dorsal digital expansions of the lateral four toes. Functionally, it assists dorsiflexion of the ankle and extends the lateral four toes, to clear the ground during the swing-through phase.

Peroneus tertius (L5, S1), a divorced part of extensor digitorum longus, arises from the lower anterolateral aspect of the fibula and inserts into the base of the fifth metatarsal. It functions as a weak dorsiflexor of the ankle and an evertor of the foot.

The peroneal muscles pass under two rectinacula to reach the lateral side of the foot. The principal function of the lateral muscles is to evert the foot, controlling side-to-side movements in standing and acting as the primary lateral dynamic stabilizers of the ankle (Frey and Shereff, 1988). Peroneus longus, together with tibialis anterior, forms a stirrup for the foot, maintaining and supporting the arches. Both peroneus longus and brevis are supplied by the superficial peroneal nerve.

Peroneus longus (L5, S1–2), the more superficial of the two peroneal tendons, arises from the head and upper lateral two-thirds of the fibula. It becomes tendinous just above the ankle and passes behind the lateral malleolus in a sheath common to it and peroneus brevis. Continuing on, it crosses the lateral surface of the calcaneum, passing below the peroneal tubercle, where it leaves peroneus brevis. It occupies a groove on the lateral and plantar surfaces of the cuboid and crosses the sole of the foot obliquely to insert into the lateral side of the base of the first metatarsal and adjacent medial cuneiform.

Peroneus brevis (L5, S1–2) arises from the lower lateral surface of the fibula. It lies in front of peroneus longus as the tendons pass behind the lateral malleolus in the common sheath. It crosses the calcaneum above the peroneal tubercle to insert into the base of the fifth metatarsal.

Generally, the more superficial posterior muscles are concerned mainly with plantarflexion of the ankle, whilst the deep muscles flex the toes. Both groups are supplied by the tibial nerve.

Gastrocnemius (S1–2) is the most superficial of the posterior muscles and gives the calf its characteristic shape. It has two heads of origin from the appropriate posterior femoral condyle. The medial head is larger, extends more distally and is a common site for muscle belly injuries. The two muscle heads come together in a broad tendon which is joined on the anterolateral side by soleus, forming the Achilles tendon. Functionally, gastrocnemius flexes the knee and plantarflexes the ankle.

Soleus (S1–2) lies deep to the gastrocnemius, arising from the upper posterior aspect of the fibula and soleal line of the tibia. The muscle fibres pass to a membranous tendon which lies deep to the gastrocnemius, allowing both muscles to function individually. These tendon fibres blend with the Achilles tendon.

Plantaris (S1–2) arises from the posterior aspect of the lateral supracondylar ridge of the femur and descends medially to blend with the Achilles tendon. Its function is to assist the gastrocnemius.

Gastrocnemius, soleus and plantaris form a functional group known as the *triceps surae*, but they also have independent functions. Gastrocnemius works with plantaris to flex the knee and plantarflex the foot, providing propulsion to the push-off phase of gait. Soleus works continuously as a postural muscle through its slow-twitch muscle fibres which maintain the upright posture (McMinn *et al.*, 1995). In standing, the ankle is in a loose-packed position with the centre of gravity falling anterior to the joint. Soleus counteracts the tendency for body weight to move forwards over the stationary foot (Williams *et al.*, 1989).

The *Achilles tendon* is a long tendon which receives the fibres of gastrocnemius and soleus. The insertion of the Achilles tendon is cushioned by two bursae – the retrocalcaneal bursa on its deep surface and the subcutaneous Achilles bursa on its superficial surface (Smart *et al.*, 1980). The tendon fibres twist as they pass down to their insertion into the middle of the posterior surface of the calcaneum. This twist in the tendon fibres is understood to be responsible for the tendon's elastic properties, the stored energy providing propulsion to lift the heel during walking, running and jumping activities (Norris, 1993). The tendon has a zone of relatively poor vascularity 2–6 cm above its insertion and is prone to overuse, degeneration and rupture, particularly at this site (Smart *et al.*, 1980; Chandnani and Bradley, 1994).

Tibialis posterior (L4–5) arises from the upper posterolateral surface of the tibia. It passes behind the medial malleolus in its own sheath, crosses the deltoid ligament and inserts into the tuberosity of the navicular. It sends tendinous slips on to every tarsal bone except the talus. Functionally it is the main invertor of the foot, working with tibialis anterior. It gives support to the arches of the foot through its many tendinous insertions. It decelerates subtalar pronation after heel contact (Blake *et al.*, 1994). Activities which involve rapid changes in direction, e.g. soccer, tennis and hockey, place increased stress on the tibialis posterior and make it vulnerable to injury in these situations (Frey and Shereff, 1988).

Flexor digitorum longus (S2–3) arises from the middle of the posterior surface of the tibia and passes downwards, becoming tendinous above the ankle joint. Behind the medial malleolus it is medial to tibialis posterior and occupies the groove under the sustentaculum tali. Dividing into four tendons, it inserts into the base of the distal phalanx of the lateral four toes. Functionally, flexor digitorum longus works with the lumbricals to keep the pads of the toes in contact with the ground, increasing the weight-bearing surface. It also acts to assist plantarflexion during the toe-off phase of gait and repeated push-off activity may cause injury of this tendon (Frey and Shereff, 1988).

The *lumbricals* (S2–3) arise from flexor digitorum longus tendons and insert into the dorsal digital expansions. They flex the metatarsophalangeal joints and extend the interphalangeal joints; this counteracts the clawing tendency of the flexor digitorum longus. Together they maintain the medial arch.

Flexor hallucis longus (S2–3) arises from the lower posterior surface of the fibula and passes behind the medial malleolus and under the sustentaculum tali to insert into the base of the distal phalanx of the big toe. It functions to provide the final thrust for toe-off and is important in supporting the medial longitudinal arch. Activities which involve repeatedly pushing off from the forefoot, e.g. ballet, may cause lesions in this tendon (Frey and Shereff, 1988).

A guide to surface marking and palpation

Medial aspect (Fig. 12.2)

Palpate the short, thick, *medial tibial malleolus*, appreciating that the apex, anterior and posterior borders are all subcutaneous. Compare this with the longer, slender, *lateral fibular malleolus* which tends to project further distally and lie slightly more posteriorly.

It is difficult to palpate the tendons lying behind the medial malleolus, but from medial to lateral they are *t*ibialis posterior,

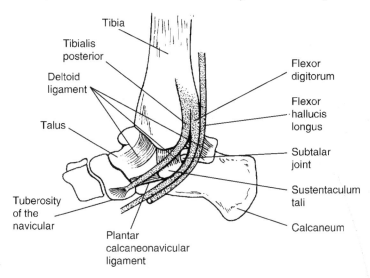

Fig. 12.2 Medial aspect of the ankle.

flexor *d*igitorum longus and flexor *h*allucis longus (*T*om, *D*ick and *H*arry). You can palpate the *posterior tibial artery* by applying light pressure behind the medial malleolus, approximately halfway between it and the Achilles tendon.

Consider the triangular *medial (deltoid) collateral ligament* which fans down from the medial malleolus to attach by a broad base from the navicular in front, to the talus behind.

Palpate the *sustentaculum tali* lying approximately one thumb's width directly below the medial malleolus, where it feels like a horizontal, bony shelf.

Move directly forwards from the sustentaculum tali to the next palpable bony bump, the *tuberosity of the navicular*. This gives insertion to *tibialis posterior* and lies at the level of the lip of a slip-on shoe. Move directly forwards from the navicular to palpate the *medial cuneiform* and the *base of the first metatarsal*.

Anterior aspect (Fig. 12.3)

Place the ankle joint into plantarflexion and inversion, making the *talus* both visible and palpable anterior to the lateral malleolus. Palpate along from the anterior aspect of the lateral malleolus and the lower margin of the tibia to identify the *joint line of the ankle*.

Move to the front of the lateral malleolus and feel the depression on the lateral side of the talus; this marks the entrance of the *sinus tarsi*.

Palpate the *tibialis anterior, extensor hallucis longus, extensor digitorum longus and peroneus tertius tendons* (from medial to lateral) as they cross the ankle joint anteriorly.

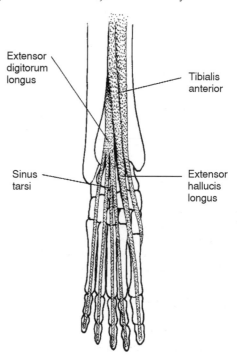

Fig. 12.3 Anterior aspect of the ankle.

Palpate the *dorsalis pedis pulse* approximately halfway between the malleoli on the dorsum of the foot, just lateral to the tendon of extensor hallucis longus.

Posterior aspect (Fig. 12.4)

Palpate the *calcaneum*, the largest of the tarsal bones, which forms the bony prominence of the heel.

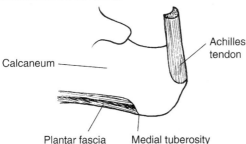

Fig. 12.4 Posterior structures of the ankle.

Palpate the *medial tuberosity of the calcaneum*, which can be located at the posteromedial edge of the plantar surface of the calcaneum; deep palpation may be necessary. This marks the insertion of the plantar fascia (Fig. 12.5).

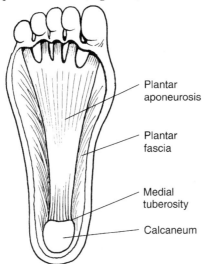

Fig. 12.5 Plantar fascia.

Locate the insertion of the *Achilles tendon* into the middle third of the posterior surface of the calcaneum. Palpate the Achilles tendon, appreciating its thickness, and follow it up to the two fleshy bellies of the gastrocnemius; the medial belly should be felt to extend further distally than the lateral.

Lateral aspect (Fig. 12.6)

Palpate the *lateral malleolus*. Move approximately one finger's width below it and slightly anteriorly to locate the *peroneal tubercle*.

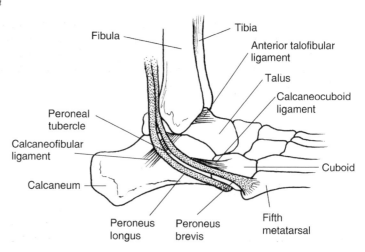

Fig. 12.6 Structures of the lateral aspect of the ankle.

This tubercle varies in size and position so may not be obvious. It divides the tendons of peroneus longus and brevis.

Consider the individual components of the lateral collateral ligament which take origin from the lateral malleolus. The *anterior talofibular ligament* is approximately the width of an index finger and it passes deeply, anteromedially to the talus. Its fibres run roughly parallel to the sole of the foot and it may be palpated in the region of the sinus tarsi. The *calcaneofibular ligament* passes obliquely downwards and backwards, under the peroneal tendons. The *posterior talofibular ligament* passes horizontally backwards to attach to the posterior talus; it is difficult to palpate.

Palpate the *base of the fifth metatarsal* and appreciate its prominent tubercle which gives attachment to peroneus brevis. Placing a thumb vertically behind the base of the fifth metatarsal will indicate the approximate position of the calcaneocuboid joint line. Placing another thumb or finger transversely across the tip of the thumb forms a T and the cross-bar of the T is resting over the dorsal aspect of the joint, indicating the approximate position of the *calcaneocuboid ligament*.

Position your hand to resist eversion of the foot, to aid identification of the two lateral tendons, *peroneus longus and brevis*. Behind the lateral malleolus, peroneus brevis lies in front of longus. They divide at the peroneal tubercle, with brevis running above the tubercle and longus below.

Commentary on the examination

Observation

Before proceeding with the history, a general observation of the patient's *face, posture and gait* will alert the examiner to abnormalities, particularly of the gait pattern. A limp usually indicates abnormal weight-bearing, but a 'short leg' can produce a limp through functional discrepancies of hyperpronation and a flattened medial arch (Kannus, 1992).

The most common injury to the ankle involves the lateral ligaments, but other injuries include lesions of the contractile units, subluxation of the peroneal tendons, damage to the subtalar and midtarsal joints (Marder, 1994). Fractures and dislocations at the ankle are outside the scope of this book.

History (subjective examination)

The age, *occupation, sports, hobbies and lifestyle* of the patient may give an indication of the cause of the lesion and alert the examiner to possible biomechanical or postural problems.

The *site and spread* of pain help to localize the lesion, but as a peripheral joint, pain is usually well-localized. The presence of paraesthesia in the foot or pain in the calf or shin could suggest a more proximal lesion.

The *onset* of the symptoms may be sudden, due to trauma, or gradual, associated with overuse or arthritis. If the onset is traumatic in nature, the mechanism of injury should be deduced, particularly to give an indication of the ligaments involved.

A minor injury is indicated by minimal pain and localized swelling, with the ability to continue weight-bearing activities. More severe injuries will produce diffuse swelling and an inability to weight-bear, suggesting ligamentous rupture or fracture.

The *duration* of symptoms indicates the stage of the lesion in the inflammatory process. A history of recurrent episodes indicates possible functional instability, requiring in-depth biomechanical assessment.

The *symptoms and behaviour* need to be considered. The behaviour of the pain indicates the nature of the lesion: mechanical lesions are eased by rest and aggravated by activity and weight-bearing.

Other symptoms described by the patient could include the ankle giving way; this is a symptom of functional instability. Functional instability can be due to ligamentous laxity or a neuromuscular component due to proprioceptive deficit. A clicking or snapping sensation on the lateral aspect of the ankle could be due to disruption of the peroneal retinaculum, allowing subluxation of the tendons.

An indication of *past medical history, other joint involvement* and *medications* will aid diagnosis and establish whether contraindications to treatment techniques exist. Rheumatoid arthritis may affect the small joints of the foot.

Inspection

This should be conducted in weight-bearing and non-weight-bearing postures.

Bony deformity and functional abnormalities, of the medial arch in particular, will usually manifest themselves in the weight-bearing position (Fig. 12.7).

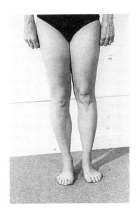

Fig. 12.7 Inspection in weight-bearing for postural deformity.

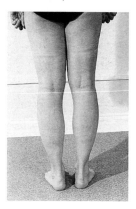

Fig. 12.8 Position of the Achilles tendon.

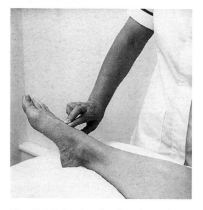

Fig. 12.9 Palpation for dorsalis pedis pulse.

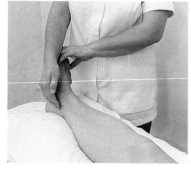

Fig. 12.10 Palpation for posterior tibial artery.

Check the height of the medial and longitudinal arches. Pes planus is a structural flat foot which is visible in both weight-bearing and non-weight-bearing positions, whilst a functional flat foot is only observed on weight-bearing.

The presence of functional flat foot can be generally estimated by looking for a difference in the height of the medial longitudinal arch in the non-weight-bearing and weight-bearing positions. Estimate the distance between the tuberosity of the navicular and the ground, first in a non-weight-bearing sitting position and second in the standing weight-bearing position (Evans, 1990).

Observe the position of the Achilles tendon from behind for any deviations in the normal straight alignment, which would indicate postural deformity (Fig. 12.8). Also notice if there is any angulation of the forefoot relative to the hindfoot.

Although it is important to note postural abnormalities of the foot, this should be kept relevant to the patient's presenting signs and symptoms. A detailed biomechanical assessment is not necessary for uncomplicated lesions, but recurrent symptoms or failure to resolve the patient's symptoms may require referral to a podiatrist.

It is worth inspecting the patient's shoes for abnormal areas of weight-bearing. This is particularly relevant to athletes and should include their training shoes. In a normal gait pattern, wear is seen on the lateral side of the heel and the medial side of the forefoot (Kannus, 1992). Camber running or worn-out or incorrect training shoes can alter angles of contact between the foot and the ground and be an external cause of overuse (Evans, 1990). Advice will need to be given regarding the type of shoe best suited to the patient's activities (Anthony, 1987). Abnormal callus formation indicates abnormal weight-bearing.

Colour changes may indicate circulatory involvement and a change in colour in transferring from the weight-bearing to the non-weight-bearing position should be further investigated by palpating for the presence of arterial pulses (Figs 12.9 and 12.10). Bruising is often associated with a recently sprained ankle and several days after a sprain the bruising often tracks peripherally. A severe sprain of the ankle can cause traction injury of the superficial peroneal nerve (Acus and Flanagan, 1991) and vascular structures. Consideration should be given to these possibilities if changes in skin colour persist.

Muscle wasting may be seen in the calf or peroneal muscles.

Swelling, together with bruising, on the lateral aspect of the ankle may be diffuse, indicating a moderate or major ligamentous lesion. Often a rounded mottled egg-shell-like swelling lies in front of the lateral malleolus: this is known as the *signe de la coquille d'oeuf* (Litt, 1992).

Minor swelling may be indicated by loss of the hollows behind the malleoli. Local swellings and ganglia should also be noted.

Palpation

As peripheral joints, the ankle and foot are palpated for signs of activity within the joint. The presence of *heat* is assessed (Fig. 12.11) and *synovial thickening* is palpated most easily along the anterior joint line (Fig 12.12). *Swelling* is usually observed, but it is possible to palpate for swelling, particularly around the malleoli. If the history indicates major lateral ligament sprain, the lower end of the shaft of the fibula can be palpated for tenderness, which may indicate a fracture.

State at rest

Before any movements are performed, the state at rest is established to provide a baseline for subsequent comparison.

The suggested sequence for the objective examination will now be given, followed by a commentary including the reasoning in performing the movements and the significance of the possible findings.

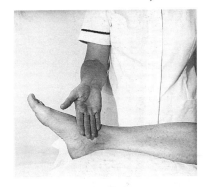

Fig. 12.11 Palpation for heat.

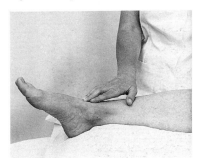

Fig. 12.12 Palpation for synovial thickening.

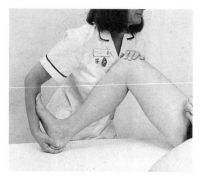

Fig. 12.13 Passive dorsiflexion.

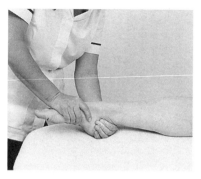

Fig. 12.14 Passive plantarflexion.

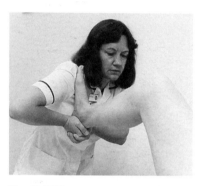

Fig. 12.15 Varus stress.

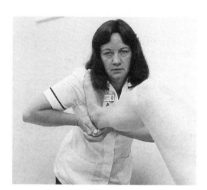

Fig. 12.16 Valgus stress.

Examination by selective tension (objective examination)

Ankle joint:

- Passive dorsiflexion (Fig.12.13)
- Passive plantarflexion (Fig. 12.14)

Subtalar joint:

- Passive varus to produce supination of the calcaneum (Fig. 12.15)
- Passive valgus to produce pronation of the calcaneum (Fig. 12.16)

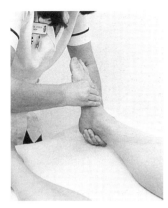

Fig. 12.17 Passive dorsiflexion.

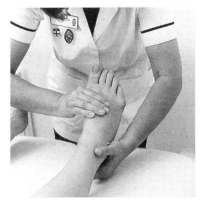

Fig. 12.18 Passive plantarflexion.

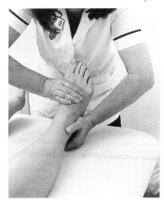

Fig. 12.19 Passive abduction.

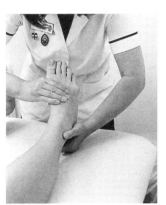

Fig. 12.20 Passive adduction.

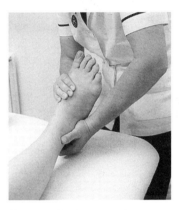

Fig. 12.21 Passive pronation plantarflexion and eversion.

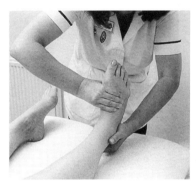

Fig. 12.22 Passive supination.

Midtarsal joints:
- Passive dorsiflexion and plantarflexion (Figs 12.17 and 12.18)
- Passive abduction and adduction (Figs 12.19 and 12.20)
- Passive pronation and supination (Figs 12.21 and 12.22)

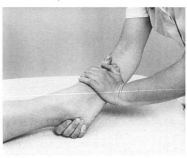

Fig. 12.23 Passive plantarflexion and inversion.

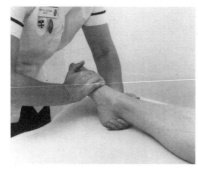

Fig. 12.24 Passive pronation.

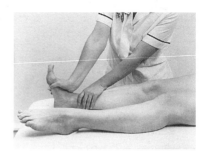

Fig. 12.25 Resisted dorsiflexion.

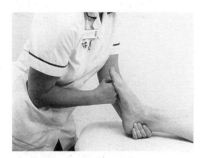

Fig. 12.26 Resisted plantarflexion.

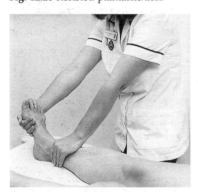

Fig. 12.27 Resisted inversion.

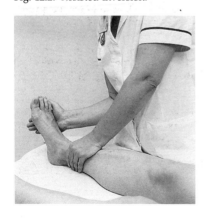

Fig. 12.28 Resisted eversion.

Gross ligament tests:

- Passive plantarflexion and inversion for lateral collateral ligament (Fig.12.23)
- Passive plantarflexion and eversion for medial (deltoid) ligament (Fig.12.24)

Contractile structures:

- Resisted dorsiflexion (Fig. 12.25)
- Resisted plantarflexion (Fig. 12.26)
- Resisted inversion (Fig. 12.27)
- Resisted eversion (Fig. 12.28)

Accessory ligament tests:

- Drawer test for the anterior talo-fibular ligament
- Talar tilt test for the lateral collateral ligament and integrity of the mortise
- Test for calcaneocuboid ligament

Toes:

- Passive and resisted testing of the toes is not performed routinely, but is included if appropriate

Palpation

Once a diagnosis has been made, the structure at fault is palpated for the exact site of the lesion

The objective examination is carried out in non-weight-bearing with the patient positioned comfortably in supine lying. The joints are examined first, assessing the range of movement, pain and end-feel. Passive dorsiflexion normally has 'hard' end-feel and to achieve end range it must be performed with the knee in flexion to take the tension off the gastrocnemius muscle complex, which spans both the knee and ankle joints. Passive plantarflexion normally has an 'elastic' end-feel due to tension in the tissues on the dorsal aspect of the foot. The presence of the capsular pattern should be noted.

Although individual passive movements can be produced at the ankle joint, it is difficult to produce isolated passive movements at the subtalar and midtarsal joints. In practice the three joint complex contributes to the composite functional movements occurring at the ankle and foot. To assess the small range of movement available at the subtalar joint, grasp the calcaneum with both hands. Flex the knee to allow relaxation of the gastrocnemius complex and push the ankle joint into the close packed position. The varus and valgus stress is then applied to the calcaneum through the heels of both hands, using body weight. The amount of passive movement available at the subtalar joint is limited to a few degrees and the normal end-feel is 'hard' for both.

To assess movements occurring at the midtarsal joints, pull down on the calcaneum to place the ankle joint into dorsiflexion. Place fingers and thumb on either side of the first metatarsal and move the midtarsal joint through its range of passive movements. These movements are minimal, difficult to produce in isolation and do not have an appreciable end-feel.

Assessing passive movements of the toes is not part of the routine ankle examination, but the movements can be applied as necessary to assess for the presence of the capsular pattern.

The main ligaments are tested by two gross composite movements, passive plantarflexion and inversion for the lateral collateral ligament and passive plantarflexion and eversion for the medial collateral ligament. Should it be necessary, the ligaments can be assessed individually, and accessory tests applied for joint instability (see below).

The contractile structures are assessed by resisted tests for pain and power. The joints are placed in the mid position and maximum resistance applied. Resisted dorsiflexion tests mainly tibialis anterior and resisted plantarflexion tests gastrocnemius and the Achilles tendon. Testing the gastrocnemius group in lying may not produce symptoms, and the test may need to be repeated in standing against the resistance of body weight. Resisted inversion tests mainly tibialis posterior and resisted eversion tests the peroneal tendons.

Accessory ligament and instability tests are applied if appropriate. The gross ligament test of passive plantarflexion and inversion mainly tests the anterior talofibular ligament which crosses the ankle joint and is the most common ligamentous injury found at the ankle. It is further assessed by the *drawer test* which assesses its integrity (Marder, 1994). Flex the leg to allow the foot to rest plantargrade on the couch. Position yourself to view movement of the fibula on the lateral side of the ankle. Place one hand over the

---

Capsular pattern of the ankle joint:

- **More limitation of plantarflexion than dorsiflexion**

Capsular pattern of the subtalar joint:

- **Increasing limitation of supination**
- **Eventual fixation of the joint in pronation**

Capsular pattern of the midtarsal joints:

- **Limitation of adduction**
- **Limitation of supination**
- **Forefoot fixes in abduction and pronation**

Capsular pattern of the first metatarsophalangeal joint:

- **Gross limitation of extension**
- **Some limitation of flexion**

Capsular pattern of the other metatarsophalangeal joints (may vary):

- **More limitation of flexion than extension**
- **Joints fix in extension**
- **Interphalangeal joints fix in flexion**

talus to fix it and the other just above the ankle joint. Apply pressure backwards against the fibula and tibia, comparing the degree of posterior movement of the fibula with the other side. Increased posterior movement of the fibula is a positive sign and indicates laxity or rupture of the anterior talofibular ligament.

The calcaneofibular ligament crosses both the ankle joint and subtalar joint. Injury to this ligament does not often occur in isolation, but in conjunction with the anterior talofibular ligament. Combined rupture of these ligaments results in an increased *talar tilt* (Boruta *et al.*, 1990, Wilkerson, 1992, Marder, 1994). With the knee straight, passively dorsiflex the ankle (this allows it to fall just short of the close packed position) and apply a strong varus stress to the calcaneum, compare the range of movement with the other side.

Disruption of the inferior tibiofibular joint may be due to a forced dorsiflexion injury which can cause widening (diastasis) of the ankle mortise (Marder, 1994). In clinical practice such an injury would only usually occur in conjunction with other major ligamentous damage, but the talar tilt test can also be applied to test the integrity of the mortise. Apply the talar tilt test as above (it can only be accurately applied if the lateral collateral ligaments are intact). If there is any widening of the mortise, pain and excessive movement will be appreciated. A 'click' may be felt as the talus tilts excessively in the enlarged mortise (Cyriax and Cyriax, 1983).

The *calcaneocuboid ligament* crosses the calcaneocuboid joint, part of the midtarsal complex, and may be involved in a lateral collateral ligament sprain or injured in isolation. To assess its involvement, apply passive adduction and supination of the mid-tarsal joints looking for increased pain.

Lesions at the ankle and foot

Capsular lesions

The presence of a capsular pattern at any of the joints in the ankle and foot indicates arthritis. The history will have established the cause of the arthritis.

Osteoarthrosis is uncommon at the ankle unless predisposed by fracture, repetitive postural overuse or instability caused by recurrent sprain. An alteration in lower limb biomechanics may predispose any of the joints to degenerative osteoarthrosis. Localized degenerative osteoarthrosis of the subtalar joint may follow fractures of the talus or calcaneum (Evans, 1990). Occasionally, a lateral ligament sprain produces a traumatic arthritis in the subtalar and midtarsal joints and, if unresolved, the joint can be injected with corticosteroid. Rheumatoid arthritis is more common in the smaller joints of the foot. Arthritis and gout of the first metatarsophalangeal joint cause a loss of the functional range of extension essential to gait activities. Corticosteroid injection may be given for symptomatic osteoarthrosis or the principles of mobilization may be applied. Rheumatoid arthritis may respond to corticosteroid injection.

Capsular pattern of the ankle joint

- **More limitation of plantarflexion than dorsiflexion**

Injection of the ankle joint

Adcortyl 10 mg/ml 2 ml	Total steroid 20 mg	Lignocaine 1% 1 ml	Total volume 3 ml

23G × 1 in (0.6 × 25 mm) blue needle or a 21G × 1½ in (0.8 × 40 mm) green needle

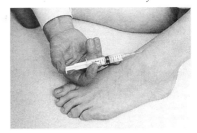

Fig. 12.29 Injection of the ankle joint.

Position the patient in supine with the foot plantargrade on the couch. This places the ankle in a degree of plantarflexion and opens the joint. Several needle entry points are possible and it may be necessary to palpate for a suitable opening over either malleolus, or between the tibialis anterior and extensor hallucis longus tendons, which avoids the dorsalis pedis artery (Figs 12.29 and 12.30). Having selected a needle entry point, give the injection as a bolus. The patient is advised to maintain a period of relative rest for approximately 2 weeks following injection.

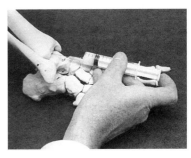

Fig. 12.30 Injection of the ankle joint showing direction of approach and needle position.

Injection of the subtalar joint (Cyriax and Cyriax, 1983; Cyriax, 1984)

Adcortyl 10 mg/ml 1 ml	Total steroid 10 mg	Lignocaine 1% 1 ml	Total volume 2 ml

23G × 1 in (0.6 × 25 mm) blue needle

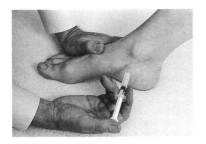

Fig. 12.31 Injection of the subtalar joint.

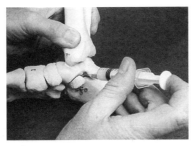

Fig. 12.32 Injection of the subtalar joint showing direction of approach and needle position.

The subtalar joint is divided into two compartments by the sinus tarsi and its interosseous ligaments. Locate the joint line immediately above the sustentaculum tali and insert the needle approximately halfway along the joint line, angling it anteriorly to inject the anterior compartment first (Figs 12.31 and 12.32). Withdraw the needle a little and reinsert it posteriorly to inject the posterior compartment secondly. Give the injection as a bolus. The patient is advised to maintain a period of relative rest for approximately 2 weeks following injection.

Capsular pattern of the subtalar joint

- Increasing limitation of supination
- Eventual fixation in pronation

Injection of the midtarsal joint (Cyriax and Cyriax, 1983; Cyriax, 1984)			
Adcortyl 10 mg/ml 1 ml	Total steroid 10 mg	Lignocaine 1% 0.5 ml	Total volume 1.5 ml
23G × 1 in (0.6 × 25 mm) blue needle			

Capsular pattern of the midtarsal joints

- Limitation of adduction
- Limitation of supination
- Forefoot fixes in abduction and pronation

The injection site will depend on the joint or joints affected. Locate the appropriate joint line dorsally by palpation, avoiding the tendons and the dorsalis pedis artery (Figs 12.33 and 12.34). Insert the needle and, once intracapsular and experiencing little resistance, give the injection as a bolus. The patient is advised to maintain a period of relative rest for approximately 2 weeks following injection.

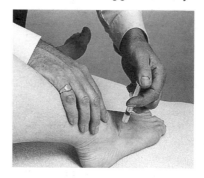

Fig. 12.33 Injection of the midtarsal joint.

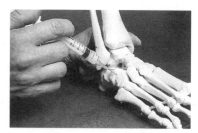

Fig. 12.34 Injection of the midtarsal joint showing direction of approach and needle position.

Capsular pattern of the first metatarsophalangeal joint

- Gross limitation of extension
- Some loss of flexion

Injection of the first metatarsophalangeal joint (Cyriax and Cyriax, 1983; Cyriax, 1984)			
Kenalog 40 mg/ml 0.25 ml	Total steroid 10 mg	Lignocaine 1% 0.25 ml	Total volume 0.5 ml
25G × $\frac{5}{8}$ in (0.5 × 16 mm) orange needle			

Identify the joint line dorsally by palpation and distract it to allow easier access; choose a point of entry to one side of the extensor tendon (Fig. 12.35). The injection is given as a bolus. The patient is advised to maintain a period of relative rest for approximately 2 weeks following injection.

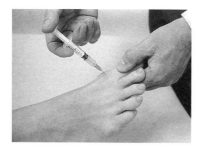

Fig. 12.35 Injection of the first metatarsophalangeal joint.

Injection of the other metatarsophalangeal joints			
Kenalog 40 mg/ml 0.25 ml	Total steroid 10 mg	Lignocaine 1% 0.25 ml	Total volume 0.5 ml
25G × $\frac{5}{8}$ in (0.5 × 16 mm) orange needle			

Identify the joint line dorsally by palpation. Insert the needle avoiding the extensor tendons, and give the injection as a bolus. The patient is advised to maintain a period of relative rest for approximately 2 weeks following injection.

Non-capsular lesions

Lateral collateral ligament sprain

Sprain of the lateral collateral ligament is the most common ankle injury, accounting for approximately 85–90% of ankle sprains (Stanley, 1991; Liu and Jason, 1994). The basic mechanism for lateral ligament sprain is a plantarflexion/inversion injury, but other forces may also be involved, for example, rotation, supination, pronation and vertical compression (Sartoris, 1994). Injury occurs commonly in sport, when a player may land on another player's foot, stumble on uneven ground; or, apart from sport, the patient may simply have tripped or slipped.

Diagnosis of sprain can be made on clinical grounds and X-ray investigation is only necessary if there is clear clinical evidence of fracture, e.g. marked bony tenderness to palpation (Auletta *et al.*, 1991; Litt, 1992). Forced inversion may cause avulsion of lateral structures or undisplaced fracture of the lateral malleolus, whilst impactive forces may stress medial structures (Sartoris, 1994).

Lateral collateral ligament sprains always involve the anterior talofibular ligament (Black *et al.*, 1978; Litt, 1992; Liu and Jason, 1994), with more severe injuries also involving other ligaments and structures on the lateral side of the ankle. Lateral collateral ligament sprains are graded according to the severity of the signs and symptoms (Boruta *et al.*, 1990; Stanley, 1991; Litt, 1992; Wilkerson, 1992; Liu and Jason, 1994).

Grade I

The lateral collateral ligament is overstretched just beyond its elastic limit, causing microfailure of a few fibres of the anterior talofibular ligament. The patient presents with mild swelling and tenderness over the ligament, little or no haemorrhage, some limitation of movement and some difficulty in weight-bearing. On examination, no clinical instability is noted and prognosis is good. The injury takes approximately 8–10 days to resolve with early mobilization.

Grade II

The lateral collateral ligament is overstretched well beyond its elastic limit, causing major tearing of the anterior talofibular ligament, the lateral capsule and often a part of the calcaneofibular ligament. The patient presents with moderate to severe swelling, bruising, pain, local tenderness, a limited range of movement and great difficulty in weight-bearing. There is limitation of movement in the capsular pattern if the lateral joint capsule is torn, and a mild degree of

---

Capsular pattern of the other metatarsophalangeal joints (may vary)

- More limitation of flexion than extension
- Joints fix in extension
- Interphalangeal joints fix in flexion

ligamentous instability may be detected clinically. Prognosis remains good, taking approximately 15–21 days to resolve with early mobilization.

Grade III

The lateral ligament is overstretched into its plastic range with macrofailure, or complete rupture, of the anterior talofibular ligament and possibly the calcaneofibular ligament, together with rupture of the ankle joint capsule. Involvement of the posterior talofibular ligament and the syndesmosis would indicate major ankle dislocation. The patient presents with diffuse swelling and marked evidence of haemorrhaging. There is severe pain and tenderness, loss of movement and great difficulty with weight-bearing. It may be difficult to assess for ligamentous laxity clinically as this may be masked by the swelling and the protective reflex muscle spasm produced by the pain.

Both operative and non-operative treatment options could be considered, but with conservative management prognosis is still good, providing the patient is not required to function at high levels of performance (Stanley, 1991; Karlsson and Lansingeer, 1992; Liu and Jason, 1994). Recurrent sprains of the ankle with clinical laxity may need stress X-ray to measure the laxity before proceeding to eventual surgical repair. In general, surgical intervention for grade III sprains is only considered in the élite athlete, or where recurrent injury has failed to respond to conservative management and is producing functional disability. Otherwise, all grades of sprain are treated conservatively (Karlsson and Lansingeer, 1992; Liu and Jason, 1994; Ogilvie-Harris and Gilbart, 1995).

Early mobilization is the key to the restoration of function in all grades of ligamentous sprain, giving a better overall result and a faster rate of recovery (Brooks *et al.*, 1981; Roycroft and Mantgani, 1983; Stanley, 1991; Ogilvie-Harris and Gilbart, 1995; Shrier, 1995). Non-steroidal anti-inflammatory drugs and ice, used early on in the inflammatory phase, seem to achieve an earlier recovery, but do not alter the overall outcome (Ogilvie-Harris and Gilbart, 1995). Corticosteroid injection is not recommended for acute ankle sprains since collagen synthesis may be suppressed (Boruta *et al.*, 1990).

Treatment is directed at all components involved in the sprain and depends on the stage reached in the inflammatory process.

Acute lateral collateral ligament sprain

A complete examination of the ankle and foot is not usually possible following an acute lateral collateral ligament sprain as the swelling and muscle spasm prevent movement. The history will indicate the mechanism of the injury and the amount of heat and swelling will give an indication of the severity. The principles of treatment for acute ligament sprain are applied.

Rest, ice, compression and elevation are applied immediately after the onset. Ice applied during the first 3 days after injury has been shown to shorten the recovery period. It is generally applied for 15–20 min three times daily (Hocutt *et al.*, 1982; Stanley, 1991; Swain and Holt, 1993).

Gentle transverse friction massage is begun as early as possible together with Grade A mobilization, aiming to encourage alignment of collagen fibres and maintain function. Treatment is delivered on a daily basis during the early acute phase and the patient is encouraged to maintain a normal heel–toe gait, possibly with the aid of crutches. Ankle supports (O'Hara *et al.*, 1992) or tape may be applied to provide compression during the early acute phase.

From days 3 to 5 onwards there should be sufficient tensile strength in the wound to allow an increasing depth of transverse friction massage and a greater range of Grade A mobilization to be applied. Treatment continues until a full range of painfree movement is attained.

Depending on the severity of the injury, the patient should be relatively painfree and walking normally within 8–21 days, if seen within a day or two from the onset. Functional rehabilitation should involve muscle balance, peroneal strengthening and proprioceptive work to re-establish normal balance and coordination (Cornwall and Murrell, 1991; Karlsson and Lansingeer, 1992). Progression to running, sprinting, jumping, figure-of-eight running, twisting and turning follows, depending on the functional requirements of the patient. The lateral ligaments require the support of the peroneal tendons to resist inversion stresses; rehabilitation aims to restore muscle strength and to re-establish the protective reflexes (Boruta *et al.*, 1990).

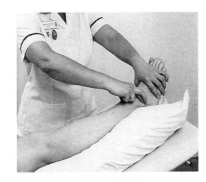

Fig. 12.36 Transverse friction massage of the anterior talofibular ligament, acute sprain.

Transverse friction massage of the lateral collateral ligament components (Cyriax and Cyriax, 1983; Cyriax, 1984)

The anterior talofibular ligament is usually involved at its fibular end, but palpation will establish the exact site of the lesion.

Stand on the patient's good side, placing an index finger reinforced by the middle finger on to the anterior edge of the malleolus. Direct the friction massage up against the malleolus and sweep transversely across the fibres (Fig. 12.36). In the acute case begin the friction massage very gently to gain some numbing. Progress to apply the friction massage more deeply and, once on the ligament, apply approximately six effective sweeps. The friction massage is followed immediately by Grade A mobilization (Figs 12.37 and 12.38) together with gait correction.

If the calcaneofibular ligament is involved, the friction massage is directed up under the apex of the lateral malleolus and immediately followed by Grade A mobilization.

Treatment of any involvement of the peroneal tendons will be covered under contractile lesions.

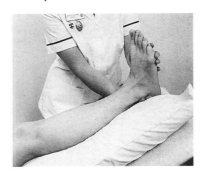

Fig. 12.37 Grade A mobilization into dorsiflexion.

Chronic lateral collateral ligament sprain

The patient has a history of a past sprained ankle which may have resolved without treatment. He or she complains of pain and some

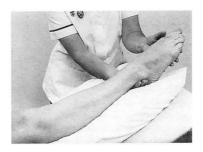

Fig. 12.38 Grade A mobilization into plantarflexion.

swelling on the lateral side of the ankle after exertion. Symptoms of recurrent giving way may indicate functional or structural instability which must be assessed using the drawer and talar tilt tests, as described above. The treatment approach for residual chronic ankle instability should be based on functional rehabilitation, with an emphasis on proprioceptive re-education and taping for sporting activities. Surgery is only considered if rehabilitation fails (Liu and Jason, 1994).

On examination there is usually pain on full passive plantarflexion and inversion, indicating involvement of the anterior talofibular ligament. Pain on passive dorsiflexion with a varus stress to the calcaneum (talar tilt test) indicates involvement of the calcaneofibular ligament. Pain on passive adduction and supination applied to the midtarsal joints indicates involvement of the calcaneocuboid ligament.

The ligament fibres have become adherent to the underlying bone and the principle of treatment is to rupture the unwanted adhesions with one Grade C manipulation at each session, once the ligament has been prepared by deep transverse friction massage. Following manipulative rupture, the patient is instructed to mobilize vigorously, in order to maintain the movement gained through manipulation. Functional or structural instability is addressed by proprioceptive exercises and balance work (Lentell *et al.*, 1990). Treatment is usually successful and requires one to three sessions.

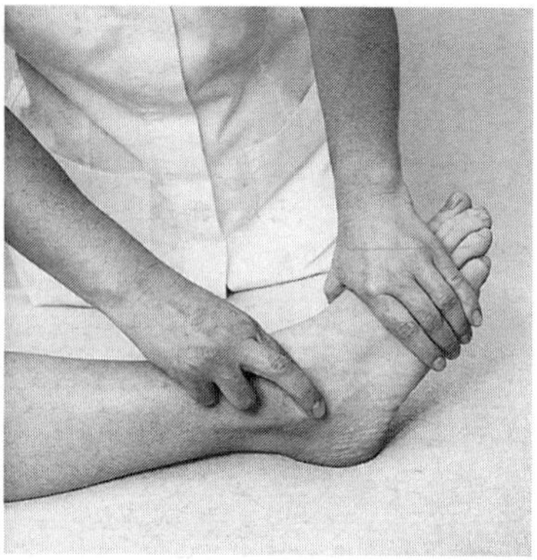

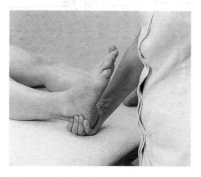

Fig. 12.39 Transverse friction massage of the anterior talofibular ligament, chronic sprain.

Fig. 12.40 Grade C manipulation: calcaneum grasped and placed into varus.

> **Transverse friction massage of the lateral collateral ligament components involved in a chronic sprain (Cyriax and Cyriax, 1983; Cyriax, 1984)**

Transverse friction massage of the anterior talofibular and calcaneofibular ligament is applied as described above (Fig. 12.39). If the calcaneocuboid ligament is involved, the friction massage is applied from the patient's good side; massage is delivered by the index finger reinforced by the middle, directed on to the ligament, which is located over the dorsal aspect of the calcaneocuboid joint. The friction massage is applied to all involved ligaments, gently to begin with to gain the numbing effect, then followed by 10 min of deep transverse friction massage, aiming to soften and numb the ligament prior to the Grade C manipulation, which follows immediately.

> **Grade C manipulation for chronic lateral collateral ligament sprain (Cyriax and Cyriax, 1983; Cyriax, 1984)**

With the patient lying supine on the couch, stand at the foot of the bed. The treatment described is for the right ankle:

- Grasp the patient's right calcaneum with your right hand and pull it into varus (Fig. 12.40).

- With a 'flipper' grip, wrap your left hand around the base of the first metatarsal (Fig. 12.41) and pull the foot into maximum plantarflexion (Fig. 12.42). Be careful not to put your thumb round on to the sole of the foot, as this is uncomfortable for the patient and makes the technique less efficient.
- Maintain the maximum plantarflexion whilst you step to the right, turning your body to the left, through 90°.
- This step and turn automatically pulls the forefoot into maximum adduction and supination, taking up the slack.
- Apply a minimal-amplitude, high-velocity thrust by a sharp adduction movement of your left arm (Fig. 12.43).

The increased range of movement must be maintained by vigorous exercise.

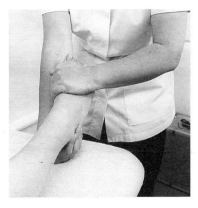

Fig. 12.41 Grade C manipulation: 'flipper' grip hand hold.

Medial collateral ligament sprain

Eversion sprains of the ankle are not common and represent 5–15% of all ankle injuries. The mechanism of injury involved is dorsiflexion and eversion, with possible damage to the syndesmosis, or fracture of the malleoli, as well as injury to the medial ligament (Roberts *et al.*, 1995).

The treatment principles are applied as for the acute and chronic stages of the lateral collateral ligament if the injury is traumatic. The various directions of the ligament fibres need to be borne in mind, to be able to apply the friction massage transversely. A Grade C manipulation is not applied in the chronic stage, due to the multidirectional nature of the fibres.

A secondary medial ligament sprain may develop through postural overuse. This is especially evident with flattening of the medial arch in the elderly. A biomechanical assessment of the foot may be indicated, together with orthotic correction.

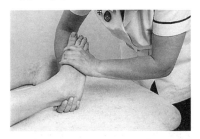

Fig. 12.42 Grade C manipulation: pulling foot into plantarflexion and inversion.

Retrocalcaneal bursitis

The retrocalcaneal bursa is horseshoe-shaped and lies between the distal end of the Achilles tendon, near its insertion, and the superoposterior surface of the calcaneum (Stephens, 1994). Fitting like a cap over the calcaneum, it is concave anteriorly. It rests against the Achilles fat pad superiorly and blends with the Achilles tendon posteriorly (Frey *et al.*, 1992).

An abnormally large bony bump (exostosis), known as Haglund's deformity, may be present on the superoposterior surface of the calcaneum; this may predispose towards retrocalcaneal bursitis. A slight soft-tissue swelling is often associated with Haglund's deformity and is known as 'pump bumps' (Stephens, 1994).

Objectively it is difficult to diagnose a retrocalcaneal bursitis differentially from an Achilles tendinitis, with which it may coexist. It presents with posterior heel pain and may produce pain on

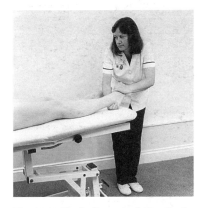

Fig. 12.43 Grade C manipulation: body turned pulling the foot into maximum adduction and supination before application of the final thrust.

passive dorsiflexion, which squeezes the inflamed bursa between the Achilles tendon and the calcaneum. Swelling and tenderness to palpation may be present, just anterior and to either side of the insertion of the Achilles tendon. Retrocalcaneal bursitis may be a manifestation of rheumatoid arthritis or one of the spondylarthropathies such as Reiter's disease (Hutson, 1990; Frey *et al.*, 1992; Baxter, 1994).

Frey *et al.* (1992) demonstrated the existence of the retrocalcaneal bursa on X-ray using an injection of contrast medium. Patients suffering from retrocalcaneal bursitis accepted less of the contrast medium than normal subjects, leading the authors of the paper to propose that inflammatory fluid, thickened oedematous bursal walls, hypertrophic synovial infoldings and pain prevented the inflamed bursa from accepting the normal amount of contrast medium.

Treatment consists of a local corticosteroid injection.

Injection of the retrocalcaneal bursa			
Kenalog 40 mg/ml 10 mg	Total steroid 0.25 ml	Lignocaine1% 0.50 ml	Total volume 0.75 ml
23G × 1 in (0.6 × 25 mm) blue needle			

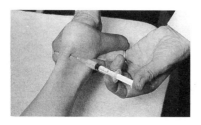

Fig. 12.44 Injection of the retrocalcaneal bursa.

Position the patient in the prone position with the foot in a degree of plantarflexion over a pillow. Palpate for the tender area anterior to the distal end of the Achilles tendon and insert the needle from either the medial or lateral aspect, running parallel to the anterior aspect of the Achilles tendon (Fig. 12.44). Give the injection as a bolus if possible, or pepper it if you feel the resistance of the synovial folds. The patient is advised to maintain a period of relative rest for approximately 2 weeks following injection.

Subcutaneous Achilles bursitis

The subcutaneous Achilles bursa lies between the skin and insertion of the Achilles tendon. It may be an adventitious bursa developing as a result of external friction (Gibbon and Cassar-Pullicino, 1994). Inflammation of this bursa presents with subcutaneous swelling and tenderness over the heel and may be due to abnormal pressure from heel counters. Treatment consists of relative rest and advising the patient about footwear, with particular regard to the height and rigidity of the heel counter (Stephens, 1994).

Plantar fasciitis

Plantar fasciitis produces a typical history of a gradual onset of pain felt over the medial plantar aspect of the heel. Its particular characteristic is pain under the heel when the foot is first put to the floor in the morning, easing after a few steps have been taken

(Kibler *et al.*, 1991; Karr, 1994). It is worse after prolonged periods of standing and on initial exercise, easing as the foot warms up.

Plantar fasciitis usually occurs in middle age, with obesity as a predisposing factor (Gibbon and Cassar-Pullicino, 1994). It may be precipitated by an alteration in footwear, e.g. wearing flip-flops or other similar unsupporting shoes, or seen as a relatively common injury in the running athlete, where it constitutes approximately 10% of running injuries seen (Kibler *et al.*, 1991).

Postural foot deformity such as pes planus and overpronation lowers the medial longitudinal arch and may overstretch the plantar fascia. Tightness of the Achilles tendon limits dorsiflexion and may contribute to the overpronation (Evans, 1990; Karr, 1994). Due to the constant-length phenomenon, extension of the toes increases the height of the longitudinal arch – the 'windlass' effect of the plantar fascia (Canoso, 1981; Sellman, 1994) – so that activities involving long-term tip-toe standing, e.g. high heels, may excessively stress the plantar fascia. It may also be associated with rheumatoid arthritis or the spondylarthropathies.

Diagnosis is made on the typical history and the absence of other findings on examination of the foot and ankle. Passive extension of the toes may reproduce the pain by its 'windlass' effect on the plantar fascia and tenderness to palpation is usually found over the medial calcaneal tuberosity.

The mechanism of the lesion is thought to be repetitive microtrauma through overloading of the longitudinal arch, which produces focal tears and chronic inflammation at the insertion of the plantar fascia at the bone–fascia interface (Kibler *et al.*, 1991; Karr, 1994; Gibbon and Cassar-Pullicino, 1994). It may be a traction injury occurring through repeated intrinsic muscle contraction against a stretched plantar fascia during the push-off phase of gait (Gibbon and Cassar-Pullicino, 1994), the plantar fascia acting as an aponeurotic attachment for the first layer of the plantar muscles. Both mechanisms could possibly lead to the development of calcaneal spurs.

Plantar fasciitis usually responds to conservative management. However, if this fails, surgery may be an option, with careful consideration paid to maintaining the load-bearing capacity of the longitudinal arch (Kulthanan, 1992; Kim and Voloshin, 1995). Tissue examined at the time of surgery has shown a hypercellular inflammatory response, reactive fibrosis and degenerative areas (Kibler *et al.*, 1991).

The chronic nature of the condition produces changes in the strength of the plantar flexors with loss of range of dorsiflexion and there may be alterations in the length of the stride (Kibler *et al.*, 1991; Chandler and Kibler, 1993). All components of dysfunction should be considered when planning a rehabilitation programme.

Treatment of plantar fasciitis is local corticosteroid injection or transverse friction massage. Either treatment is combined with rest from overuse activities, intrinsic muscle exercises and correction of foot posture if appropriate.

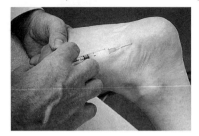

Fig. 12.45 Injection of the plantar fascia.

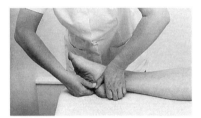

Fig. 12.46 Transverse friction massage for the plantar fascia.

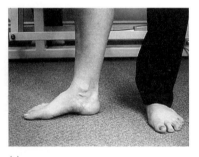

(a)

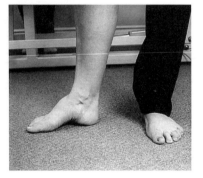

(b)

Fig. 12.47 (a, b) Intrinsic muscle exercises.

Injection of the plantar fascia (Cyriax and Cyriax, 1983; Cyriax, 1984)			
Kenalog 40 mg/ml 0.5 ml	Total steroid 20 mg	Lignocaine 1% 1 ml	Total Volume 1.5 ml
21G × 1½ in (0.8 × 40 mm) green needle			

Position the patient in prone lying with the knee flexed and the lower leg resting on a pillow. Hold the foot in dorsiflexion to apply some tension to the plantar fascia. Insert the needle at the medial border of the heel, anterior to the point of tenderness, and angle it posteriorly towards the site of tenderness (Fig. 12.45). Deliver the injection to the origin of the plantar fascia by a peppering technique with the needle point in contact with bone at the anterior edge of the medial tubercle. The patient is advised to maintain a period of relative rest for approximately 2 weeks following injection.

Dasgupta and Bowles (1995) conducted bone scans on 15 patients with a diagnosis of plantar fasciitis, to localize the inflammatory focus. In 80% of patients, an area was localized to the medial aspect of the plantar surface of the calcaneum. An accurately placed injection into this area abolished the pain and tenderness. An accurate injection technique is important to prevent the need for repeated injection, as cases of plantar fascia rupture associated with corticosteroid injection have been reported (Sellman, 1994).

Transverse friction massage technique for the plantar fascia

Position the patient in supine lying with the foot supported on a pillow, the leg in lateral rotation. Standing on the affected side, direct the pressure posteromedially against the origin of the plantar fascia, with one thumb reinforced by the other, and friction transversely across the fibres (Fig. 12.46). Maintain the friction for 10 min after achieving the numbing effect. It is important to assess foot posture and to instruct the patient in intrinsic foot exercises (Fig. 12.47). Care should be taken when teaching intrinsic foot exercises to avoid any clawing of the toes, which reinforces the activity of the long plantar flexors. Relative rest is advised where functional movements may continue, but no overuse or stretching until the structure is painfree on resisted testing.

Other techniques including taping and supports may be applied and a heel raise may help to reduce the stretch on the fascia.

Loose bodies

Although relatively rare, loose bodies can occur in the ankle or subtalar joints. The patient presents with a history of twinging pain with giving way or a momentary inability to weight-bear. On examination, a non-capsular pattern may be present. The principle of treatment for a loose body is applied – strong traction and Grade A mobilization. The direction selected for the mobilization is not important.

Loose body mobilization technique for ankle joint (Cyriax and Cyriax, 1983; Cyriax, 1984)

Position the patient in supine with the foot level with the end of the couch. Grasp the calcaneum and hold it to act as a fulcrum. Grasp the dorsum of the foot with the web of the other hand and lean back to apply strong traction. Allow the traction to establish, then apply a circumduction movement with the hand placed around the dorsum of the foot.

Loose body mobilization technique for subtalar joint (Cyriax, 1984)

Position the patient prone with the foot just off the end of the couch. Cross your thumbs over the posterosuperior aspect of the calcaneum and wrap your hands around the talus anteriorly. Lean back to apply strong traction and apply a varus and valgus movement to the calcaneum with the heels of your hands by rotating your body from side to side.

Contractile lesions

The following contractile lesions have been chosen for discussion since they occur relatively commonly in clinical practice. However, the principles of diagnosis and treatment can be applied to any other lesion.

Peroneal tendinitis and tenosynovitis

Peroneal tendinitis or tenosynovitis may have an acute onset if the tendons are involved in an inversion sprain of the ankle. A chronic onset may be due to overuse, e.g. walking or training on unaccustomed surfaces, or predisposed by altered foot biomechanics.

On examination pain is felt on the lateral side of the ankle on resisted eversion of the foot. Acute tenosynovitis may also produce pain on passive inversion. The exact site of the lesion is determined by palpation and may be at the musculotendinous junction, the tendons above, behind or below the malleolus, or at the insertion of peroneus brevis into the base of the fifth metatarsal.

Transverse friction massage is the treatment of choice, with the tendons on stretch if a tenosynovitis exists. If the lesion lies in the common sheath below the malleolus, corticosteroid injection can be applied.

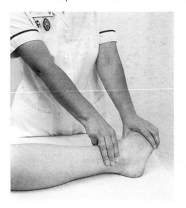

Fig. 12.48 Transverse friction massage of the peroneal tendons, above the malleolus.

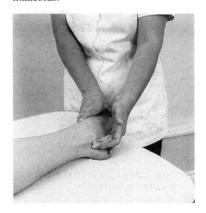

Fig. 12.49 Transverse friction massage of the peroneal tendons, behind the malleolus.

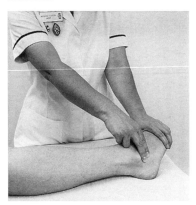

Fig. 12.50 Transverse friction massage of the peroneal tendons, below the malleolus.

> **Transverse friction massage technique for peroneal tendons (Cyriax and Cyriax, 1983; Cyriax, 1984; Figs 12.48–12.51)**

Stand on the patient's good side and apply treatment to the appropriate site:

Musculotendinous junction

Locate the site of the lesion and apply the transverse friction massage with the index finger, re-inforced by the middle finger. Maintain downward pressure as the friction massage is applied transversely across the fibres.

Above the malleolus (Fig. 12.48)

Three fingers are required to cover the extent of the lesion. Maintain downward pressure over the tendons as the transverse friction massage is applied.

Behind the malleolus (Fig. 12.49)

Here the tendons run in a common sheath so they must be put on a stretch. Use the middle finger, re-inforced by the index and apply the friction massage by pronation and supination of the forearm.

Below the malleolus (Fig. 12.50)

Two fingers are required to cover the extent of the lesion. The tendons here continue in their common sheath, therefore they are treated on the stretch. Maintain downward pressure over the tendons as the transverse friction massage is applied.

At the insertion of peroneus brevis into the base of the fifth metatarsal (Fig. 12.51)

An index finger, re-inforced by the middle is applied to the insertion and the friction massage is delivered transversely across the fibres.

Acute lesions are frictioned gently for approximately six effective sweeps after the numbing effect is achieved. Chronic lesions require deep transverse friction massage for approximately 10 min after the numbing effect is achieved. Relative rest is advised where functional movements may continue, but no overuse or stretching until the structure is painfree on resisted testing.

Injection technique for tenosynovitis of the peroneal tendons in the common sheath

Kenalog 40 mg/ml	Total steroid	Lignocaine 1%	Total volume
0.25 ml	10 mg	0.75 ml	1 ml

25G $\times \frac{5}{8}$ in (0.5 × 16 mm) orange needle or 23G × 1 in (0.6 × 25 mm) blue needle

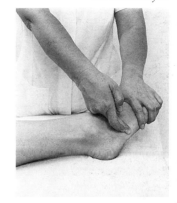

Fig. 12.51 Transverse friction massage at the insertion of peroneus brevis into the base of the fifth metatarsal.

Locate the peroneal tubercle, which indicates the distal end of the common sheath. Insert the needle into the sheath at the point of diversion of the tendons, aiming the needle towards the malleolus, parallel to the tendons (Fig. 12.52). Give the injection as a bolus into the sheath. The patient is advised to maintain a period of relative rest for approximately 2 weeks following injection.

The peroneal muscles act as dynamic stabilizers of the ankle joint and contract eccentrically to prevent inversion sprains (Shrier, 1995). If the peroneal tendinitis or tenosynovitis is the result of an inversion sprain, proprioception is most likely to have been altered; this may lead to functional instability and recurrent giving way. Rehabilitation must include peroneal strengthening and proprioceptive re-education, once the tendinitis or tenosynovitis has been appropriately managed.

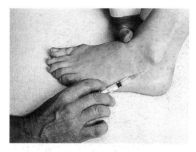

Fig. 12.52 Injection technique for tenosynovitis of the peroneal tendons in the common sheath.

Achilles tendinitis

The Achilles tendon is the longest tendon in the body; it is up to 1.5 cm wide and less than 1 cm in anteroposterior thickness (Chandnani and Bradley, 1994). Lesions of the Achilles tendon usually occur about 2–6 cm proximal to its insertion, which is the zone considered to be of relatively poor vascularity (Lagergren and Lindholm, 1958; Smart *et al.*, 1980; Chandnani and Bradley, 1994).

Lesions of the Achilles tendon can be a tendinitis, which may be reversible, a tendinosis, i.e. focal degenerative lesions within the tendon itself which may be irreversible (Williams, 1986; Mahler and Fritschy, 1992), or involve partial or complete rupture. The condition has been considered to be a continuum of a degenerative process which may eventually progress to total rupture (Fox *et al.*, 1975; Read and Motto, 1992).

Several aetiological mechanisms are suggested for Achilles tendinitis – altered biomechanics, overpronation, incorrect or worn-out footwear, pressure from heel counters, inappropriate training surfaces, excessive training, training errors or indirect trauma. Achilles tendinitis may also be associated with rheumatoid arthritis and the spondylarthropathies (Smart *et al.*, 1980). As the fibres of gastrocnemius and soleus do not insert into the Achilles tendon in a parallel direction, abnormal sheer stresses may be set up, creating an area of weakness and making it susceptible to injury (Frey and Shereff, 1988).

Patients present with a history of a gradual onset of pain felt locally at the back of the heel. They may or may not recall the causative factors. The pain is worse when the foot is first put to the floor in the morning (the different location of the pain distinguishes it from plantar fasciitis), easing after several steps. Pain is increased by activity and the tendon itself may show some thickening. It is tender to palpation.

On examination, pain is felt on resisted plantarflexion, which should be performed against gravity with body-weight resistance to reproduce the symptoms in minor or chronic lesions. If the history indicates Achilles tendinitis, but pain cannot be reproduced on examination, the patient may have to perform some sort of provocative exercise to produce symptoms before assessment, to allow accurate diagnosis.

Rupture of the Achilles tendon rarely occurs if the tendon is healthy, but may occur if there is existing tendinitis or tendinosis with fibrous degeneration (Smart *et al.*, 1980). Rupture, whether partial or complete, may occur through indirect violent trauma, e.g. push-off with knee extension during weight-bearing as in sprinting, unexpected forced dorsiflexion, e.g. missing a step, or stumbling or forced dorsiflexion of the plantarflexed foot, as in falling from a height (Smart *et al.*, 1980; Mahler and Fritschy, 1992).

Total rupture presents with a history of intense pain at the time of injury, but little pain since. Function is disrupted and the patient is unable to tip-toe stand. A gap may be palpable immediately after injury, and the foot fails to plantarflex passively when the gastrocnemius/soleus muscle bulk is squeezed – Thompson's test (Frey and Shereff, 1988).

X-ray can be used to confirm complete rupture of the Achilles tendon. Kager's triangle is a triangular space filled with fatty tissue bordered posteriorly by the inner contour of the Achilles tendon, anteriorly by the deep flexor tendons and inferiorly by the upper border of the calcaneum (Grisogono, 1989; Cetti and Andersen, 1993). In total rupture, Kager's triangle loses its normal contours on the X-ray picture (Smart *et al.*, 1980). Ultrasound and magnetic resonance imaging scanning have since become much more commonly used to confirm diagnosis.

The condition is treated by immobilization in plaster, usually after surgical repair, followed by early mobilization to achieve rapid recovery and to return to normal strength (Saw *et al.*, 1993).

Transverse friction massage of the Achilles tendon (Cyriax and Cyriax, 1983; Cyriax, 1984)

The most common sites for Achilles tendinitis are the anterior aspect, the sides of the tendon and the insertion into the calcaneum. The affected site is identified by palpation.

Anterior aspect of the tendon

Position the patient in prone lying with the foot plantarflexed on a pillow. Push the relaxed Achilles tendon laterally with a finger, placing your middle finger reinforced by the index against the

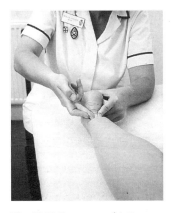

Fig. 12.53 Transverse friction massage of the anterior aspect of the Achilles tendon, lateral.

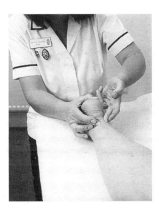

Fig. 12.54 Transverse friction massage of the anterior aspect of the Achilles tendon, medial.

exposed anterolateral surface of the tendon (Fig. 12.53). Apply the friction massage by a pronation/supination movement of your forearm. Repeat the same procedure with the tendon pushed medially to gain access to the anteromedial side (Fig. 12.54).

Sides of the tendon

Position the patient in prone lying with the foot resting on a pillow over the edge of the couch. Rest your leg against the patient's foot to place it in a degree of dorsiflexion, applying enough tension to the Achilles tendon to stabilize it for treatment (Fig. 12.55). Grasp the tendon between your fingers and thumb, depending on the extent of the lesion, and friction transversely across the fibres.

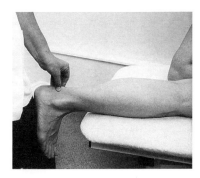

Fig. 12.55 Transverse friction massage of the sides of the Achilles tendon.

Insertion of the Achilles tendon into the calcaneum

Position the patient in prone lying, with the head of the couch slightly elevated and a pillow under the foot to relax it into plantarflexion. This provides you with a 'ledge' of the calcaneum against which to friction the insertion. Make a ring formed by the index fingers, one reinforced by the other, and the thumbs. Rest your index fingers on the calcaneal 'ledge' and wrap your thumbs around the heel. Direct the pressure through your index fingers down on to the calcaneal 'ledge' and impart the friction massage transversely across the fibres (Fig. 12.56).

Relative rest is advised where functional movements may continue, but no overuse or stretching until the structure is painfree on resisted testing.

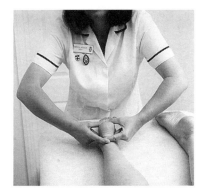

Fig. 12.56 Transverse friction massage of the insertion of the Achilles tendon into the calcaneum.

Injection of the Achilles tendon

Controversy exists over corticosteroid injections and their relationship to tendon rupture (Kennedy and Baxter Willis, 1976;

Smart *et al.*, 1980; Kleinman and Gross, 1983; Mahler and Fritschy, 1992; Read and Motto, 1992). Corticosteroid injections tend to be used for chronic long-standing lesions in which it is difficult to assess the degree of degeneration present in the tendon and to qualify whether the complication of rupture occurred due to injection or the underlying degeneration. Uncomplicated tendinitis may respond well to an early corticosteroid injection to relieve the inflammation, whilst tendinosis, i.e. focal degeneration of the tendon, may not benefit from corticosteroid injection. It seems that studies based on animal experiments show that intratendinous injections cause a reduction in the tensile strength of the Achilles tendon, whilst studies relating to peritendinous injections have not shown these adverse effects (Kleinman and Gross, 1983; Mahler and Fritschy, 1992; Read and Motto, 1992).

Peritendinous* injection of the Achilles tendon (Cyriax and Cyriax, 1983; Cyriax, 1984)

Kenalog 40 mg/ml 0.5 ml	Total steroid 20 mg	Lignocaine 1% 1.5 ml	Total volume 2 ml

21G × 1½ in (0.8 × 40 mm) green needle

* Note: the injection is peritendinous, aiming to bathe the sides of the tendon, and is *not* placed directly into the tendon.

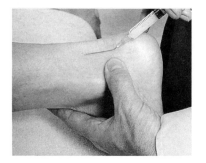

Fig. 12.57 Peritendinous injection of the Achilles tendon.

Position the patient prone on the couch with the ankle resting in dorsiflexion. Bend the hub of the needle to facilitate entry alongside the tendon. Two insertions are made, one on each side of the tendon. Advance the needle to its full length adjacent to the tendon and inject half of the solution as a bolus on each side, as the needle is withdrawn (Fig. 12.57). The patient is advised to maintain a period of relative rest for approximately 2 weeks following injection.

Gastrocnemius muscle belly

Strain of the gastrocnemius muscle belly often has an acute onset following a sudden sprinting action and is sometimes called tennis leg (Cyriax, 1982). Patients feel as though they have been kicked or hit in the calf, the pain is acute and weight-bearing is difficult. The limb becomes swollen and bruising develops within 24–48 h. The diagnosis is conclusive from the history and palpation often localizes the lesion to the medial head of the gastrocnemius muscle belly.

A chronic strain of the gastrocnemius muscle belly may be the result of a past acute lesion or chronic overuse.

Treatment of acute gastrocnemius muscle belly lesion

Apply the principles of treatment for acute lesions, with rest, ice, compression and elevation being applied as soon as possible after the onset. Gentle transverse friction massage is given to the full extent of the lesion with the muscle belly in a relaxed position (Fig. 12.58). This imitates the normal function of the muscle belly fibres, which is to broaden as the muscle contracts. Transverse friction massage is followed immediately by Grade A mobilizations. The patient is taught to maintain a normal heel–toe gait, with the aid of crutches if necessary. A heel raise takes the pressure off the muscle belly and can be gradually reduced as movement is regained.

The patient is seen on a daily basis. An increasing depth of transverse friction massage and greater range of Grade A mobilization is applied until full painless function is restored.

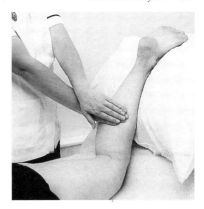

Fig. 12.58 Transverse friction massage of the acute and chronic gastrocnemius muscle belly lesion.

Treatment of chronic gastrocnemius muscle belly lesion

Deep transverse friction massage is applied with the muscle belly in a relaxed position, to facilitate the broadening of the fibres (Fig. 12.58). Vigorous Grade A exercises are performed. The patient is treated every 2–3 days until normal painless function is restored. Should the muscle need to be stretched, it is applied once the muscle is painfree on resisted testing.

References

Acus, R.W., Flanagan, J.P. (1991) Perineural fibrosis of superficial peroneal nerve complicating ankle sprain: a case report. *Foot and Ankle* **11**: 233–235.

Anthony, R.J. (1987) The functional anatomy of the running training shoe. *Chiropodist* 451–459.

Auletta, A.G., Conway, W.F., Hayes, C.W. *et al.* (1991) Indications for radiography in patients with acute ankle injuries. Role of the physical examination. *American Journal of Roentgenology* **157**: 789–791.

Baxter, D.E. (1994) The heel in sport. *Clinics in Sports Medicine* **13**: 683–693.

Black, H.M., Brand, R.L., Eichelberger, M.R. (1978) An improved technique for the evaluation of ligamentous injury in severe ankle sprains. *American Journal of Sports Medicine* **6**: 276–282.

Blake, R.L., Anderson, K., Ferguson, H. (1994) Posterior tibial tendinitis. *Journal of the American Podiatric Medical Association* **84**: 141–149.

Boruta, P.M., Bishop, J.O., Braly, W.G., Tullos, H.S. (1990) Acute lateral ankle ligament injuries: a literature review. *Foot and Ankle* **11**: 107–113.

Boytim, M.J., Fischer, D.A., Neumann, L. (1991) Syndesmotic ankle sprains. *American Journal of Sports Medicine* **19**: 294–298.

Brooks, S.C., Potter, B.T., Rainey, J.B. (1981) Treatment for partial tears of the lateral ligament of the ankle: a prospective trial. *British Medical Journal* **282**: 606–607.

Canoso, J.J. (1981) Bursae, tendons and ligaments. *Clinics in Rheumatic Diseases* **7**: 189–221.

Cetti, R., Andersen, I. (1993) Roentgenographic diagnosis of ruptured Achilles tendons. *Clinical Orthopaedics and Related Research* **286**: 215–221.

Chandler, T.J., Kibler, W.B. (1993) A biomechanical approach to the prevention, treatment and rehabilitation of plantar fasciitis. *Sports Medicine* **15**: 344–352.

Chandnani, V.P., Bradley, Y.C. (1994) Achilles tendon and miscellaneous lesions. *MRI Clinics of North America* **2**: 89–96.

Cornwall, M.W., Murrell, P. (1991) Postural sway following inversion sprain of the ankle. *Journal of the American Podiatric Medical Association* **81**: 243–247.

Cyriax, J. (1982) *Textbook of Orthopaedic Medicine*, vol. 1, 8th edn. Baillière Tindall.

Cyriax, J. (1984) *Textbook of Orthopaedic Medicine*, vol. 2, 11th edn. Baillière Tindall.

Cyriax, J., Cyriax, P. (1983) *Illustrated Manual of Orthopaedic Medicine*. Butterworths.

Dasgupta, B., Bowles, J. (1995) Scintigraphic localisation of steroid injection site in plantar fasciitis. *Lancet* **346**: 1400–1401.

Edwards, G.S., DeLee, J.C. (1984) Ankle diastasis without fracture. *Foot and Ankle* **4**: 305–312.

Evans, P. (1990) Clinical biomechanics of the subtalar joint. *Physiotherapy* **76**: 47–81.

Fox, J.M., Blanzina, M.E., Jobe, F.W. *et al.* (1975) Degeneration and rupture of the Achilles tendon. *Clinical Orthopaedics and Related Research* **107**: 221–224.

Frey, C., Shereff, M.J. (1988) Tendon injuries about the ankle in athletes. *Clinics in Sports Medicine* **7**: 103–118.

Frey, C., Rosenberg, Z., Shereff, M.J., Kim, H. (1992) The retrocalcaneal bursa: anatomy and bursography. *Foot and Ankle* **13**: 203–207.

Gibbon, W.W., Cassar-Pullicino, V.N. (1994) Heel pain. *Annals of the Rheumatic Diseases* **53**: 344–348.

Grisogono, V. (1989) Physiotherapy treatment for Achilles tendon injuries. *Physiotherapy* **75**: 562–572.

Hocutt, J.E., Jaffe, R., Rylander, C.R., Beebe, J.K. (1982) Cryotherapy in ankle sprains. *American Journal of Sports Medicine* **10**: 316–319.

Hutson, M.A. (1990) *Sports Injuries – Recognition and Management*. Oxford Medical Publications.

Kannus, P., Renstrom, P. (1991) Treatment for acute tears of the lateral ligaments of the ankle. *Journal of Bone and Joint Surgery* **73-A**: 305–312.

Kannus, V.P.A. (1992) Evaluation of abnormal biomechanics of the foot and ankle in athletes. *British Journal of Sports Medicine* **26**: 83–89.

Kapandji, I.A. (1985) *The Physiology of the Joints: Lower Limb*, vol. 2, 2nd edn. Churchill Livingstone.

Karlsson, J., Lansingeer, O. (1992) Lateral instability of the ankle joint. *Clinical Orthopaedics and Clinical Research* **276**: 253–261.

Karr, S.D. (1994) Subcalcaneal heel pain. *Orthopedic Clinics of North America* **25**: 161–175.

Kennedy, J.C., Baxter Willis, R. (1976) The effects of local steroid injections on tendons: a biomechanical and microscopic correlative study. *American Journal of Sports Medicine* **4**: 11–21.

Kibler, W.B., Goldberg, C., Chandler, T.J. (1991) Functional biomechanical deficits in running athletes with plantar fasciitis. *American Journal of Sports Medicine* **19**: 66–71.

Kim, W., Voloshin, A.S. (1995) Role of plantar fascia in the load bearing capacity of the human foot. *Journal of Biomechanics* **28**: 1025–1033.

Kleinman, M., Gross, A.E. (1983) Achilles tendon rupture following steroid injection. *Journal of Bone and Joint Surgery* **65-A**: 1345–1347.

Kulthanan, T. (1992) Operative treatment of plantar fasciitis. *Journal of the Medical Association of Thailand* **75**: 337–340.

Lagergren, C., Lindholm, A. (1958) Vascular distribution in the Achilles tendon. *Acta Chirurgica Scandinavica* **116**: 491–495.

Lentell, G.L., Latzman, L.L., Walters, M.R. (1990) The relationship between muscle function and ankle stability. *Journal of Orthopaedic and Sports Physical Therapy* **11**: 605–611.

Litt, J.C.B. (1992) The sprained ankle: diagnosis and management of lateral ligament injuries. *Australian Family Physician* **21**: 447–457.

Liu, S.H., Jason, W.J. (1994) Lateral ankle sprains and instability problems. *Clinics in Sports Medicine* **13**: 793–809.

McMinn, R.M.H., Gaddum-Rosse, P., Hutchings, R.T., Logan, B.M. (1995) *Functional and Clinical Anatomy*. Mosby.

Mahler, F., Fritschy, D. (1992) Partial and complete ruptures of the Achilles tendon and local corticosteroid injections. *British Journal of Sports Medicine* **26**: 7–13.

Marder, R.A. (1994) Current methods for the evaluation of ankle ligament injuries. *Journal of Bone and Joint Surgery* **76-A**: 1103–1111.

Nordin, M., Frankel, V.H. (1989) *Basic Biomechanics of the Musculoskeletal System*, 2nd edn. Lea & Febiger.

Norris, C.M. (1993) *Sports Injuries: Diagnosis and Management for Physiotherapists*. Butterworth-Heinemann.

Ogilvie-Harris, D.J., Gilbart, M. (1995) Treatment modalities for soft tissue injuries of the ankle: a critical review. *Clinical Journal of Sports Medicine* **5**: 175–186.

O'Hara, J., Valle-Jones, J.C., Walsh, H. *et al.* (1992) Controlled trial of an ankle support (Malleotrain) in acute ankle injuries. *British Journal of Sports Medicine* **26**: 139–142.

Read, M.T.F., Motto, S.G. (1992) Tendo Achillis pain: steroids and outcome. *British Journal of Sports Medicine* **26**: 15–21.

Roberts, C.S., DeMaio, M., Larkin, J.J., Paine, R. (1995) Eversion ankle sprains. *Sports Medicine Rehabilitation Series* **18**: 299–304.

Roycroft, S., Mantgani, A.B. (1983) Treatment of inversion injuries of the ankle by early active management. *Physiotherapy* **69**: 355–356.

Rule, J., Yao, L., Seegar, L.L. (1993) Spring ligament of the ankle: normal MR anatomy. *American Journal of Roentgenology* **161**: 1241–1244.

Sartoris, D.J. (1994) Diagnosis of ankle injuries: the essentials. *Journal of Foot and Ankle Surgery* **33**: 102–107.

Saw, Y., Baltzopoulos, V., Lim, A. *et al.* (1993) Early mobilisation after operative repair of ruptured Achilles tendon. *International Journal of the Care of the Injured* **24**: 479–484.

Sellman, J.R. (1994) Plantar fascia rupture associated with corticosteroid injection. *Foot and Ankle International* **15**: 376–381.

Shrier, I. (1995) Treatment of lateral collateral sprains of the ankle: a critical appraisal of the literature. *Clinical Journal of Sports Medicine* **5**: 187–195.

Smart, G.W., Taunton, J.E., Clement, D.B. (1980) Achilles tendon disorders in runners – a review. *Medicine and Science in Sports and Exercise* **12**: 231–243.

Stanley, K.L. (1991) Ankle sprains are always more than 'just a sprain'. *Postgraduate Medicine* **89**: 251–255.

Stephens, M.M. (1994) Haglund's deformity and retrocalcaneal bursitis. *Orthopedic Clinics of North America* **25**: 41–46.

Swain, R.A., Holt, W.S. (1993) Ankle injuries: tips from sports medicine physicians. *Postgraduate Medicine* **93**: 91–100.

Wilkerson, L.A. (1992) Ankle injuries in athletes. *Primary Care* **19**: 377–392.

Williams, J.G.P. (1986) Achilles tendon lesions in sport. *Sports Medicine* **3**: 114–115.

Williams, P.L., Warwick, R., Dyson, M., Bannister, L.H. (1989) *Gray's Anatomy*, 37th edn. Churchill Livingstone.

13 The lumbar spine

Summary

Low back pain presents a challenge to the clinician. Diagnosis is not simple and the clinical data collected may indicate complicated lesions, with several factors contributing to the signs and symptoms. One possible cause of back pain is lumbar disc displacement, the mechanism of which is still poorly understood. Mechanical, chemical and ischaemic factors are currently under investigation.

This chapter outlines the relevant anatomy to enable discussion of evidence for the causes of back pain and differential diagnosis. The clinical examination procedure will be outlined and interpreted, and the models used in orthopaedic medicine will be identified to act as a guide to treatment.

Emphasis will be placed on the selection of patients suitable for treatment and the contraindications to treatment will be discussed. Treatment techniques will be described and guidelines for safety in the application of treatment techniques will be suggested.

Anatomy

There are five lumbar vertebrae, each with a large vertebral body designed for weight-bearing (Fig. 13.1). Each *vertebral body* consists of a shell of cortical bone surrounding a cancellous cavity of

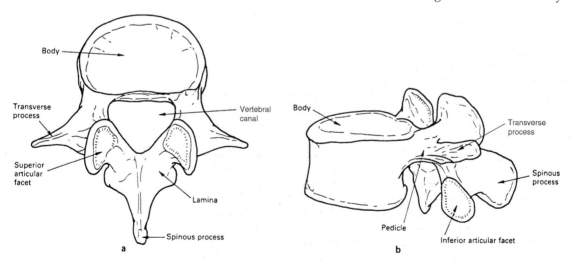

Fig. 13.1 Typical lumbar vertebra. Adapted from Palastanga *et al.* (1989) with permission.

supporting struts and cross-beams called trabeculae. This provides a light-weight box with the strength to support longitudinally applied loads. The intervening *intervertebral disc* provides a mechanism for shock absorption, distribution of forces and movement (Jensen, 1980).

The stabilizing function of the lumbar spine is achieved by the various bony processes that make up the posterior elements of the lumbar vertebrae, i.e. the pedicles and laminae, and the articular, spinous and transverse processes. The position and direction of the *articular processes* that form the synovial, *zygapophyseal joints* prevent forward sliding and rotation of the vertebral bodies, whilst the *spinous and transverse processes* act as leverage and provide attachment for muscles.

The *vertebral foramen* is surrounded by the vertebral body in front and the posterior elements behind. It is triangular in the lumbar spine and is larger than that in the thoracic spine but smaller than that in the cervical spine. Together the vertebral foramina form the *vertebral canal* which contains the termination of the spinal cord opposite the L1–2 disc, and the *cauda equina*. The vertebral canal can vary in shape and this may be relevant to pathology.

The *lumbar lordosis*, the posterior postural concavity, compensates for the inclination of the sacrum and maintains the upright posture. The wedge-shaped lumbosacral disc and vertebral body of L5 contribute to the lordosis as well as the antigravity effect of the constant activity in the erector spinae muscles that prevent the trunk from falling forwards (Oliver and Middleditch, 1991).

The intervertebral disc

The intervertebral disc has special biomechanical requirements. It is strong to sustain weight and transmit loads whilst being able to deform to adjust to movement. The intervertebral disc has three parts: a central nucleus pulposus surrounded by a peripheral annulus fibrosus which blends above and below into vertebral end-plates.

The *nucleus pulposus* accommodates to movement and transmits compressive loads from one vertebral body to another. Its consistency has been likened to that of toothpaste. It is composed of irregularly arranged collagen fibres and cartilage cells scattered within amorphous ground substance. The collagen fibres are composed of type II collagen, suited to accept pressure and compression (see Chapter 2). The nucleus in particular has great water-binding capacity through its proteoglycan content. The fluid nature of the nucleus allows it to deform under pressure whilst the vertebral end-plates prevent its superior and inferior deformation. In this way the intervertebral disc supports and transmits loads.

Although it has long been recognized for its fluid properties, the nucleus also behaves as a viscoelastic solid under dynamic conditions. Iatridis *et al.* (1996) investigated the viscoelastic properties of the healthy nucleus pulposus, showing it to be sensitive to different loading rates. The higher loading rates produced failure of the end-plate and vertebral body, whilst slower loading rates produced progressive failure of the annulus and disc herniation.

The ***annulus fibrosus*** consists of a geometrically organized arrangement of collagen and elastic fibres bound together by a proteoglycan gel, allowing it to support weight without buckling. Type I and II collagen exists in the annulus fibrosus, but the majority of fibres are type I, suited to withstand tensile forces. The fibres are arranged in concentric lamellae around the central nucleus. In each lamella, the collagen fibres lie parallel to each other, inclined at an angle of approximately 65–70° to the vertical (Fig. 13.2). The direction of fibres alternates in adjacent lamellae (Bogduk and Twomey, 1991). Marchand and Ahmed (1990) noted a number of irregularities within the laminate structure of the annulus, particularly at the posterolateral corners, where a number of incomplete layers were seen. Increased stresses applied to the annulus in this region could produce fissuring and provide the nuclear material with an escape route.

The annulus fibrosus acts like a ligament, restraining excessive movement to stabilize the intervertebral joint, whilst allowing flexibility to permit normal movement. The alternating oblique annular fibres resist horizontal and vertical forces, allowing the annulus to oppose movements in all directions (Bogduk, 1991).

The outer half of the annulus at least is known to have a nerve supply (Cavanaugh *et al.*, 1995). The main source of the supply is believed to be the sinuvertebral nerve and branches of the ventral rami and grey rami communicantes. The sinuvertebral nerve supplies the disc at one level and the disc above (Bogduk and Twomey, 1991).

The ***vertebral end-plates*** are thin layers of cartilage, approximately 1 mm thick, covering the superior and inferior surfaces of the discs. They form a permeable barrier for diffusion, mainly between the nucleus and the cancellous bone of the vertebral bodies. They fail relatively easily under excessive compressive loading.

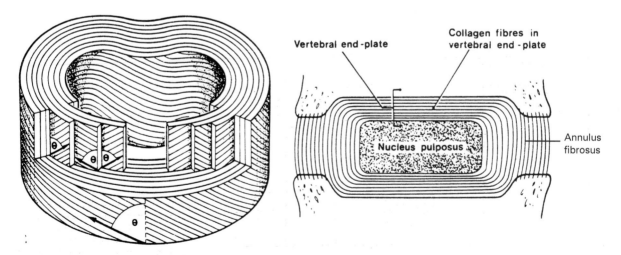

Fig. 13.2 Laminate structure of the disc. Adapted from Bogduk and Twomey (1991) with permission.

Properties of the intervertebral disc

The intervertebral disc at rest possesses an intrinsic pressure due to the compressive effect of the elastic ligamentum flavum (Oliver and Middleditch, 1991). This preloaded or prestressed state provides it with an intrinsic stability to resist applied forces such as body weight (Jensen, 1980). The resting pressure is affected by posture and loading, being lowest in the lying position and highest in the sitting position, with a further increase if external loading is applied (Nachemson, 1966). In the sitting position the spine usually rests in a degree of flexion and the activity in psoas major contributes a compressive effect on the disc as it stabilizes the spine.

Clinically, somatic back pain and radicular pain are affected by movements and posture, as well as being increased by straining,

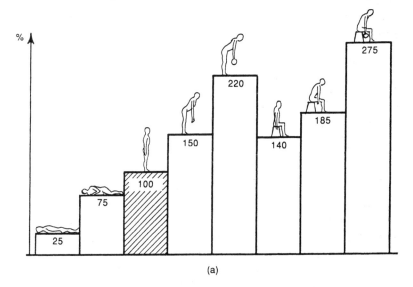

(a)

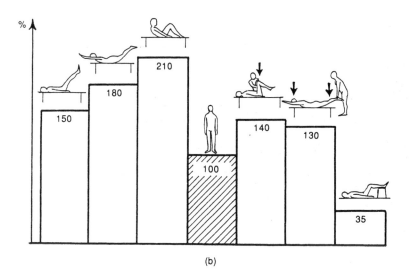

(b)

Fig. 13.3 Discal pressures. Relative change in pressure (or load) in the third lumbar disc: (a) in various positions; (b) in muscle-strengthening exercises. From Nachemson (1966) with permission.

coughing or laughing. An increase in intradiscal pressure of about 50% was noted when straining was performed in standing, due to the increase in loading produced by muscle activity (Nachemson and Elfstrom, 1970). The chart originating from the investigations of Nachemson (1966) has been reproduced in several publications as a useful guide to the variation in intradiscal pressure with different postures and activities (Fig. 13.3).

Movement of the spine involves simultaneous tension, compression and shear at different locations of the disc affecting intradiscal pressure and fluid flow. Flexion, extension and side flexion produce tension resulting in stretching of the annulus on one side, and compression on the other side through body weight (Jensen, 1980). Flexion includes a component of forward translation that is stabilized by the zygapophyseal joints, whilst extension is limited by bony impaction of the inferior articular processes against the lamina of the vertebra below. Axial rotation produces torsion in the intervertebral discs, with tension in half of the annular fibres that are inclined towards the direction of the rotation, and impaction of the zygapophyseal joints. Side flexion is a composite movement which includes side flexion and rotation (Bogduk and Twomey, 1991).

As a viscoelastic material, the intervertebral disc is subjected to the phenomena of creep, hysteresis and set (Twomey and Taylor, 1982; Bogduk and Twomey, 1991; Oliver and Twomey, 1995), as discussed in Chapter 2. The creep behaviour of flexion and extension is similar, with the amount of creep increasing with load and progressing with time. Creep also increases with age when hysteresis recovery is slower. Flexion creep, in particular, has implications for occupations that require a constant flexed posture, e.g. brick layers. It may also be responsible for fatigue in the disc, making it vulnerable to a sudden applied force – the 'straw that breaks the camel's back'.

Nutrition of the intervertebral disc

Nutrition of the intervertebral disc occurs through two routes: the blood vessels situated around the peripheral annulus and those in the central portion of the vertebral end-plate. The mechanisms involved are diffusion and fluid flow and are interrelated. Both are affected by posture and motion (Adams and Hutton, 1986).

The water content of the disc varies and represents a balance between two opposing osmotic and hydrostatic pressures, i.e. a swelling pressure (imbibition) which hydrates the disc, and a mechanical pressure (posture, movement, loading and creep) which dehydrates the disc. Diurnal decrease in the total length of the spine is offset by its recovery in the supine position overnight (Parke and Schiff, 1971; Porter, 1995). Flexion postures cause a larger fluid outflow from the disc than erect or lordotic postures, with this outflow being further reduced when the spine is unloaded by lying down. Alternating between rest and activity will enhance fluid flow (Adams and Hutton, 1983, 1986). Factors that influence the nutrition of the disc are increased loading, vibration or spinal deformity.

Factors that compromise the vascular supply include smoking, vascular disease and diabetes (Buckwalter, 1995).

Zygapophyseal joints

The zygapophyseal joints are synovial joints that provide stability of the spine, control of movement and protection of the intervertebral discs (Fig. 13.4) (Taylor and Twomey, 1994). The articular facets are covered with articular cartilage and the joints are surrounded by a fibrous capsule and lined with synovium. The *superior articular facets* face posteromedially and grasp on to the *inferior articular facets* of the vertebra above, that face anterolaterally. The resultant plane of the joint facilitates flexion and extension movements, but prevents rotation. It also restricts translation in healthy joints, helping to protect the lumbar disc from the shearing forces responsible for fissuring (Bogduk, 1991; Taylor and Twomey, 1994).

The *fibrous capsule* consists of an outer layer of regularly arranged connective tissue and an inner layer of yellow elastic fibres. Anteriorly the capsule is replaced by the *ligamentum flavum*, whilst some of the deep fibres of *multifidus* give the capsule reinforcement

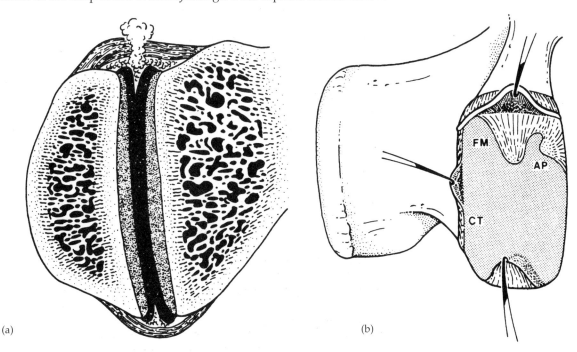

(a) (b)

Fig. 13.4 Intra-articular structures of the lumbar zygapophyseal joints. (a) Coronal section of a left zygapophyseal joint showing fibroadipose meniscoids projecting into the joint cavity from the capsule over the superior and inferior poles of the joint. (b) Lateral view of a right zygapophyseal joint, in which the superior articular process has been removed to show intra-articular structures projecting into the joint cavity across the surface of the inferior articular facet.

The superior capsule is retracted to reveal the base of a fibroadipose meniscoid (FM) and an adipose tissue pad (AP). Another fibroadipose meniscoid at the lower pole of the joint is lifted from the surface of the articular cartilage. A connective tissue (CT) rim has been retracted along the posterior margin of the joint. From Bogduk and Twomey (1991) with permission.

medially (Yamashita *et al.*, 1996). The superior and inferior aspects of the capsules are loose and contain *intra-articular structures* consisting of fat and meniscoid structures (Bogduk and Twomey, 1991). Fine nerve fibres thought to conduct nociceptive and proprioceptive sensations have been found (Yamashita *et al.*, 1996).

The zygapophyseal joints cannot be discounted as a cause of back pain since, as synovial joints, they may be subjected to trauma or arthritis. Degenerative changes usually coexist in the intervertebral joint of the same segment and increased torsion results in fissuring of the intervertebral disc.

Authors have looked at the pattern of pain referral of the zygapophyseal joints in an attempt to establish a recognized syndrome and pain referral patterns (Mooney and Robertson, 1976; Bogduk, 1994). Schwarzer *et al.* (1994a) acknowledged this joint as a possible source of pain, but questioned the existence of a facet syndrome. Some authors suggest that the zygapophyseal joint is responsible for the acute locked back as the intra-articular structures become trapped between the articular surfaces (Bogduk and Twomey, 1991; Twomey and Taylor, 1994), whilst Kuslich *et al.* (1991) demonstrated that stimulation of the zygapophyseal joint capsule very rarely generated back pain. In a study of the relative contributions of the disc and zygapophyseal joint in chronic low back pain, pain was noted to arise more commonly from the disc than the zygapophyseal joint (Schwarzer *et al.*, 1994b).

Ligaments

Anterior and posterior longitudinal ligaments are well-developed in the lumbar region where both stabilize the vertebral bodies and control movement (Fig. 13.5). The *anterior longitudinal ligament* is widest in the lumbar spine where it covers most of the anterior and lateral surfaces of the vertebral bodies and intervertebral discs. The *posterior longitudinal ligament* has a denticulate arrangement that permits the passage of vascular structures. Superficial fibres bridge several vertebrae whilst deeper fibres pass over two joints and have lateral extensions intimately related to the intervertebral disc (Parke and Schiff, 1971). The strong central portion of the posterior longitudinal ligament provides resistance to central disc displacement, deflecting it laterally where the lateral extensions are deficient and offer a space for posterolateral displacement.

The *ligamenta flava* consist of predominantly yellow elastic fibres and connect adjacent laminae. They control lumbar flexion by braking the separation of the laminae and assisting the return to the upright posture. They also restore the ligament to its normal length after stretching, to prevent buckling into the spinal canal and compression of the spinal cord. Such pathology may arise in the degenerate ligament.

The *iliolumbar ligament* provides stability for the lumbosacral junction (Yamamoto *et al.*, 1990), attaching the L5 transverse process to the pelvis. Sometimes a band also passes from the transverse

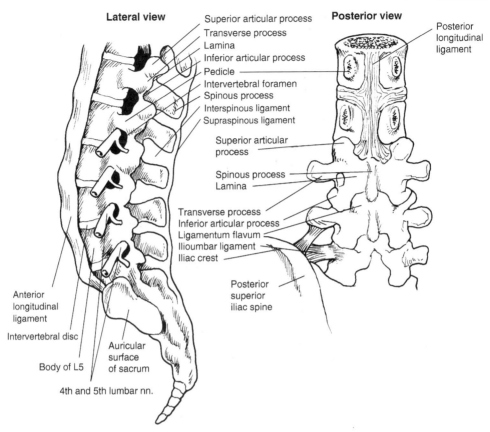

Fig. 13.5 The ligaments of the lumbar spine.

process of L4. This anchorage of L5 to the pelvis may restrict the amount of accommodation possible for disc displacement and disc displacement at the L5, S1 level may produce pain with the patient fixed in flexion, whereas displacement above this level, usually L4–5, may be accommodated more readily by a lateral shift.

Lumbar spinal nerves

The termination of the *spinal cord* lies approximately level with the L1–2 disc, and the lumbar and sacral nerve roots descend vertically in the *cauda equina*, surrounded by the dural sac, to exit via their appropriate lumbar or sacral intervertebral foramina.

Dorsal (sensory) and ventral (mainly motor) nerve roots join to form the relatively short *spinal nerve* that is situated in the intervertebral foramen, together with the dorsal root ganglion. The *dorsal root ganglion* is the collected cell bodies of all sensory nerve fibres related to that segment. The cell bodies of the motor axons are located in the anterior horns of the grey matter in the spinal cord. In the intervertebral foramen the spinal nerve is surrounded by the dural nerve root sleeve, that eventually blends with the epineurium of the nerve. Immediately after leaving the intervertebral foramen the spinal nerve divides into ***dorsal and ventral rami***.

Spinal nerves do not possess the same protective connective tissue sheaths as peripheral nerves and are therefore vulnerable to direct mechanical injury (Rydevik and Olmarker, 1992).

There are five pairs of lumbar nerves, five pairs of sacral nerves and one pair of coccygeal nerves. Their dorsal and ventral nerve roots pass in the cauda equina in an inferolateral direction to reach their appropriate level, before joining to emerge through the intervertebral foramina as the spinal nerves. Until the coccygeal level is reached there are several nerve roots passing vertically in the cauda equina (Fig. 13.6).

The clinical implications of this should be recognized as it is possible for a displaced lumbar disc to encroach on more than one nerve root. It also explains how a lumbar disc displacement can compress the S4 nerve root to affect bladder function.

Lumbar pathology

Degenerative changes

There is a suggestion that the intervertebral discs degenerate first, causing secondary osteoarthritic changes in the zygapophyseal joints (Acaroglu *et al.*, 1995). Degeneration in the zygapophyseal joints involves fibrillation of the articular cartilage that occurs as vertical tears and tangential splits. 'Wrap-around bumpers' appear at the edge of the articular cartilage protecting the articular processes from repeated rotary stresses, whilst osteophyte formation is thought to increase the load-bearing area of these joints (Bogduk and Twomey, 1991).

The most marked ageing or degenerative changes occur in the nucleus of the intervertebral disc. There is a reduction in the water and proteoglycan content and a change in the number and nature of the collagen fibres, with the typical type II fibres of the nucleus changing to resemble the type I fibres of the annulus (Bogduk and Twomey, 1991; Umehara *et al.*, 1996). The water content of the nucleus reduces from 90% at birth to approximately 65–71% by the age of 75 and reduces the preloaded state of the disc (Jensen, 1980; Bogduk and Twomey, 1991; Taylor and Twomey, 1994).

The nucleus, in losing some of its fluid properties, is less able to exert a radial pressure on the annulus. Therefore, a greater portion of vertical load is supported by the annulus; the greater stresses contribute to circumferential tears and radial fissures. The lumbar discs become stiffer and less resilient and overall there is reduced mobility in the lumbar spine.

Degeneration affects the structure of the annulus, with a decrease in the number of lamellae. Individual lamellae become thicker and there is fraying, splitting and breakdown of the laminate structure with less evidence of a transitional zone between annulus and nucleus (Marchand and Ahmed, 1990; Bernick *et al.*, 1991; Holm, 1993; Acaroglu *et al.*, 1995). This degenerative process causes a

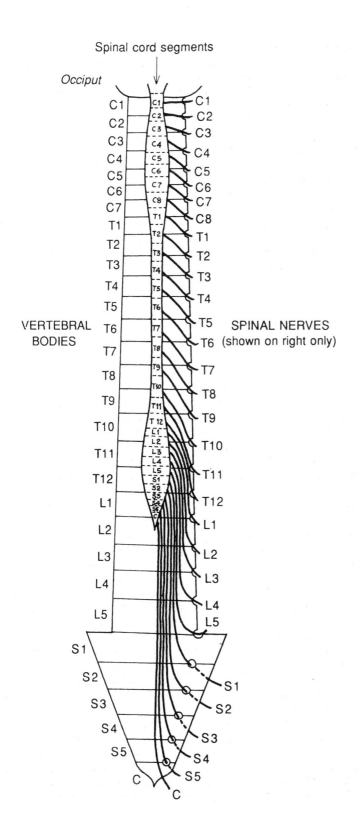

Spinal cord segments

Occiput

VERTEBRAL
BODIES

SPINAL NERVES
(shown on right only)

Fig. 13.6 The cauda equina and emerging nerve roots. From Oliver and Middleditch (1991) with permission.

change in the tensile properties of the annulus that affect its mechanical properties, as well as rendering it vulnerable to failure at lower stresses (Acaroglu *et al.*, 1995).

Three types of annular defects are noted (Osti and Cullum, 1994):

- Rim lesions – discrete defects between the outer annulus and the vertebral body.
- Circumferential tears – more common in the lateral and posterior layers.
- Radial fissures – commonly seen in degenerating discs, extending from the nucleus.

Bone density in the vertebral bodies reduces with age, causing weakening of the trabecular system, a loss of the horizontal trabeculae and a gradual collapse of the vertebral end-plate (Taylor and Twomey, 1994). This results in the intervertebral disc bowing into the concavity of the weakened end-plate, with consequences for the nutrition of the disc via this route. A loss of overall height with ageing is not therefore thought to be due to a loss in disc height, but a loss in vertebral body height due to the collapse of the vertebral end-plate (Bogduk and Twomey, 1991; Taylor and Twomey, 1994).

Lumbar pain syndromes

Any structures in the lumbar region that receive a nerve supply can be a primary source of somatic pain. Congenital or acquired disorders of a single component of the motion segment cannot exist without affecting the functions of other components of the same segment and the functions of other segmental levels of the spine (Parke and Schiff, 1971). However, Schwarzer *et al.* (1994b) consider zygapophyseal joint pain to be uncommon, with discogenic pain a singular, independent disorder.

The zygapophyseal joints, as synovial joints, can be affected by arthritis and the presence of intra-articular structures makes derangement of the joint a possibility. The intervertebral disc is known to degenerate and since the outer annulus receives a nerve supply it can be a primary source of pain. Displacements of nuclear material are well-recognized and are a secondary cause of pain, affecting other pain-sensitive structures.

Traction exerted on the dura and noxious stimulation of the back muscles, ligaments and lumbar zygapophyseal joints have provoked a pain response (Bogduk, 1994). Compression of normal nerves does not provoke a pain response whilst stimulation of swollen, stretched or compressed nerve roots has been shown to produce leg pain, with the dorsal root ganglion tending to be more tender than other parts of the nerve (Kuslich *et al.*, 1991). In the same study, stimulation of the outer annulus fibrosus and the posterior longitudinal ligament produced back pain whilst there was tenderness on stimulation of the capsule of the zygapophyseal joint, also associated with localized back pain. Pain may be produced in any pain-sensitive structure through chemical, mechanical or ischaemic mechanisms, although it seems more than likely that all factors coexist in disc pathology or displacement.

Chemical pain is the result of irritation of the nociceptive nerve endings by the products of inflammation, generally following tissue damage. The products of inflammation can either sensitize nerve endings so that they respond to a lower threshold of stimulus, or activate silent nociceptors (see below) to provoke a response.

Mechanical pain occurs through stretching, compression or distortion of connective tissue structures stimulating the intervening nociceptors. Mechanical stress ultimately produces vascular changes and ischaemia, which activates nociceptors.

Whilst acknowledging the existence of all pain-sensitive structures within the spinal joints, diagnosis of disc displacement is central to the concepts of treatment in orthopaedic medicine. With evidence from scans more readily available, the disc would seem to be a major contributor to spinal pain, but the mechanisms of internal derangement, disc displacement and the recovery from disc pathology, often spontaneously, remain unknown. More recent work has concentrated on the chemical effects of displaced nuclear material whilst the exact mechanism of pain produced by mechanical compression is unclear.

Primary disc pain

The outer part of the annulus fibrosus receives a nerve supply, thought to be nociceptive. Pressure exerted on the outer annulus and injection of contrast medium into the disc have each provoked a pain response (Bogduk, 1994). Roberts *et al.* (1995) found sensory nerve endings in the form of mechanoreceptors in intervertebral discs and the posterior longitudinal ligament. Golgi tendon organs were the most frequently seen. These may directly elicit pain or modulate muscle activity, perhaps in the form of muscle spasm that is often associated with acute disc displacement.

As with all connective tissue structures, the elastic property of the collagen fibres in the annulus, enhanced by 'crimp', allows it to tolerate tensile forces. When placed under excessive mechanical tension the annulus deforms and may directly squeeze or distort pain-sensitive nerve endings, producing pain of mechanical origin. Once forces exceed normal limits microtrauma occurs, producing pain of chemical origin. The most vulnerable position for the annulus is when it is placed under rotational strains in flexion, ultimately resulting in circumferential splits (Bogduk and Twomey, 1991). Shear and tensile forces initiate damage at the peripheral portion of the disc but not at the centre, since fibre strain is always minimal at the centre and maximal at the periphery (Brinckmann, 1986).

With consideration for the chemical contribution to low back pain, substance P causes the release of inflammatory mediators that affect the local environment and may sensitize nociceptors, resulting in chronic pain (Zimmermann, 1992; Beaman *et al.*, 1993; Palmgren *et al.*, 1996). Substance P immunoreactive nerve fibres have been identified in the zygapophyseal joint capsule and synovial folds, the supraspinous ligament, posterior longitudinal ligament and the annulus fibrosus. Some fine unmyelinated and small myelinated fibres in the annulus are thought to serve as a type of pain fibre, termed silent nociceptor, that is not excited by mechanical stress, but responds to algesic chemicals produced at times of tissue damage or inflammation (Cavanaugh, 1995).

There is no evidence as yet to support a nerve supply to the nucleus pulposus and pathological processes can occur internally within the nucleus without provoking a pain response.

Secondary disc pain

Mixter and Barr (1934) suggested that a displaced fragment of the intervertebral disc into the vertebral canal causes mechanical compression of the lumbar nerve roots and sensory root ganglia. However, the mechanism by which back or leg pain is produced by this mechanical compression is still not fully understood. Kuslich *et al.* (1991) demonstrated that stimulation of a normal nerve root did not produce a pain response, whilst stimulation of an already swollen, stretched or compressed nerve root produced leg pain. However, no suggestion was made for how much, or for how long, mechanical stress should be applied to a previously undamaged nerve root before changes occur to make it sensitive.

The extruded disc material in disc prolapse usually consists of nuclear material, sometimes with end-plate material and occasionally elements of the annulus (Bogduk, 1991; Brock *et al.*, 1992). However, normal disc material does not usually rupture and the nucleus is thought to undergo some process of deterioration or degradation, in order for it to be displaced (Bogduk, 1991). Hormonal, nutritional or viral factors or simply an acceleration of the degenerative process have been proposed as possible reasons for the degradation of the nucleus.

Bogduk and Twomey (1991) offer a plausible explanation of mechanical trauma together with an autoimmune reaction within the nucleus. Proteins in the nucleus may act as an antigen which, when exposed to the circulation for the first time, trigger an autoimmune response. Intrinsically, this can occur via contact with the circulatory plexus associated with the vertebral end-plate through microfracture due to compressive loading. The provoked autoimmune inflammatory response causes degradation of the nucleus which continues once the microfractures heal. Degrading the nuclear material in this way renders it capable of displacement. Changes must also occur within the annulus since displacement of nuclear material can only occur through a radial fissure in a weakened annular wall (Brinckmann, 1986).

The posterolateral corners of the annulus are irregular, thin and potentially weak (Umehara *et al.*, 1996). Radial fissures and circumferential splits commonly develop here, providing an escape route for the degraded nuclear material, when a force is applied sufficient to expel it. Flexed postures, especially combined with rotation, trigger backwards displacement of the nuclear material through a weakened annular wall (Bogduk and Twomey, 1991).

The effects of disc prolapse into the vertebral or intervertebral canal

As well as being a primary source of pain, the disc, through displacement, can have a secondary effect on any pain-sensitive structure lying within the canal or intervertebral foramen. This effect can be mechanical through compression and distortion, chemical through the inflammatory process and ischaemic through the pressure of oedema.

Once nuclear material enters the vertebral canal it may again be treated as foreign and stimulate an extrinsic autoimmune inflammatory response as it comes into contact with the circulation in the vertebral canal. The resulting chemical mediators affect adjacent pain-sensitive structures. If the displaced fragment is small, it will be dealt with by the macrophage system; if large, the inflammatory process continues until the fragment is eventually organized into scar tissue (Hirabayashi *et al.*, 1990).

Both mechanical and inflammatory mechanisms can produce ischaemia. The inflammatory mediators produced are thought to have a role in somatic pain (McCarron *et al.*, 1987; Bogduk, 1994) and in radicular pain (Doita *et al.*, 1996; Kang *et al.*, 1996; Takahashi *et al.*, 1996).

The quality of pain seems to be instrumental in distinguishing somatic and radicular pain. Somatic and somatic referred pain is produced when any sensitive structure is stimulated and is deep, aching and hard to localize. Radicular pain is produced when a nerve root is compressed and was described by Smyth and Wright as shooting, lancinating pain felt in a relatively narrow band, approximately 4 cm wide, into the limb (Bogduk, 1994).

Compression of undamaged nerves produces numbness, paraesthesia and muscle weakness. Under some circumstances, which are not well-understood, compression alters nerve root conduction and compromises their nutritional support (Garfin *et al.*, 1995), causing them to become pain-sensitive through inflammation, ischaemia or both. Recent studies suggest that the products of the autoimmune inflammatory process stimulated by the displaced nuclear material may increase the sensitivity of the nerve root to bradykinin and be involved in the pathophysiology of radiculopathy (Saal, 1995; Kang *et al.*, 1996; Takahashi *et al.*, 1996).

For referred leg pain to be radicular in origin, arising from compression of a nerve root, it must be accompanied by the other signs of compression – paraesthesia and muscle weakness. If these are absent, pain referred to the limb must be somatic in origin (Bogduk, 1994).

However, in clinical practice, signs and symptoms of somatic and radicular pain coexist since, for a disc displacement to compress a nerve root, it must first compress and stimulate nerve endings in its dural nerve root sleeve. Thus the dural nerve root sleeve produces somatic referred pain, either mechanical or chemical in origin.

As well as objective neurological signs, the compressed nerve root becomes pain-sensitive. The mechanical effects of compression of a nerve root may be direct or more probably indirect through ischaemia. A sequence of events may be induced involving impairment of nutrition and increased microvascular permeability, leading to intraneural oedema, blockage of axonal transport and altered function (Rydevik and Olmarker, 1992).

In studies on peripheral nerves, a critical level of pressure is significant for structural and functional changes to occur and longer periods of compression would seem to be responsible for more damage. Prolonged compression may produce changes in axonal transport impairing the transport of proteins from the nerve cell body to the distal parts of the body and resulting in compression-induced effects in the distal axonal segment (double crush syndrome).

The trauma evoked by compression may alter the permeability of the intraneural vessels, resulting in oedema. The oedema usually persists after removal of the compression and therefore may adversely affect the nerve root for longer. The presence of intraneural oedema is thus related to intraneural fibrosis and adhesion formation.

Unfortunately, at the time of writing, there do not appear to have been many experimental studies on spinal nerves, but they are known to be more susceptible to compression than peripheral nerves since they do not have the same protective connective tissue sheaths. The critical pressure levels for compression to induce impairment of nerve nutrition or function are not known, or the length of time that compression needs to be applied before changes occur.

Differential diagnosis at the lumbar spine

The mechanism by which the lumbar intervertebral disc produces pain is probably complicated, with several factors contributing to the diagnosis. It is important to understand the anatomy and the possible mechanisms for pain production.

Patients with non-mechanical causes of back pain can present with signs and symptoms that mimic those of disc pathology. It is important to recognize those features that allow them to be identified, since manual techniques are either contraindicated or not appropriate, and the patient needs to be referred to the appropriate specialist. The following section is divided into two parts. The first covers lumbar disc lesions; the second covers the non-mechanical causes of back pain and associated signs and symptoms.

A recap of the terminology used to describe disc displacement is provided on page 401 to add clarity to the following discussion.

In contrast to the cervical spine, where the degenerate disc tends to displace as a central bar-like protrusion of the annulus, the degenerate lumbar disc involves degradation and displacement of nuclear material through a weakened annular wall. This displacement may occur as a protrusion into the weakened annulus where it may produce primary disc pain, or as a prolapse where nuclear material moves into the vertebral canal. Here it can have a secondary effect on any pain-sensitive structure by mechanisms involving compression, inflammation and ischaemia.

Disc protrusion

- Central disc material passes into the weakened laminate structure of the annulus, where it can produce primary disc pain since the outer annulus receives a nerve supply.

Disc prolapse

- Discal material passes through a ruptured annulus into the vertebral canal where it has a secondary effect on the pain-sensitive structures in the vertebral canal. The sequela of this is sequestration of the disc.

A central prolapse affects central structures, in particular the posterior longitudinal ligament and the dura mater. Pain arising from compression of the dura mater is extrasegmental in nature (see Chapter 1). A posterolateral prolapse affects unilateral structures, mainly the dural nerve root sleeve and nerve root, which tend to produce segmental pain.

A disc displacement, either protrusion or prolapse, produces a pattern of signs and symptoms that are progressive, with a history of increasing, worsening episodes. Often the precipitating factor is trivial. The dural nerve root sleeve and nerve root are vulnerable in the lumbar spine to posterolateral prolapse, with pain and other associated symptoms referred into the leg. A set of clinical models has been established to aid diagnosis and to establish treatment programmes. These are outlined in the treatment section later in this chapter, since they relate directly to treatment selection.

Other causes of back pain, leg pain and associated signs and symptoms

Non-mechanical lesions, including serious pathology, have features that do not 'fit'. Since they represent contraindications to manual orthopaedic medicine treatments, they must be recognized and the patients referred appropriately.

Arthritis, in any form, presents with the capsular pattern which is demonstrated by the lumbar spine as a whole.

Degenerative osteoarthrosis affects the intervertebral joint and the zygapophyseal joint. The consequences of degeneration and degradation of the intervertebral disc lead to increased possibility of disc displacement. Disruption of the intervertebral joint affects the zygapophyseal joint, causing the joint surfaces to bear increased weight.

Osteophytes may form at the peripheral margins of the disc, possibly in association with rim lesions of the annulus, as well as at the zygapophyseal joints. Overall the degenerative changes may lead to spinal stenosis.

Spinal stenosis is a term that has become synonymous with *neurogenic* or *spinal claudication*. It should be used to define any

Capsular pattern of the lumbar spine:

- Limitation of extension
- Equal limitation of side flexions
- Usually full flexion

symptomatic condition in which limited space in the vertebral canal is a significant factor (Porter, 1992). Lateral stenosis affects the nerve root; central stenosis affects the spinal cord or cauda equina and may coexist with lateral stenosis.

Some patients have a developmental abnormality where the spinal canal has a trefoil shape in cross-section (Vernon-Roberts, 1992) and spinal stenosis is particularly prevalent in this group. Narrowing can also occur as a result of degenerative changes through ageing, injury, disease, or as a result of surgery (Lee *et al.*, 1995). Irrespective of cause, a small vertebral canal can have clinical significance for back pain (Porter and Oakshot, 1994).

Degenerative spinal stenosis can be associated with osteophyte formation at the vertebral body or zygapophyseal joints, with reactive proliferation of capsular and soft tissues, and fibrous scarring around the nerve roots. The vertebral canal can be compromised by thickening of the ligamentum flavum, that shows a 50% increase in thickness with ageing over a normal life span (Twomey and Taylor, 1994). Degenerative spondylolisthesis may also narrow the canal (Osborne, 1974; Rauschning, 1993).

A bulging disc may significantly reduce the size of both the vertebral and intervertebral foramina and Porter *et al.* (1978) noted that the risk of developing disabling symptoms from disc displacement is inversely related to the size of the spinal canal. The anterior margin of the canal can be indented to compress the cauda equina by a lax posterior longitudinal ligament overlying degenerate bulging discs. Cyriax (1982) termed this the 'mushroom phenomenon'.

Spinal stenosis can produce neurogenic or spinal claudication which was recognized by Verbiest, in 1954, as due to structural narrowing of the vertebral canal compressing the cauda equina and producing claudication symptoms (Porter, 1992). Men over the age of 50 with a lifestyle that has involved heavy manual work are affected. The entire cauda equina can be compressed centrally causing bilateral symptoms, or the emerging nerve root can be affected (Osborne, 1974). The patient complains of discomfort, pain, paraesthesia and heaviness in one or both legs whilst standing or walking. There may be night cramps and restless legs. A long history of back pain may be present and the patient may have undergone back surgery at some time. The symptoms are usually of several months' duration. There is usually a threshold distance when the symptoms develop and a tolerance when they have to stop; the tolerance distance is about twice the threshold (Porter, 1992). These symptoms are similar to those of the ischaemic pain associated with intermittent claudication of peripheral vascular disease and with the age group affected, the two conditions can coexist, making diagnosis difficult.

With neurogenic claudication, stooping or bending forwards relieves the symptoms and allows the patient to continue. Flexion increases the space in the canal and tightens the ligaments, straightening out the buckling that tends to occur with degeneration. The patient can usually walk uphill, which involves a flexed posture, easier than walking downhill, which involves an extended posture.

On examination, the patient often stands with a stooped posture, with flexed hips and knees and a flattened lumbar spine with loss of the lordosis. This posture becomes more evident on walking. The capsular pattern is present with marked loss of spinal extension. Extension may produce the pain as it decreases the calibre of the spinal canal whilst, conversely, flexion relieves the pain (Osborne, 1974). Dynamic variations in flexion and extension are related to changes in the buckling of the ligamentum flavum and the bulging of the intervertebral discs (Rauschning, 1993). The rest of the examination may be unremarkable and back pain itself may not be a feature. Neurological signs are often absent.

Management may involve spinal decompressive surgery or advice on how to live with the condition. Symptoms do not usually resolve, but they do not always get worse.

Rheumatoid arthritis can affect the spinal joints and this has been covered in Chapter 8. Ankylosing spondylitis is discussed in Chapter 14.

Structural abnormalities can be completely asymptomatic or may produce pain, inflammation and neurological signs, or coexist with disc displacement.

Spondylolysis is a defect in the neural arch between the lamina and the pedicle (pars interarticularis) of L5 and sometimes L4. *Spondylolisthesis* is an anterior shift of one vertebral body on another, usually involving slippage of L5 on S1. It may be congenital, acquired through degeneration, trauma, or as a sequela to spondylolysis. It is commonly associated with over-training in such sports as gymnastics involving hyperextension, and the rotational stresses involved in fast bowling (Bush, 1994). If symptomatic, the main symptom is back pain that may be referred to the buttocks. The pain is aggravated by exercise and standing and is eased by sitting. Inspection may reveal excessive skin folds above the defect and a step defect may be felt on palpation (Norris, 1993). On examination, extension is limited and painful and passive overpressure of the affected vertebra produces the pain. Diagnosis is confirmed by oblique X-rays that show the typical 'Scottie dog' with its collar representing fracture of the pars articularis.

X-ray assesses the degree of spondylolisthesis that is measured by the distance the slipped upper vertebra moves forward on its lower counterpart. Slippage is divided into four degrees, progressing from a first-degree slip, which is a forward displacement of one-quarter of the anteroposterior diameter of the vertebral body, to a fourth-degree slip with a full anteroposterior diameter displacement (Corrigan and Maitland, 1983).

A particular feature of *serious non-mechanical conditions* is an unwell patient with possible weight loss. Neoplasm of the lumbar spine, although relatively uncommon, should be considered as a possible cause of low back and leg pain. Metastases may be secondary to carcinoma of the bronchus, breast, ovary, prostate, thyroid or kidney. Metastatic invasion may involve bone or may be intradural. Primary bone tumours occasionally affect the posterior elements of the vertebrae and multiple myeloma can produce backache due to vertebral involvement.

Neoplasm involving the lumbar spine may be clinically silent or may produce pain in isolation or cause associated neurological deficit (Findlay, 1992). The pain may be due to compression or distortion of pain-sensitive structures and or to destructive changes in the bone. Neurological deficit is usually of a lower motor neuron type and it may begin either at the same time as the pain, or prior to it.

The pain of neoplastic disease has characteristic features. It is usually deep-seated, boring, relatively constant, steadily worsening and often persistent at night. If there is collapse of the vertebral body, the pain will be associated with movement and activity due to the spinal instability (Findlay, 1992). Aside from night pain, symptoms of weakness, fatigue and weight loss should be considered to be serious in a patient complaining of back pain.

The signs and symptoms of a tumour can mimic a disc lesion. Palma *et al.* (1994) reported three cases of neurinoma of the cauda equina initially misdiagnosed as a disc lesion. Pain which worsens during recumbency and improves in sitting and walking together with bilateral, multiple root involvement is more indicative of an expanding lesion in the cauda equina than sciatica. Unusual cases of a primary extraosseous Ewing sarcoma in a 15-year-old girl with a history of chronic back and leg ache (Allam and Sze, 1994) and primary Hodgkin's disease of the bone presenting clinically with an extradural tumour (Moridaira *et al.*, 1994) exist in the literature.

Infection may cause osteomyelitis or discitis and epidural abscess is possible. Pyogenic organisms, e.g. *Staphylococcus aureus*, *Myobacterium tuberculosis* or, rarely, *Brucella* may be responsible (Kumar and Clark, 1994). The clinical presentation of spinal infection varies from a complaint of back pain only to being very ill, emaciated and febrile, and with a raised erythrocyte sedimentation rate. On examination tenderness is elicited on percussion of the affected vertebra and widespread muscle spasm may be present. X-ray may show loss of bony contour, cavitation and collapse and possibly an associated paravertebral abscess (Kemp and Worland, 1974).

Aortic aneurysms are commonly abdominal (Kumar and Clark, 1994). When they rupture they may present with epigastric pain that radiates through to the back. The patient is shocked and a pulsatile mass is felt. This situation is a medical emergency. Dissecting aortic aneurysm also presents as severe central pain often radiating to the back. Galessiere *et al.* (1994) presented three cases of chronic, contained rupture of aortic aneurysms associated with vertebral erosion. The patients presented with a history of chronic backache.

Non-organic back pain should be considered at the lumbar spine, although true psychogenic back pain is rare. Back pain begins as a physical problem, but if it becomes chronic, psychological factors are relevant. As clinicians, the physical and psychological factors that coexist in chronic pain must be understood in order to provide care. Anxiety tends to be associated with acute back pain whilst depression is associated with chronic back pain; both are indicators of the patient's distress.

The diagnostic approach to back pain involves a recognized set of signs and symptoms. If this recognizable pattern is absent, with mutually contradictory signs, a psychogenic element to the patient's pain is probably present.

Waddell *et al.* (1980) and Waddell (1992) identified a group of symptoms and signs that are physically inappropriate to benign musculoskeletal back pain and are indicators of the patient's emotional reaction to pain. The group of symptoms should be taken as a whole rather than in isolation. The following symptoms and physical signs may occur in serious pathology, e.g. tumour or infection, and these should be eliminated before being attributed to a behavioural pattern. These symptoms and signs are based on the patterns described by Waddell.

Behavioural symptoms

- Tailbone pain not related to trauma.
- Whole leg pain or numbness in a stocking distribution.
- Whole leg giving way: this is incompatible with the usual neurological deficit associated with back pain.
- Never free of pain, often persisting for years.
- Intolerance and side-effects to numerous treatments.
- Emergency admissions to hospital: this is a measure of the patient's distress and emotional reaction to the pain.

Behavioural responses to examination

- Tenderness which is superficial and non-anatomical.
- Simulation tests which give the impression that a manoeuvre has been performed when it has not (e.g. passive rotation of the shoulders and pelvis in the same direction).
- Tests which distract the patient's attention (e.g. comparing the consistency of the ranges of straight leg raise and lumbar flexion).
- Regional disturbances producing inconsistent signs, e.g. weakness of many muscle groups, or jerky 'giving way' (juddering) on resisted testing which appears to be a behavioural response.

Commentary on the examination

Observation

A general observation of the *patient's face, posture and gait* will alert the examiner to the seriousness of the condition. Patients in acute pain will generally look tired and worn. They may have adopted an antalgic posture of flexion or lumbar scoliosis that is generally indicative of an acute locked back, probably due to a displaced disc. A shift is pathognomonic of a disc lesion (Porter, 1995). Patients may not be able to sit during the examination due to discomfort from this particular posture. Their gait may be uneasy with steps taken cautiously, obviously wary of provoking twinges of pain by sudden movements or pain on weight-bearing. A dropped foot may be evident on walking and will lead you to consider involvement of the L4 nerve root affecting the tibialis anterior muscle and interfering with function.

History (subjective examination)

The history is particularly important at the spinal joints. Selection of patients for orthopaedic medicine treatment techniques relies on a diagnosis of a displaced intervertebral disc and certain aspects of the history will assist in this diagnosis. There is a close relationship between signs and symptoms from the lumbar spine, sacroiliac joint and hip joint. The history will help with the differential diagnosis but conditions at each of these areas can coexist. Major pathology can affect the spine, such as malignancy, infection, spondylo-arthropathy or fracture, but these represent a small percentage of the problems compared with mechanical lesions of the lower back (Swezey, 1993). X-ray findings can be misleading, particularly when showing the degenerative changes of osteoarthrosis which may or may not be painful. Similarly, spondylolysis progressing to spondylolisthesis occurs in approximately 5% of adults but is symptomatic in only half of them (Swezey, 1993).

The *age, occupation, sports, hobbies and lifestyle* of the patient may give an indication of provoking mechanisms. Often the incident precipitating the episode of back pain may be relatively minor, whilst factors predisposing to the event may have been continuing for some time. Whilst cure will be the initial aim of treatment, ultimately the management of the condition and prevention of recurrence will become the patient's responsibility. Patients will require advice and guidance on management of their back condition.

Many occupations involve a flexion lifestyle, e.g. sedentary office work and brick-laying apply postural stress to the intervertebral joint. These patients require advice about changing postures to minimize the stress inflicted by work. Directives on the manual handling of loads are in existence and patients should receive advice about this in their place of work. The vibration of motor vehicle driving may have an influence, as well as the sitting posture involved, which is known to increase intradiscal pressure (Osti and Cullum, 1994).

Assessment of patients with chronic low back pain presents a particular challenge to the clinician. Emotional, environmental and industrial factors may influence pain perception, whilst monotony or dissatisfaction at work or home is relevant (Osti and Cullum, 1994). Distinction will need to be made between the true physical symptoms of the presenting condition and those relating to psychological factors that influence the way the patient reacts to the pain (see above). Inquiry should be made about the possibilities of secondary gain factors relating to disability, or the presence of psychological or social stresses that might predispose the patient to chronic pain disorders (Swezey, 1993). Standard questions on quality of sleep, tiredness levels, concentration, appetite, etc. may establish whether the patient is depressed.

The *site* of the pain will give an indication of its origin. Lumbar pain is generally localized to the back and buttocks or felt in the limb in a segmental pattern. Sacroiliac pain may be unilateral, felt in the buttock, or more commonly in the groin, and occasionally referred into the leg. The hip joint may produce an area of pain in the buttock consistent with the L3 segment, pain in the groin, or pain referred down the anteromedial aspect of the thigh and leg to the medial aspect of the ankle. Dural pain is extrasegmental and will be central or bilateral. Pressure on the dural nerve root sleeve will be referred segmentally to the relevant dermatome. Pressure on the nerve root will refer pain to the relevant limb with accompanying symptoms of paraesthesia at the distal end of the dermatome.

Vucetic *et al*. (1995) considered the difficulty that patients have in giving a precise verbal description of pain. They support the use of a pain drawing, which may take a few minutes to obtain, but the result can be grasped at a glance. Waddell (1992) warns that how a patient draws pain is influenced by emotional distress and that non-anatomical, widespread and magnified drawings tell of the patient's distress rather than the physical characteristics of the pain.

The *spread* of pain will not only give an indication of its origin, but also the severity or irritability of the lesion. Generally, the more peripherally the pain is referred, the greater the source of irritation. A mechanical lesion due to a displaced lumbar disc produces central or unilateral back or buttock pain. If pain shifts into the leg, it generally ceases or is reduced in the back. Pain of non-musculoskeletal origin does not follow this pattern and serious lesions produce an increasing spreading pain, with pain in the back remaining as severe as that felt peripherally.

The *onset and duration* of the pain can assist the choice of treatment. In very general terms, a sudden onset of pain is likely to respond to manipulation whilst a gradual onset of pain may respond better to traction. The whole clinical picture will need to be reasoned through in order to make a decision about treatment which may contradict these rules of thumb.

The nature and mode of onset are important. The patient may remember the exact time and mode of onset that may have involved a flexed and rotated posture. If lifting was involved in the precipitating episode, it may only have been a trivial weight. If the patient reports a gradual onset of pain, it is worth questioning further for details of previous activity. A minor traumatic incident some time before the onset of back pain or the maintenance of a sustained flexion posture may have been sufficient to provoke the attack.

The gradual onset of degenerative osteoarthrosis is common in the zygapophyseal joints and hip joints, whilst a subluxation of the sacroiliac joint can occur with a sudden onset. Serious pathology develops insidiously.

If trauma is involved, the exact nature of the trauma should be ascertained and any possible fracture eliminated. Direct trauma may produce soft-tissue contusions, whilst fracture may involve the spinous process, transverse process, pars interarticularis, vertebral body or vertebral end-plate. Compression fractures of the vertebral body are common in horse riders and those falling from a height, and involve the vulnerable cancellous bone of the vertebral body (Hartley, 1995). Hyperflexion injuries may cause ligamentous lesions or involve the capsule of the zygapophyseal joint, whilst hyperextension injuries compress the zygapophyseal joints. Both forces can injure the intervertebral disc.

The **symptoms and behaviour** need to be considered. The behaviour of the pain will give an indication of the irritability of the patient's condition and provide clues to differential diagnosis. The pattern of all previous episodes of back pain should be ascertained, as in disc lesions a pattern of gradually worsening and increasing episodes of pain usually emerges.

The mechanisms whereby the displaced disc material can cause pain have been discussed earlier in this chapter. The typical pattern of pain from disc displacement is usually one of a central pain that moves laterally. As the pain moves laterally, the central pain usually ceases or reduces. A gradually increasing central pain accompanied by increasing leg pain is indicative of serious pathology and this pain is usually not altered by either rest or activity.

The daily pattern of pain is important and typically a disc lesion produces a pattern of pain that is better first thing in the morning after rest, becoming worse as the day goes on. Patients can sleep reasonably well at night as they are usually able to find a position of ease. However, as the disc imbibes water overnight, the patient may experience increased pain on weight-bearing first thing in the morning due to increased pressure on sensitive tissues.

Mechanical pain can cause an on/off response through compression or distortion of pain-sensitive structures. This can involve the annulus itself or structures in the vertebral canal. The patient with a displaced disc usually complains of pain on movement easing with rest. Changing pressures in the disc affect the pain and it tends to be worse with sitting and stooping postures than when standing or lying down. In an acute locked back, small movements can create exquisite twinging pain.

Displaced disc material produces an inflammatory response resulting in chemical pain. Chemical pain is characteristically a constant ache associated with morning stiffness. Sharper pain can also be associated with chemical irritation as the nerve endings become sensitized and respond to a lower threshold of stimulation. It is important to differentiate mechanical back pain from inflammatory arthritis and sacroiliac joint lesions through consideration of other factors, since it also produces pain associated with early-morning stiffness.

Radicular pain (see above) is generally a severe lancinating pain, often burning in nature, which is felt in the distribution of the dermatome associated with the nerve root. Sciatica is commonly associated with lumbar disc pathology and will occur if the L4–5,

S1 or 2 nerve roots are involved. The most common levels affected are the L4–5 or L5, S1 discs affecting the lower sciatic nerve roots. If the higher levels are involved, pain will similarly be referred into the relevant segment.

The words used by patients to describe the quality of their pain will indicate the balance between the physical and emotional elements of their pain. 'Throbbing', 'burning', 'twinging' and 'shooting' pain describe the sensory quality of the pain whilst emotional characteristics are expressed in such words as 'sickening', 'miserable', 'unbearable' and 'exhausting' (Waddell, 1992).

The other symptoms described by the patient provide evidence for differential diagnosis, contraindications to treatment and the severity or irritability of the lesion. An increase in pressure through coughing, sneezing, laughing or straining can increase the back pain and this is the main dural symptom. Paraesthesia is usually felt at the distal end of the dermatome and is a symptom of nerve root compression. Confirmation of this is made through the objective compression signs of muscle weakness, altered sensation and reduced or absent reflexes.

Specific questions must be asked concerning pain or paraesthesia in the perineum and genital area as well as bladder and bowel function. The presence of any of these symptoms indicates compression of the S4 nerve root at the preganglionic extent which could produce irreversible damage, and indicates immediate referral for surgical opinion. Manipulation is absolutely contra-indicated in these cases. The symptoms of difficulty in passing water, inability to retain urine or lack of sensation when the bowels are opened are important. It is not unusual to find urinary frequency or difficulty in defecating associated with effort in hyperacute lumbar pain.

Bilateral sciatica with objective neurological signs and bilateral limitation of straight leg raise suggest a massive central protrusion compressing the cauda equina through the posterior longitudinal ligament, with possible rupture of the ligament (Cyriax, 1982). It is an absolute contraindication to manipulation, since a worsening of the situation could lead to irreversible damage to the cauda equina, as mentioned above. The symptoms of cauda equina compression should be distinguished from extrasegmental, dural reference of pain into both legs, where there may be bilateral limitation of straight leg raise but no neurological signs.

Questioning the patient about *other joint involvement* will indicate whether inflammatory arthritis exists or if there is a tendency towards degenerative osteoarthrosis.

The *past medical history* and the patient's current general health will help to eliminate possible serious pathology, past or present. An unexplained recent weight loss may be significant in systemic disease or malignancy. Visceral lesions can refer pain to the back, e.g. kidney, aortic aneurysm or gynaecological conditions. Infections should be obvious, with an unwell patient showing a fever. Malignancy can affect the lumbar and pelvic region, but the pattern of the pain behaviour does not generally fit that of musculoskeletal origin. Serious conditions produce an unrelenting pain, therefore night pain is usually a feature and is responsible for the patient looking tired and ill.

The *medications* taken by the patient will indicate their current medical state as well as alerting the examiner to possible contraindications to treatment, e.g. tamoxifen. Anticoagulant therapy and long-term oral steroids are contraindications to manipulation. It is useful to know what analgesics are being taken and how frequently. This gives an indication of the severity of the condition and can be used as a marker for progression of treatment, with the need for less analgesia indicating a positive improvement. If patients are currently taking antidepressant medication, this may indicate their emotional state and possibly exclude them from manipulation. Care is needed in making this decision, however, since antidepressants can be used in low doses as an adjunct to analgesics in back pain.

Inspection

The patient should be adequately undressed down to underwear and in a good light. The difficulty in undressing, especially of socks and shoes, is associated with disc pathology and indicates the irritability of the lesion. A general inspection from behind, each side, and in front will reveal any *bony deformity* (Figs 13.7–13.9). The general spinal curvatures are assessed, i.e. the cervical and lumbar lordosis and the thoracic kyphosis. The level of the shoulders, inferior angles of the scapulae, buttock and popliteal creases, the position of the umbilicus and the posture of the feet can all be assessed for relevance to the patient's present condition. Any structural or acquired scoliosis is noted. In disc pathology, the patient may have shifted laterally to accommodate the protrusion and this is evident in standing. Small deviations can be noted by assessing the distance between the waist and the elbow in the standing position. In hyperacute back pain, the patient may be fixed in a flexed posture and unable to stand upright, and any attempt to do so produces twinges of pain.

The level of the iliac crests and the posterior and anterior superior iliac spines gives an overall impression of leg length discrepancy or pelvic distortion. If these are considered relevant, they can be investigated further. Postural asymmetry and malalignment are not necessarily indicative of symptoms. It is worth noting them, since imbalances can be explained to the patient and addressed in the final rehabilitation programme, in an attempt to prevent recurrence. If structural abnormalities are considered responsible for the present condition, a full biomechanical assessment will need to be conducted.

Colour changes and *swelling* would not be expected in the lumbar spine unless there has been a history of direct trauma. Any marks on the skin, lipomata, 'faun's beards' (tufts of hair), birthmarks or café-au-lait spots may indicate underlying spinal bony or neurological defects (Hoppenfeld, 1976; Hartley, 1995). An isolated 'orange-peel' appearance of the skin that is tough and dimpled

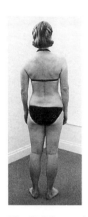

Fig. 13.7 Inspection for posture.

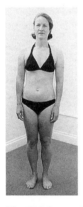

Fig. 13.8 Inspection for bony deformity.

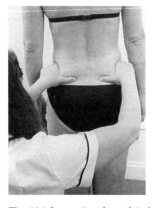

Fig. 13.9 Inspection for pelvic levels.

may indicate spondylolisthesis at that level (Hartley, 1995). Patients with low back pain often apply a hot water bottle to the skin which produces an erythematous reaction called erythema ab igne (redness from the fire). Swelling is not usually a feature but muscle spasm may give the appearance of swelling, especially to the patient.

Muscle wasting may not be obvious if the attack of low back pain is recent. Chronic or recurrent episodes of pain may show wasting in the calf muscles or possibly the quadriceps or gluteal muscles.

Palpation may be conducted to assess changes in skin temperature and sweating suggestive of autonomic involvement. Palpation for swelling is not usually necessary at the spinal joints. In standing, the lumbar spine is palpated for a 'shelf' that would indicate spondylolisthesis. In sitting, the level of the posterior superior iliac spines is assessed, according to the history, to differentiate between a lumbar and sacroiliac lesion. Piedallu's sign (see Chapter 14) assesses sacroiliac dysfunction when the sacrum and the ilium on the painful side move together rather than independently (Grieve, 1981).

State at rest

Before any movements are performed, the state at rest is established to provide a baseline for subsequent comparison.

The suggested sequence for the objective examination will now be given, followed by a commentary including the reasoning in performing the movements and the significance of the possible findings.

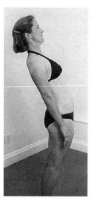

Fig. 13.10 Active extension.

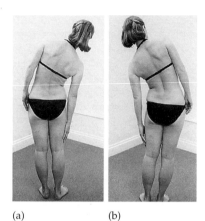

(a)   (b)

Fig. 13.11 (a, b) Active side flexions.

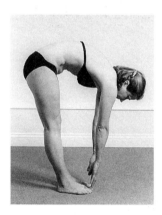

Fig. 13.12 Active flexion.

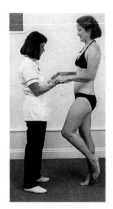

Fig. 13.13 Resisted plantarflexion in standing.

Examination by selective tension

Articular signs:

- Active lumbar extension (Fig. 13.10)
- Active lumbar right side flexion (Fig. 13.11a)
- Active lumbar left side flexion (Fig. 13.11b)
- Active lumbar flexion (Fig. 13.12)
- Tip toe standing, gastrocnemius (Fig. 13.13) **S1, 2**

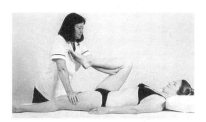

Fig. 13.14 Passive hip flexion.

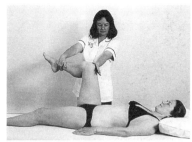

Fig. 13.15 Passive hip medial rotation.

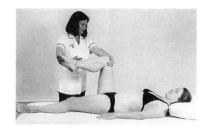

Fig. 13.16 Passive hip lateral rotation.

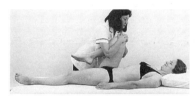

(a)

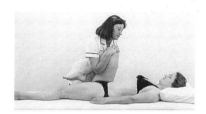

(b)

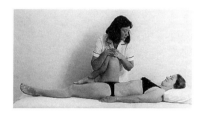

(c)

Fig. 13.17 (a–c) Shear tests to assess the sacroiliac joint.

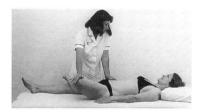

Fig. 13.18 FABER test to assess the sacroiliac joint.

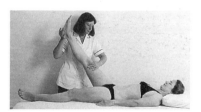

Fig. 13.19 Straight leg raise.

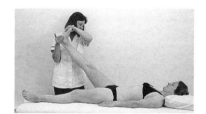

(a)

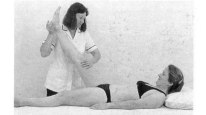

(b)

Fig. 13.20 (a, b) Straight leg raise with sensitizing components.

> *Supine lying*:
> - Passive hip flexion (Fig. 13.14)
> - Passive hip medial rotation (Fig. 13.15)
> - Passive hip lateral rotation (Fig. 13.16)
> - Sacroiliac joint shear tests (Fig 13.17a,b,c)
> - FABER test (Fig. 13.18)
> - Straight leg raise (Fig. 13.19 and 13.20a,b)   L*4, 5, S1, 2*, 3

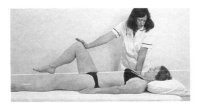

Fig. 13.21 Resisted hip flexion.

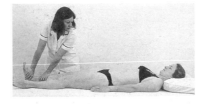

Fig. 13.22 Resisted ankle dorsiflexion.

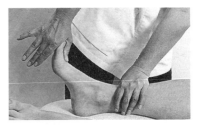

Fig. 13.23 Resisted extension of the big toe.

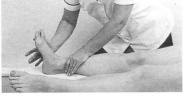

Fig. 13.24 Resisted ankle eversion.

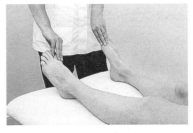

Fig. 13.25 Checking skin sensation.

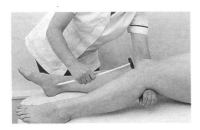

Fig. 13.26 Knee reflex.

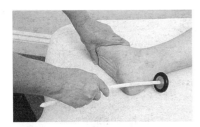

Fig. 13.27 Ankle reflex.

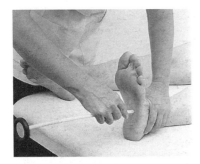

Fig. 13.28 Assessing for Babinski reflex.

Resisted tests for objective neurological signs and alternative causes of leg pain:

- Resisted hip flexion, psoas (Fig. 13.21)   **L*1, 2*, 3**
- Resisted ankle dorsiflexion, tibialis anterior (Fig. 13.22)   **L*4*, 5**
- Resisted big toe extension, extensor hallucis longus (Fig. 13.23)   **L*5, S1***
- Resisted eversion, peroneus longus and brevis (Fig. 13.24)   **L*5, S1*, 2**

Skin sensation (Fig. 13.25):

- Big toe only: L4
- First, second and third toes: L5
- Lateral two toes: S1
- Heel: S2

Relexes:

- Knee reflex (Fig. 13.26)   **L2, *3, 4***
- Ankle reflex (Fig. 13.27)   **S*1, 2***
- Babinski reflex (Fig. 13.28)

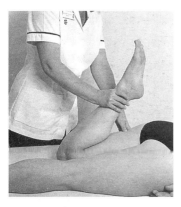

Fig. 13.29 Femoral stretch test.

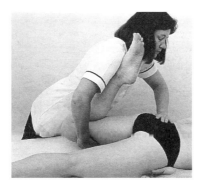

Fig. 13.30 Femoral stretch test with sensitizing component.

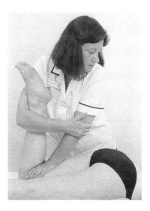

Fig. 13.31 Resisted knee extension.

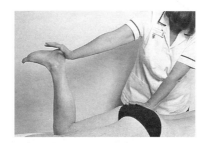

Fig. 13.32 Resisted knee flexion.

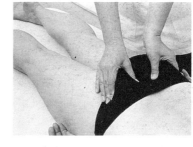

Fig. 13.33 Gluteal contraction, squeezing muscle bulk to assess wasting.

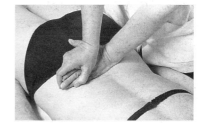

Fig. 13.34 Palpation.

Prone lying:

- Femoral stretch test (Fig. 13.29, 13.30) L2, *3*, 4
- Resisted knee extension, quadriceps (Fig. 13.31) L2, *3*, 4
- Resisted knee flexion, hamstrings (Fig. 13.32) *L5*, *S1*, *2*
- Static contraction of the glutei (Fig. 13.33) *L5*, *S1*, *2*

Palpation

- Spinous processes (Fig.13.34)

Capsular pattern of the lumbar spine:

- **Limitation of extension**
- **Equal limitation of side flexions**
- **Usually full flexion**

Active movements are tested in the lumbar spine since, in common with the other spinal regions and shoulders, it can be a focus for 'emotional' symptoms. The active movements indicate the 'willingness' to perform the movements as well as determining the presence of the capsular or non-capsular pattern. End-feel is not routinely assessed since the information gathered from the 'active' movements is generally sufficient. The presence of a painful arc on any movement should be noted and Cyriax (1982) considered this to be pathognomic of disc displacement. Look for apprehension, guarding or exaggerated movements. The presence of the capsular pattern indicates arthritis and it is typically found in degenerative osteoarthrosis of the more mature spine.

An important finding is the non-capsular pattern, usually presenting as an asymmetrical limitation of lumbar movements, indicating a mechanical lesion. The hypothesis is that this is due to a displacement of the intervertebral disc, either as a disc protrusion where the nuclear material has passed into the weakened annulus causing primary disc pain, or as a disc prolapse which has ruptured through an annular fissure into the vertebral canal to have a secondary effect on other pain sensitive structures.

Gastrocnemius is assessed for objective signs of nerve root compression. Testing the muscle group against gravity in standing is convenient at this point, in terms of sequence, before lying the patient down.

The resisted tests are not part of the routine examination at the lumbar spine, but should be applied if there is a history of trauma, e.g. for a muscle lesion or suspected serious pathology, e.g. fracture, metastases or pyschogenic pain (see Chapter 9).

In supine lying, other joints are eliminated from the examination to confirm that the site of the lesion is in the lumbar spine. Passive flexion, medial and lateral rotation are conducted at the hip, to assess the hip joint for the capsular pattern or other hip pathology. The sacroiliac joint is assessed by three shear tests and the FABER test (see Chapter 14). To limit these tests to the hip and sacroiliac joint it may be necessary to place the patient's forearm under the lumbar spine to increase the lordosis and to stabilize the spine. If the lesion in the lumbar spine is very irritable, it may not be possible to conduct these tests adequately.

The straight leg raise or Lasègue's test is applied passively to each leg in turn, keeping the knee straight (Karbowski and Radanov, 1995). If positive, this may be interpreted as a dural sign, or as an indicator of neural tension affecting the L4, 5, S1, 2, 3 nerve roots. It is an important clinical test for assessing nerve root tension due to a disc lesion (Supik and Broom, 1994; Jönsson and Strömqvist, 1995). Increased pain on the addition of neck flexion incriminates the dura mater. Further sensitising components such as passive ankle dorsiflexion, passive ankle plantarflexion and inversion, and passive hip medial rotation and adduction can also be added to explore the mobility of the nervous system further as appropriate.

The normal range of movement for the straight leg raise is between 60–120°, with movement being limited by tension in the hamstrings. The range of the straight leg raise should be consistent with the range of lumbar flexion, which is also limited to a certain degree by tension in the hamstrings. A disc protrusion does not always produce a positive sign on straight leg raise. If the nerve root exits high up in the intervertebral foramen, it may escape compression by a posterolateral disc protrusion.

The limited range of the straight leg raise is dependent upon the compression on the dura mater or dural nerve root sleeves and the greater the compression the greater the limitation. A painful arc may be found which is indicative of a small disc protrusion and is a 'useful' finding since, empirically, it usually implies that manipulation will be beneficial.

A bilateral limitation of straight leg raise is usually due to a central disc protrusion compressing the dura mater and is accompanied by an extrasegmental distribution of pain.

Bilateral sciatica from the same level producing bilateral limitation of straight leg raise and objective neurological signs is indicative of cauda equina compression. It is an absolute contraindication to manipulation and requires urgent specialist opinion.

A 'crossed' or 'well leg raise' describes the production of the pain in the back or leg on the painful side on straight leg raise of the painless limb. The intensity of the pain induced by the crossed straight leg raise is usually less than that produced on the painful side (Karbowski and Dvorak, 1995). Its explanation lies in the suggestion that if a posterolateral protrusion is sitting in the 'axilla' of the nerve root or directly anterior to the root, straight leg raise on the painless side will pull the root against the protrusion and give a positive sign. It usually occurs at the L4 level (Cyriax, 1982, Khuffash and Porter, 1989).

The patient is assessed for root signs and alternative causes of pain by the selective application of resisted tests. Objective signs of muscle weakness, altered skin sensation and absent or reduced reflexes will indicate compression of the nerve root.

The Babinski reflex, the extensor plantar response, is assessed by stroking up the lateral border of the sole of the foot and across the metatarsal heads. The response is extensor, i.e. upgoing, if extension of the big toe, sometimes with fanning of the other toes and withdrawal of the leg occurs (Bassetti, 1995). It is indicative of an upper motor neuron lesion, although this is not likely to occur with lumbar lesions since the spinal cord ends at approximately the level of the L1, 2 disc. The normal response is flexor.

The femoral stretch test (prone knee bending) is applied to assess the dura mater and the L2–4 dural nerve root sleeves. The knee is passively flexed and if positive, pain is usually produced at approximately 90°. A sensitising component of hip extension can be added. Pain is usually felt in the back and the test is limited by tension in the quadriceps. If positive unilaterally it implicates the nerve roots, if positive bilaterally the dura mater is at fault. It is theoretically possible to produce a crossed or well leg femoral stretch test but this is not as commonly found in practice.

The remaining resisted tests for the quadriceps and hamstrings are conducted in prone lying. A static contraction of the gluteal muscles is performed to assess for muscle bulk and palpation is conducted, using the ulnar border of the hand on the spinous processes, for pain, range of movement and end-feel.

Any other tests can be superimposed on this basic routine examination of the lumbar spine, including repeated, combined and accessory movements and neural tension testing as appropriate.

If serious pathology is suspected, further tests and specialist investigations will need to be implemented. Standard X-ray investigation provides little useful information for mechanical lesions over and above that gleaned from the clinical examination. However, if the patient fails to respond in the expected way further investigation may be indicated, including computed tomography or magnetic resonance imaging.

From the examination a working hypothesis is established and a treatment plan prepared.

Management of back pain

Orthopaedic medicine aims to apply techniques of manipulation, traction and injections effectively to lumbar disc lesions as appropriate. The choice of treatment will depend on the nature of the pain or the irritability of the lesion, the reference of pain and the mode of onset.

The Clinical Standards Advisory Group Report (1994) issued management guidelines for back pain. The report emphasized the importance of early management of back pain, i.e. within the first 6 weeks from onset, since the establishment of chronic back pain makes any form of treatment difficult and less successful. The natural history of acute back pain is recovery, with a 90% chance of return to work within 6 weeks. However, 60% of these people will experience at least one recurrence of their pain within 1 year.

Primary management of acute back pain is the responsibility of the general practitioner, occupational health service, physiotherapist, osteopath or chiropractor and has two main aims:

- Symptomatic pain relief.
- Prevention of disability.

If back pain has not settled within 6 weeks it is at risk of becoming chronic and the longer patients are off work, the lower their chances of ever returning. Patients off work for 6 months have only a 50% chance of returning to their previous job. Once they have been off work for 2 years, or have lost their job because of back pain, they will have great difficulty in returning to any kind of work and any further treatment is unlikely to avoid chronic disability.

Following initial assessment the report encourages selection from a diagnostic triage that forms the basis for decisions about referral, investigation and further management. This diagnostic triage consists of:

- Simple backache in which a 90% recovery is expected within 6 weeks.
- Nerve root pain with objective neurological signs in which a 50% recovery is expected within 6 weeks.

- Possible serious pathology, e.g. cauda equina syndrome, which requires urgent referral for specialist opinion within hours, or infection, neoplasm and inflammatory arthritis which require relatively urgent referral depending on the condition.

Suggestions for management are provided in the report as follows.

Early management of simple backache

- Simple analgesia – non-steroidal anti-inflammatory drugs (NSAIDs).
- If symptoms last more than a few days, arrange therapy, including manipulation, active exercise and physical activity to modify pain mechanisms and speed recovery.
- Advise bed rest if absolutely necessary, but no more than 1–3 days maximum.
- Promote positive attitudes to work and activity.
- Reduce distress, treat depression.
- Keep patient at work or advise early return to work.

Early management of nerve root pain

- Follow the same principles as for simple backache, but recovery will be slower.
- Adequate analgesia is particularly important – paracetamol up to 3 g/day in divided doses. If inadequate, paracetamol used in combination tablets with codeine (co-codamol), dihydrocodeine (co-dydramol) or dextropropoxyphene (co-proxamol).
- NSAIDs may be used instead – the simplest and safest is ibuprofen.
- If muscle spasm is a feature, NSAIDs may be combined with a muscle relaxant, e.g. methocarbamol or baclofen.
- A higher proportion of patients will require bed rest, but there is no evidence to support bed rest for more than 2 weeks for severe root pain.

It is clear from the report that chronic back pain and disability should be prevented by early management, therefore referral to hospital departments with long waiting lists is not appropriate. A change in attitudes to back pain is needed and a redeployment of resources for physical treatment (Ellis, 1995). Teamwork in the primary care setting would seem to be the key, with general practitioner and therapist working together to relieve pain, promoting early activity and the return to work.

The psychological and social factors of chronic pain may require a more detailed biopsychosocial assessment, and physical treatments at this stage may not be sufficient. Additional therapeutic options for symptomatic relief include low-dose antidepressants, epidural and sclerosant injections as well as other physical modalities. Counselling and coping strategies may need to be implemented.

Treatments to be avoided are long-term bed rest, bed rest with traction, manipulation under anaesthetic and plaster jacket. Secondary referral may be necessary, aiming for a second opinion, rehabilitation, vocational assessment and guidance, surgery or pain management. For more detailed information the reader is referred to the report itself.

Treatment in orthopaedic medicine is traditionally aimed at the disc, to reduce displacement, relieve pain and restore movement. The treatment techniques described are by no means a cure-all for every case of back pain. However, uncomplicated lesions of recent onset may respond well to the manipulative techniques of orthopaedic medicine. The key, as in the cervical spine, is the selection of appropriate patients for treatment.

Whilst not ideal, the presentation of signs and symptoms of lumbar disc lesions has been categorized into clinical models adapted from Cyriax's original theories in the light of current research. These give guidelines for treatment choice and a rationale for treatment programmes but are not intended to be restrictive. The reader is encouraged to be inventive, to draw on other experiences and to implement the approach into their existing knowledge when putting a treatment programme together for individual patients.

Lumbar disc lesions – the five clinical models

1.   *Lumbar disc displacement of gradual onset*

History:

- short central or unilateral pain (not referred below the knee)
- gradual onset
- patient *cannot* recall the exact mode and time of onset
- may be precipitated by a period of prolonged flexion.

Examination:

- non-capsular pattern
- *may* have increased pain on side flexion *towards* the painful side
- *no* neurological signs.

The hypothesis is that gradual displacement of nuclear material has occurred. Possibly a protrusion into the annulus causing primary disc pain, or prolapse into the vertebral canal producing secondary pain through compression of other pain sensitive structures. Pain may be extrasegmental and/or segmental in distribution. Adams and Hutton (1985) suggested that a gradual prolapse is a slowly progressing injury which occurs more readily in non-degenerate discs.

Traction is the treatment of choice for gradual onset disc displacement. However, manipulation can be applied, providing there are no contraindications, since, if successful, the response is quicker. Cyriax (1982) considered this gradual presentation to be typical of soft, nuclear disc material, and a positive indication for reduction by traction.

2.   *Lumbar disc displacement of sudden onset*

History:

- short central or unilateral pain (not referred below the knee)
- sudden onset
- patient *can* recall the exact mode and time of onset.

Examination:

- non-capsular pattern
- *may* have increased pain on side flexion *away* from the painful side
- *no* neurological signs.

The hypothesis is that disc material has suddenly protruded into the outer weakened annulus causing primary disc pain, or prolapsed through the weakened annulus into the vertebral canal producing secondary pain through compression of other pain sensitive structures. Pain may be extrasegmental and/or segmental in distribution.

Manipulation is the treatment of choice for sudden onset disc displacement. Cyriax (1982) considered this sudden presentation to be typical of hard or cartilaginous disc material, i.e. annular, and a positive indication for reduction by manipulation.

3.   *Lumbar disc displacement of mixed onset*

History:

- short central or unilateral pain (not referred below the knee)
- patient *may* recall the exact mode and time of onset, but the initial pain settles
- sometime later (hours or days) a gradual onset of pain occurs.

Examination:

- non-capsular pattern
- *no* neurological signs.

The hypothesis is that the initial precipitating factors weakened the annulus followed by a gradual displacement of nuclear material. As in the previous models, pain may be primary, if the disc material protrudes into the outer annulus, or secondary if it prolapses into the vertebral canal causing compression of other pain sensitive structures. Pain may be extrasegmental and/or segmental in distribution.

The treatment of choice is manipulation as it can achieve immediate results. If manipulation fails or is only partially successful, traction may be applied.

4.   *Lumbar disc displacement – large posterolateral prolapse*

History:

- central or unilateral back or buttock pain, followed by referred leg pain (the central pain ceasing or diminishing)
- sudden or gradual onset
- often part of a history or increasing, worsening episodes, therefore a progression of the above scenarios
- patient may or may not recall the exact time and mode of onset
- patient may complain of root symptoms, i.e. paraesthesia felt at the distal end of the dermatome.

Examination:

- non-capsular pattern
- root signs may be present, i.e. muscle weakness, absent or reduced reflexes.

The hypothesis is that a large posterolateral prolapse of disc material has occurred, producing pain referred into the leg through compression of the dural nerve root sleeve or the nerve root itself. Pain, therefore, is segmental in distribution. If the nerve root is involved, there will be objective neurological signs. Since the nerve roots emerge obliquely in the lumbar spine, more than one nerve root may be involved in a disc lesion. As discussed earlier in the chapter, the quality of the pain helps to distinguish somatic and radicular pain. Acute lumbar radiculopathy most commonly affects the L5 or S1 root, less commonly the L4 root and the others uncommonly (Caplan, 1994).

Treatment is aimed at relieving pain. Manipulation may be carefully applied provided the neurological signs are minimal and stable and that no contraindications exist. However, the more peripheral the symptoms, the less likely manipulation is to be successful. Manipulation should not be attempted if the neurological deficit is severe and progressing, other modalities, e.g. traction and mobilisation, may be more effective. A caudal epidural of corticosteroid and local anaesthetic may be indicated or alternatively a mechanism of spontaneous recovery may occur (see below).

5.   *Lumbar disc displacement – primary posterolateral prolapse (Cyriax, 1982)*

History:

- young adult
- unilateral leg pain, no central pain
- gradual onset
- patient may not recall the exact mode and time of onset
- symptoms are not severe.

Examination:

- non-capsular pattern, lumbar movements provoke the leg symptoms
- *no* neurological signs.

The hypothesis is that prolapsed disc material has moved posterolaterally to compress the dural nerve root sleeve whilst the central pain sensitive structures have escaped compression. Back pain is never a feature. It is an uncommon presentation and usually affects the younger adult patient.

Treatment of choice is traction, although the condition often recovers spontaneously.

Treatment of lumbar disc lesions

Manipulation provides good short-term symptomatic relief for patients with acute back pain of less than 4–6 weeks' duration and without nerve root pain. Manipulation may also be effective in recurrent attacks.

Manipulation is the treatment of choice for uncomplicated back pain of recent onset. Ideal patients are those that fall into the clinical model groups 2 and 3; those that fall into clinical model 1 may also benefit. Manipulation can be attempted for chronic back pain and for referred leg pain of somatic origin but is not indicated in patients with the severe lancinating pain of radicular origin or severe or progressive neurological deficit.

How manipulation works is not clear and many hypotheses are proposed, including mechanical, physiological and neurophysiological mechanisms (Twomey, 1992). If successful, manipulation dramatically reduces pain and produces an increased range of movement. The principles of manipulation are described in Chapter 4.

The success of manipulation depends on the selection of suitable patients and indiscriminate manipulation will produce unsatisfactory results. Orthopaedic medicine spinal manipulation techniques aim to reduce the signs and symptoms of a disc displacement. In terms of expectations of treatment outcomes, the ideal patient for manipulation has, in summary:

- Short central or unilateral back or buttock pain (the more distal the pain, the less likely manipulation is to succeed).
- Recent onset of pain, preferably within the last 6 weeks.
- History of sudden onset of pain; the patient recalls the exact time and mode of onset.
- Non-capsular pattern on examination.
- Pain increased by side flexion away from the painful side.
- No objective neurological signs.
- No contraindications to manipulation.

The absolute contraindications to lumbar manipulation are:

- Cauda equina syndrome: S4 symptoms of saddle anaesthesia, signs of bladder or bowel dysfunction – this patient requires urgent surgical referral (Lehmann *et al.*, 1991; O'Flynn *et al.*, 1992; Dinning and Schaeffer, 1993).
- Bilateral sciatica from the same level with bilateral limitation of straight leg raise and bilateral objective neurological signs indicating a large, central disc prolapse threatening the cauda equina (Dinning and Schaeffer, 1993).
- Severe or progressive neurological deficit.
- Hyperacute pain – the patient is too irritable to manipulate.
- Symptoms of neurogenic (spinal) claudication and associated spinal stenosis.
- Anticoagulant therapy, blood-clotting disorders, long-term oral steroid intake.

Caution is required in:

- Pregnancy.
- Neurosis.
- Children, adolescents and the elderly since disc displacement is uncommon in these age groups.

Guidelines to minimize risk from lumbar manipulation

Following the recommended guidelines below, ensures maximum safety and preparation for the unexpected. The practitioner must take all due care whilst applying the treatment techniques (see *Rules of Professional Conduct*, Rules 1, 2 and 4, and the *Standards of Physiotherapy Practice*, both available from the Chartered Society of Physiotherapy, 14 Bedford Row, London WC1R 4ED).

Ensure that:

- A full history and examination have been completed and recorded, sufficient to establish indications and to exclude contraindications to treatment.

- Specific questions have been asked relating to the following and the result recorded:

  bladder and bowel symptoms
  saddle anaesthesia
  anticoagulant therapy
  blood clotting disorders
  inflammatory arthritis
  past history of trauma.

From the examination, the following factors are present:

  a non-capsular pattern of limited movement at the lumbar spine
  a normal plantar response
  no increase in lower limb reflexes.

- There are no contraindications to manipulation, but it may be attempted if minimal neurological signs exist. The more peripheral the symptoms the less likely manipulation is to work. If neurological deficit is severe and progressing, manipulation should not be attempted, but other modalities may be more effective, e.g. traction and mobilization.

- You have provided sufficient information, including possible risks and advice, if manipulation is indicated, so that the patient can give informed consent. You must respect the right of the patient to refuse manipulation.

- You re-examine the patient after the application of each technique and decisions to continue should be based on the results of the previous technique.

- Any significant adverse response to treatment will be reported immediately to the patient's doctor.

Manipulation produces immediate results, therefore treatment should be progressed on a constant reassessment process. If a technique helps, it is repeated; if it is unsuccessful, another technique or alternative modality may be chosen according to professional judgement. The principles of manipulation, described in Chapter 4, apply to lumbar manipulation.

The lumbar manipulation procedure

It is recommended that a course in orthopaedic medicine is attended before the treatment techniques described later in the chapter are applied in clinical practice (see Appendix).

Two types of manipulative techniques are used, the first incorporating a short or long lever arm according to the effect required:

- Rotational manoeuvres for unilateral pain.
- Central manoeuvres for central pain.

The techniques described below are conducted with the couch at a suitable height for the operator. Generally this should be as low as possible. The techniques may be easier to perform if the patient is asked to take in a small breath, with the technique being applied after he or she has breathed out. This encourages patient relaxation and will allow for the effective application of the overpressure with minimal tissue resistance.

Rotation manoeuvres

The following manoeuvres are described in a suggested order of progression for the novice manipulator but once experience is gained in the application of the techniques, any may be chosen as a starting point. The comparable signs are assessed after every manoeuvre and the next manoeuvre is chosen based on the outcome. As long as a technique is gaining an increase in range and/or a decrease in pain, it can be repeated. Improvement may reach a plateau or the feedback from the patient may become unclear. Only professional judgement will reliably dictate when treatment should be stopped in each treatment session. It is better to err towards the side of caution in the early stages of acquiring manipulative skill.

Distraction technique

Position the patient in side lying with the painful side uppermost. Flex the upper hip and knee to 90° to assist the rotational stress and extend the lower leg. Pull the shoulder firmly through such that the shoulder is positioned backwards and the pelvis positioned forwards. Stand behind the patient at waist level and place one hand over the greater trochanter pointing down the long axis of the femur. Put your other hand comfortably on the patient's uppermost shoulder with your fingers pointing away from your other hand. Apply rotation with the hand on the greater trochanter until the pelvis lies just forwards of the midline and the patient's waist is upwards. Apply pressure equally through both hands to impart a distraction force; you will see the patient's waist crease stretch out as you lean through your arms (Fig. 13.35). Apply a minimal-amplitude, high-velocity thrust once all of the slack has been taken up.

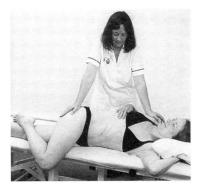

Fig. 13.35 Distraction technique.

Short-lever rotation technique – pelvis forwards

Position the patient in supine lying with the hips and knees flexed (crook lying). Ask the patient to lift and rotate the hips so that he or she is lying with the painful side uppermost and the shoulders relatively flat. Position the legs as for the distraction technique. Stand in front of the patient with one hand fixing the patient's shoulder whilst the other is placed with the heel of the hand on the blade of the ilium, with the forearm horizontal and your fingers pointing back towards you. Apply pressure through the hand on the ilium in a horizontal direction towards you to achieve a rotational strain (Fig. 13.36). Apply a minimal-amplitude, high-velocity thrust once all the slack has been taken up. If you find it difficult to apply the thrust with your hand against the ilium, place the forearm against the bone to give you better leverage.

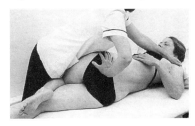

Fig. 13.36 Short-lever rotation technique – pelvis forwards.

Short-lever rotation technique – pelvis backwards (Cyriax and Cyriax, 1983; Cyriax, 1984)

Position the patient in side lying with the painful side uppermost. Take the lower arm behind the patient and place the upper arm into elevation, resting in front of the patient's face. Extend the upper leg and flex the hip and knee of the lower leg to 90°. The shoulder will now be positioned forwards and the pelvis backwards. Stand behind the patient at waist level; place one hand on the scapula to give a little distraction to take up the slack. Place the other hand on the front of the pelvis with your forearm horizontal and pointing back towards you (Fig. 13.37). Apply a minimal-amplitude, high-velocity thrust once all of the slack is taken up.

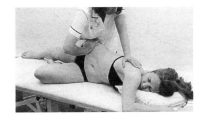

Fig. 13.37 Short-lever rotation technique – pelvis backwards.

Long-lever rotation technique (Cyriax and Cyriax, 1983; Cyriax, 1984)

This is a stronger rotational manoeuvre and care is recommended in its application to older patients to avoid placing undue strain on the neck of the femur.

Position the patient as for the short-lever rotation – pelvis forwards technique. Stand in front of the patient at waist level, facing the patient's feet to allow the arms to be placed more vertically. Fix the shoulder with one hand and place the other hand behind the knee, with your thumb in the knee crease. Lean on the knee to produce

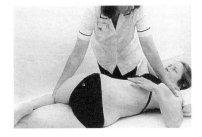

Fig. 13.38 Long-lever rotation technique.

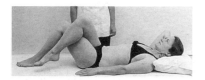

Fig. 13.39 'Pretzel' technique: starting position with knees flexed and good leg placed over the bad.

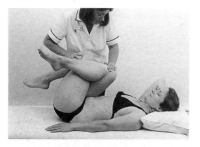

Fig. 13.40 Both hips flexed.

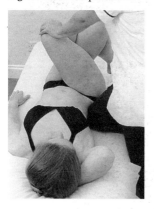

Fig. 13.41 Spine side-flexed around pivot of caudal knee placed in patient's waist.

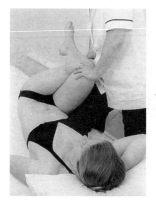

Fig. 13.42 Pelvis rotated forwards to rest patient's knees against thigh.

a rotation strain (Fig. 13.38). Apply a minimal-amplitude, high-velocity thrust once all of the slack is taken up.

> ## 'Pretzel' technique

This is a strong, long-lever rotation technique when used as a manipulation. It can be broken down into its individual stages and used as a mobilizing technique for hyperacute pain in which the lesion is too irritable for manipulation (see below). It helps in both instances to be clear on the different stages of the technique. It may be useful for correcting a lateral shift (Cyriax and Cyriax, 1983).

- Stand on the patient's painless side with the patient in supine lying. Flex the knees and cross the good leg over the bad (Fig. 13.39).
- Flex both hips (Fig. 13.40).
- Place your knee which is furthest from the patient's head at the patient's waist to act as a pivot point. Place your hands on the patient's knees and side-flex the lumbar spine to gap the affected side (Fig. 13.41).
- Rotate the pelvis towards you until the patient's knees are resting on your thigh (Fig. 13.42).
- Gently lower your thigh, taking the pelvis further into rotation ensuring that the other hand fixes the patient's shoulder flat on the couch (Figs 13.43 and 13.44). Apply a minimal-amplitude, high-velocity thrust once all of the slack is taken up. Help the patient back to the starting position.

If the patient is large, an assistant may be required to fix the patient's shoulder.

For hyperacute pain, each step is conducted individually using Grade A mobilization, constantly monitoring for improvement before progressing to the next step. Progress through the steps is made cautiously and steadily and may take 5 or 10 min to achieve in the very irritable state. The end of range will not necessarily be reached before proceeding to the next step. The technique should not aggravate the pain and the patient should be firmly and comfortably supported throughout. This is not a manipulation as such and any other mobilizing modality may be applied at each stage.

Extension manoeuvres

Extension manoeuvres are used for central pain or pain that is referred unilaterally into the back. They may be used as first-line treatment if a patient presents with central pain, or as a progression of the rotational manoeuvres as the pain centralizes.

Straight extension thrust technique (Cyriax and Cyriax, 1983; Cyriax, 1984)

This technique is indicated if a small central pain exists. Position the patient in prone lying and palpate the spinous processes to locate the painful level. Place the ulnar border of your hand over the tender spinous process and reinforce it with the other hand by placing the thumb web over your fingers. Apply pressure directly down on to the spinous process through straight arms (Fig. 13.45). Apply a minimal-amplitude, high-velocity thrust once all the slack is taken up by lifting and dropping your head down between your shoulders. Be careful not to lose the end of range by lifting your hands as you raise your head.

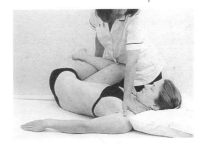

Fig. 13.43 Lowering the patient's knees by removing the thigh, to take the pelvis into rotation, stabilizing the shoulder on the couch.

Unilateral extension thrust technique (Cyriax and Cyriax, 1983; Cyriax, 1984)

If the pain centralizes to a short unilateral pain, or the patient presents with a short unilateral pain, this technique may be applied. Position the patient in prone lying, stand on the painful side and palpate the spinous process to locate the painful level. Place the ulnar border of the hand over the transverse process at the tender level on the side furthest away from you. The pisiform should be adjacent to the spinous process and the pressure is applied through the paravertebral muscles for patient comfort. Stand close to the bed with your knees hooked on to the edge to enable you to lean over the patient. Apply pressure down on to the transverse process through arms as straight as possible, directing the pressure back towards your own knees (Fig. 13.46). Apply a minimal-amplitude, high-velocity thrust once all of the slack is taken up by lifting and dropping your head between your shoulders.

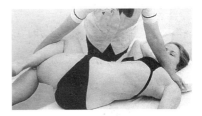

Fig. 13.44 Taking up the slack before applying the Grade C thrust.

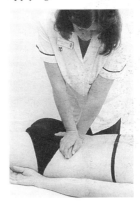

Fig. 13.45 Straight extension thrust technique.

Extension technique with leverage (Cyriax and Cyriax, 1983; Cyriax, 1984)

If the above fails to clear unilateral pain, this technique is a little stronger. Position the patient in prone lying and stand on the painless side. Position one hand flat, just above the painful level. Wrap the other hand over and under the bad leg just above the knee. Stand close to the couch, lift the bad leg into full extension and step back to apply side flexion, gapping the painful side (Fig. 13.47). Apply a minimal-amplitude, high-velocity thrust, continuing the direction of movement, once all of the slack is taken up.

Lumbar traction

The major indication for lumbar traction is the presence of disc displacement of gradual onset or clinical model 1 (see above).

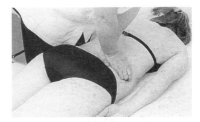

Fig. 13.46 Unilateral extension thrust technique.

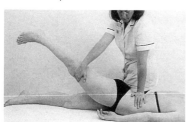

Fig. 13.47 Extension technique with leverage.

Suspicion of this pathology will be aroused following thorough assessment of the patient with consideration of the history and the presenting signs and symptoms. Traction may be applied to any of the other clinical models if other treatments have been unsuccessful or only partially successful, provided that there are no contra-indications.

Contraindications to lumbar traction

- Patients with acute lumbago or sciatica usually associated with twinges and antalgic postures: the application of traction may be quite comfortable but as the traction is released the patient will be far worse and the pain and twinges will be agonizing. It may take some hours for the pain to subside sufficiently to allow the patient to get up and the whole experience is awful for both patient and therapist alike. With patients with less irritable back pain, symptoms are often eased as traction is applied, but be particularly cautious if the history, signs and symptoms reveal an acute situation and the pain is completely relieved by traction.
- Patients with severe cardiac or respiratory problems may not be able to tolerate either the straps or the supine lying position. A bad cough also contraindicates treatment since pain will be made much worse.
- Patients with claustrophobia or other psychological disorders may become panic-stricken whilst undergoing traction, although such patients do not usually give consent to its application in the first place.

Whilst not absolute contraindications, there are several instances where traction is ill-advised or unlikely to be successful:

- S4 symptoms only may theoretically respond to traction but it is always best to exercise caution in any situation that implies a large central protrusion, including bilateral sciatica from the same level (Cyriax, 1982). Worsening of the situation could lead to increased compression on the cauda equina and possible permanent damage to bladder function.
- The pain of disc protrusions with neurological deficit is unlikely to be relieved by traction since the protrusion is too large to be reduced. Manipulation is less likely still to be effective and the treatment of choice is epidural anaesthesia.
- Sciatica which has lasted for more than 6 months is unlikely to respond to traction. The patient may be advised to await spontaneous recovery, to try epidural anaesthesia or to seek a surgical opinion, according to the severity of the symptoms and the patient's choice.

Technique

Friction-free electrically operated traction beds have been designed which may be used in conjunction with electronically operated units, that supply options for either rhythmical or static traction. Neither is an absolute necessity for the application of static traction as suggested by Cyriax and Cyriax (1983). The debate of sustained versus intermittent traction is considered in Chapter 4. Far less sophisticated apparatus may be used which is just as effective, but adjustments may then be needed to calculate the distracting force applied, on the basis of overcoming the friction forces created between the patient and the couch (see below).

A thoracic and a pelvic harness are affixed to either end of a couch, and applied to the patient. Harnesses of modern design are usually comfortable and easy to readjust since they have Velcro fastenings. A simple device is required for taking up the slack and applying a continuous pull-down through the pelvic belt, so providing traction to the intervening lumbar spine.

The principle of application is that the pull should be as strong as is comfortable. In the early stages this was the only guideline provided and there was no way of knowing the exact poundage being applied. A spring balance was then introduced in series with the pelvic rope, which gave some indication of poundage. However, Judovitch and Nobel (1957) calculated the coefficient of friction to be 0.5 and since half the body weight is distributed below the level of L3 then a force of $\frac{1}{2} \times 0.5 = \frac{1}{4}$ of the patient's body weight is required to overcome the friction between the body and the couch before the distracting force is applied to the spine. This is an important factor in calculating the actual poundages being applied when using a standard couch. When using a friction-free couch, the poundages registering on the accompanying machine are relatively faithful to the actual poundages being applied.

Feedback from the patient is just as important as in the days before a means of measuring poundages was devised, however, 'as strong as is comfortable' should still be the rule. An approximate estimate of the appropriate poundage may be made by assessing the size and weight of the patient, in the light of experience with other patients.

Before the commencement of treatment, a thorough explanation should be given to the patient on the reasons for applying the technique and the likely outcome, including any possible adverse effects such as stiffness or increased proximal pain. Consent should then be gained.

Before applying traction a selected comparable sign should be tested, such as the straight leg raise or particular lumbar movements in standing.

The patient does not need to be completely undressed for traction. Light clothing may be worn, being careful to remove belts, buckles, car keys, etc., and ensuring that clothing can separate in the middle. The patient is instructed to lie down sideways on the couch before rolling into supine lying.

The usual starting position is in supine lying but the number of pillows under head and knees may be adjusted for comfort. As the knees are lifted so the lumbar lordosis will flatten and a stool may be used to achieve Fowler's position (hips and knees flexed to 90°) if the patient is more comfortable with the spine completely flat.

The thoracic belt should be tight enough to grip the chest to prevent it from sliding up towards the axillae, which is very uncomfortable, and a little undignified for the well-endowed female. However, the grip should not be so tight as to restrict breathing, although patients will tend to find that they employ apical breathing more than diaphragmatic breathing whilst the traction is being applied.

The pelvic harness should sit comfortably above or around the iliac crests where it can pull down on the pelvis as the traction is applied but without slipping. The pelvic harness should not be so tight as to compress the abdomen uncomfortably and patients should be warned not to have a heavy meal before treatment.

If using a friction-free couch, ensure that the sliding lumbar section of the table is locked in its fixed position whilst the harnesses are being applied. The lumbar spine segment being treated should initially be placed over the division in the table.

The slack is taken up in the pelvic rope to apply tension to the system. This may be done by hand or through pulleys in the more rudimentary units, or by machine in an automatic unit.

Traction is then applied steadily, either manually by releasing ropes, turning wheels, pumping down on handles, etc., or automatically.

At the first treatment, 20 min of traction is usually sufficient and provides enough time to be effective, but not enough to overtreat, causing severe after-treatment stiffness or soreness. Feedback is encouraged from patients throughout treatment and it is essential to know if they become uncomfortable or if there is a marked increase in their pain. Simple adjustments can be made to lessen discomfort from the straps or to reduce the traction as necessary.

The patient should always be supplied with a means of summoning help such as a bell or buzzer. In subsequent treatments the time may be increased to 30 min. These timings are suggested on an empirical basis and little research has been done on this. Often the time allocated for treatment sessions in the appointment system is the limiting factor.

After treatment the traction should be released steadily and slowly, gaining feedback from the patient throughout, to be guided on the appropriate rate. The electrical units do not usually allow for this flexibility but do release steadily.

The traction belts are then released and patients are encouraged to wriggle for a minute or two. They are allowed to roll over but should not sit up until the residual stiffness following the application of traction has eased.

When ready, patients should be asked to turn onto their side, if they have not already done so, and to push themselves up sideways to avoid straining the back. Some patients need to sit for a moment or two whilst any dizziness or light-headedness arising from postural hypotension has subsided.

When dressing, patients should be advised to avoid bending, putting tights or socks on by bringing their foot up towards them and doing shoes up by bringing the foot up on to a chair rather than by bending to the floor.

Patients should be encouraged to continue with their everyday activities within the limits of pain, but prolonged sitting or lifting should be avoided whilst the treatment is continuing.

Ideally, the patient should be seen daily but it does not appear to be necessary to include weekends. Treatment should last for a period of at least 2 weeks, going into a third if improvement is continuing. Improvement should become apparent after three or four treatments and if no improvement is evident modification of the traction position may be made before abandoning the modality altogether.

Other positions such as prone lying may be tried if the patient is more comfortable in lumbar extension. Theoretically there are eight combinations of straps varying the patient's position between supine and prone, and choosing to place each of the thoracic and pelvic straps either underneath or on top of the patient. In practice, however, lying supine or prone, with the straps underneath the patient in both instances, are the two most popular and comfortable positions.

In terms of treatment frequency and duration, the ideal is rarely attained due to the various time and financial constraints of the patient in both the National Health Service and the private sector. However, in spite of this it is still worth applying traction as frequently as possible and it will not necessarily fail if the ideal conditions are not available.

The physical treatment techniques of manipulation and traction have a limited use in the treatment of back pain. As has already been emphasized, the selection of suitable patients for such techniques is essential. The treatment programme for all patients should include a positive approach to the management of back pain with an emphasis on balanced activity and rest. Patients should be involved in the management of their condition and a home treatment regime should be implemented, including postural and ergonomic advice where appropriate. The reader is recommended to the McKenzie approach for the management of lumbar disc lesions, which particularly complements the orthopaedic medicine approach, although the hypotheses on pathology and explanation of effect differ.

Lumbar injections

Caudal epidural injections

Sicard in 1901 introduced local anaesthetic into the epidural space and this technique has continued, with the addition of corticosteroid in the 1950s, to be efficacious in the management of discogenic sciatica (Dilke *et al.*, 1973; Bush and Hillier, 1991; Bush, 1994). It is a well-tolerated procedure with a high patient satisfaction rate and relatively low side-effects. Recent adverse publicity of arachnoiditis is associated with the intrathecal rather than the epidural route (Bowman *et al.*, 1993).

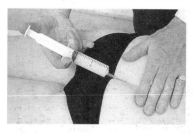

Fig. 13.48 Caudal epidural injection.

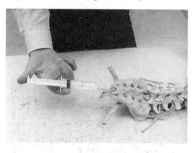

Fig. 13.49 Caudal epidural injection, showing direction of approach and needle position.

Indications for caudal epidural injection

- Hyperacute pain which fails to settle with adequate analgesia and up to 3 days' bed rest, and is too irritable for manipulation or traction.
- Radicular pain which has failed to respond to conservative management during the first 6 weeks from onset.
- Chronic back or leg pain, with or without neurological deficit, which has failed to respond to conservative measures.
- As a trial to treat pain before surgical intervention is considered.

Bush and Hillier (1991) indicated that active intervention by caudal epidural of triamcinolone plus procaine improves signs and symptoms at the 4-week follow-up, with improvement maintained at 1-year follow-up.

The mechanism by which caudal epidural produces this improvement in pain relief is still debated and several hypotheses exist (Bush and Hillier, 1991). Disc material can exert a mechanical effect through compression, a chemical effect through inflammation and an ischaemic effect through oedema. Introducing corticosteroid into the epidural space may directly affect the chemical and indirectly the ischaemic effects of pain. The introduction of fluid into a fluid-filled space can mechanically affect the relationship between the disc and the nerve root, whilst the introduction of local anaesthetic may have sufficient short-term effects to break the pain cycle.

Epidural injection via the caudal route can be carried out as an outpatient procedure. It is recommended that the procedure should only be conducted by an experienced medical practitioner, after appropriate training. The injection involves the introduction of 40–80 mg triamcinolone acetonide in 20–30 ml of 0.5% procaine hydrochloride via the sacral hiatus using a no-touch technique, with observation of blood or cerebrospinal fluid backflow (Figs 13.48 and 13.49) (Bush, 1994).

Sclerosant therapy

Sclerosant or prolotherapy is used to treat chronic spinal instability and chronic pain. It involves the injection of a chemical irritant into the ligaments surrounding an unstable spinal or sacroiliac segment. The chemical irritant produces an inflammatory response, causing fibroblast hyperplasia and subsequent increase in strength of the supporting ligaments (Ongley *et al.*, 1987).

The patient undergoes manipulation first of all to ensure that a full range of movement is achievable and to reduce the disc displacement. An injection is given of a solution called P2G comprising phenol, dextrose and glycerine. Each osseoligamentous junction is infiltrated using a peppering technique (Fig. 13.50a,b,c). Injections are given at weekly intervals with a maximum of three or four injections. The patient is instructed to avoid flexion to allow the ligamentous tissue to contract sufficiently to stabilize the joints.

Orthopaedic medicine courses include the principles of sclerosant injections for medical practitioners but a period of supervised clinical practice is recommended.

Mechanism of spontaneous recovery

Irrespective of treatment, the natural history of a disc prolapse is one of resolution (Bogduk, 1991) and the possible mechanisms for this will now be discussed.

Bush *et al.* (1992) demonstrated that a high proportion of patients with discogenic sciatica made a good recovery together with resolution of the disc herniation in a significant number. They concluded that, with good pain control, nature can be allowed to run its course. Ellenberg *et al.* (1993) prospectively studied 14 patients with definite radiculopathy and disc herniation on computed tomographic scan. They showed that the natural history of disc herniation with radiculopathy is improvement or complete recovery in 78% in 6–18 months, with non-surgical management.

Pople and Griffith (1994) suggested that a disc protrusion stretches the posterior longitudinal ligament, producing predominantly back pain, whilst a disc prolapse exiting through a tear in the posterior longitudinal ligament produces reduced tension. This explains why patients with an extruded fragment often experience a decrease or complete resolution of back pain as the root symptoms begin. According to Cyriax (1982), nerve root pain is expected to recover spontaneously provided the backache ceases when the pain shifts into the leg. This may take 8–12 months, but the older the patient, the longer or less likely the spontaneous recovery. Cyriax (1982) considered recovery to occur through mechanisms of shrinkage of the prolapsed disc material or through its accommodation by vertebral erosion. Nerve root atrophy may occur with the patient losing pain through ischaemia of the nerve root, but the neurological signs tending to take longer to recover.

With advanced technology involving magnetic resonance imaging scans, the position of the prolapse can be seen and monitored. It may be seen to disappear completely, reduce, or remain evident and is not necessarily indicative of symptomatology. In some cases the improvement in clinical findings is seen before recessive changes are observed on magnetic resonance imaging (Teplick and Haskin, 1985; Delauche-Cavallier *et al.*, 1992; Komori *et al.*, 1996), or the prolapse can persist with no symptoms at all (Bush *et al.*, 1992). A prolapsed fragment of nuclear material may be reduced through a process of disc absorption that involves neovascularization and macrophage phagocytosis (Saal *et al.*, 1990; Doita *et al.*, 1996; Ito *et al.*, 1996).

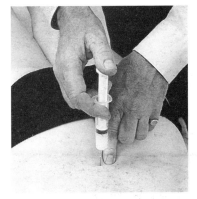

(a)

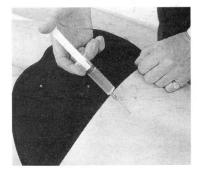

(b)

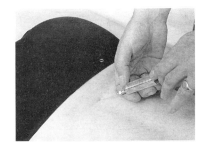

(c)

Fig. 13.50 Sclerosant injection, indicating needle placement to pepper the lumbosacral and sacroiliac ligaments.

References

Acaroglu, E.R., Iatridis, J.C., Setton, L.A. *et al.* (1995) Degeneration and aging affect the tensile behaviour of human lumbar annulus fibrosus. *Spine* **20**: 2690–2701.

Adams, M.A., Hutton, W.C. (1983) The effect of posture on the fluid content of lumbar intervertebral discs. *Spine* **8**: 665–671.

Adams, M.A., Hutton, W.C. (1985) Gradual disc prolapse. *Spine* **10**: 524–531.

Adams, M.A., Hutton, W.C. (1986) The effect of posture on diffusion into lumbar intervertebral discs. *Journal of Anatomy* **147**: 121–134.

Allam, K., Sze, G. (1994) MR of primary extraosseous Ewing sarcoma. *American Journal of Neuroradiology* **15**: 305–307.

Australian Physiotherapy Association (1988) Protocol for pre-manipulative testing of the cervical spine. *Australian Journal of Physiotherapy* **34**: 97–100.

Bassetti, C. (1995) Historical perspective: Babinski and Babinski's sign. *Spine* **20**: 2591–2594.

Beaman, D.N., Graziano, G.P., Glover, R.A. *et al.* (1993) Substance P innervation of lumbar spine facet joints. *Spine* **18**: 1044–1049.

Bernick, S., Walker, J.M., Paule, W.J. (1991) Age changes to the annulus fibrosus in human intervertebral discs. *Spine* **16**: 520–524.

Bogduk, N. (1991) The lumbar disc and low back pain. *Neurosurgery Clinics of North America* **2**: 791–806.

Bogduk, N. (1994) Innervation, pain patterns and mechanisms of pain production. In: *Clinics in Physical Therapy, Physical Therapy of the Low Back*, 2nd edn (Twomey, L.T., ed.). Churchill Livingstone, pp. 93–109.

Bogduk, N., Twomey, L.T. (1991) *Clinical Anatomy of the Lumbar Spine*. Churchill Livingstone.

Bowman, S.J., Wedderburn, L., Whaley, A. *et al.* (1993) Outcome assessment after epidural corticosteroid injection for low back pain and sciatica. *Spine* **18**: 1345–1350.

Brinckmann, P. (1986) Injury of the annulus fibrosus and disc protrusions – an *in vitro* investigation on human lumbar discs. *Spine* **11**: 149–153.

Brock, M., Patt, S., Mayer, H. (1992) The form and structure of the extruded disc. *Spine* **17**: 1457–1461.

Buckwalter, J.A. (1995) Aging and degeneration of the human intervertebral disc. *Spine* **20**: 1307–1314.

Bush, K. (1994) Lower back pain and sciatica – how best to manage them. *British Journal of Hospital Medicine* **51**: 216–222.

Bush, K., Hillier, S. (1991) A controlled study of caudal epidural injections of triacinolone plus procaine for the management of intractable sciatica. *Spine* **16**: 572–575.

Bush, K., Cowan, N., Katz, D.E., Gishen, P. (1992) The natural history of sciatica associated with disc pathology. *Spine* **17**: 1205–1212.

Caplan, L.R. (1994) Management of patients with lumbar disc herniations with radiculopathy. *European Neurology* **34**: 114–119.

Cavanaugh, J.M. (1995) Neural mechanisms of lumbar pain. *Spine* **20**: 1804–1809.

Cavanaugh, J.M., Kallakuri, S., Ozaktay, A.C. (1995) Innervation of the rabbit lumbar intervertebral disc and posterior longitudinal ligament. *Spine* **20**: 2080–2085.

Clinical Standards Advisory Group Report (1994) *Back Pain*. HMSO.

Corrigan, B., Maitland, G.D. (1983) *Practical Orthopaedic Medicine*. Butterworths.

Cyriax, J. (1982) *Textbook of Orthopaedic Medicine*, vol. 1, 8th edn. Baillière Tindall.

Cyriax, J. (1984) *Textbook of Orthopaedic Medicine*, vol. 2, 11th edn. Baillière Tindall.

Cyriax, J., Cyriax, P. (1983) *Illustrated Manual of Orthopaedic Medicine*. Butterworths.

Delauche-Cavallier, M.-C., Budet, C., Laredo, J.-D. *et al.* (1992) Lumbar disc herniation. *Spine* **17**: 927–933.

Dilke, T.W.F., Burry, H.C., Grahame, R. (1973) Extradural corticosteroid injection in management of lumbar nerve root compression. *British Medical Journal* **2**: 635–637.

Dinning, T.A.R., Schaeffer, H.R. (1993) Discogenic compression of the cauda equina – a surgical emergency. *Australian and New Zealand Journal of Surgery* **63**: 927–934.

Doita, M., Kanatani, T., Harada, T., Mizuno, K. (1996) Immunohistologic study of the ruptured intervertebral disc of the lumbar spine. *Spine* **21**: 235–241.

Ellenberg, M.R., Ross, M.L., Honet, J.C. *et al.* (1993) Prospective evaluation of the course of disc herniations in patients with proven radiculopathy. *Archives of Physical Medicine and Rehabilitation* **74**: 3–8.

Ellis, R.M. (1995) Back pain – emphasise early activity and support it with services geared to active management. *British Medical Journal* **310**: 1220.

Findlay, G.F.G. (1992) Tumours of the lumbar spine. In: *The Lumbar Spine and Back Pain*, 4th edn (Jayson, M., ed.). Churchill Livingstone, pp. 355–369.

Galessiere, P.F., Downs, A.R., Greenberg, H.M. (1994) Chronic, contained rupture of aortic aneurysms associated with vertebral erosion. *Canadian Journal of Surgery* **37**: 23–28.

Garfin, S.R., Rydevik, B., Lind, B., Massie, J. (1995) Spinal nerve root compression. *Spine* **20**: 1810–1820.

Grieve, G. (1981) *Common Vertebral Joint Problems*. Churchill Livingstone.

Hartley, A. (1995) *Practical Joint Assessment: Lower Quadrant*, 2nd edn. Mosby, pp. 1–88.

Hirabayashi, S., Kumano, K., Tsuiki, T. *et al.* (1990) A dorsally displaced free fragment of lumbar disc herniation and its interesting histologic findings. *Spine* **15**: 1231–1233.

Holm, S. (1993) Pathophysiology of disc degeneration. *Acta Orthopaedica Scandinavica* **64**: (Suppl. 251) 13–15.

Hoppenfeld, S. (1976) *Physical Examination of the Spine and Extremities*. Appleton Century Crofts.

Iatrides, J.C., Weidenbaum, M., Setton, L.A., Mow, V.C. (1996) Is the nucleus pulposus a solid or a fluid? Mechanical behaviour of the nucleus pulposus of the human intervertebral disc. *Spine* **21**: 1174–1184.

Ito, T., Yamada, M., Ikuta, F. *et al.* (1996) Histologic evidence of absorption of sequestration-type herniated disc. *Spine* **21**: 230–234.

Jensen, G.M. (1980) Biomechanics of the lumbar intervertebral disc: a review. *Physical Therapy* **60**: 765–773.

Jönsson, B., Strömqvist, B. (1995) The straight leg raising test and the severity of symptoms in lumbar disc herniation. *Spine* **20**: 27–30.

Judovitch, B., Nobel, G.R. (1957) Traction therapy, a study of resistance forces. *American Journal of Surgery* **93**: 108–114.

Kang, J.D., Georgescu, H.I., McIntyre-Larkin, L. *et al.* (1996) Herniated lumbar intervertebral discs spontaneously produce matrix metalloproteinases, nitric oxide, interleukin-6, and prostaglandin E_2. *Spine* **21**: 271–277.

Karbowski, K., Dvorak, J. (1995) Historical perspective: description of variations of the sciatic stretch phenomenon. *Spine* **20**: 1525–1527.

Karbowski, K., Radanov, B.P. (1995) Historical perspective: the history of the discovery of the sciatica stretching phenomenon. *Spine* **20**: 1315–1317.

Kemp, H.B.S., Worland, J. (1974) Infections of the spine. *Physiotherapy* **60**: 2–6.

Khuffash, B., Porter, R.W. (1989) Cross leg pain and trunk list. *Spine* **14**: 602–603.

Komori, H., Shinomiya, K., Nakai, O. *et al.* (1996) The natural history of herniated nucleus pulposus with radiculopathy. *Spine* **21**: 225–229.

Kumar, P., Clark, M. (1994) *Clinical Medicine*, 3rd edn. Ballière Tindall.

Kuslich, S.D., Ulstrom, C.L., Michael, C.J. (1991) The tissue origin of low back pain and sciatica. *Orthopedic Clinics of North America* **22**: 181–187.

Lee, H.-M., Kim, N.-H., Kim, H.-J., Chung, I.-H. (1995) Morphometric study of the lumbar spinal canal in the Korean population. *Spine* **20**: 1679–1684.

Lehmann, O.J., Mendoza, N.D., Bradford, R. (1991) Beware the prolapsed disc. *British Journal of Hospital Medicine* **46**: 52.

McCarron, R.F., Wimpee, M.W., Hudkins, P.G., Laros, G.S. (1987) The inflammatory effect of the nucleus pulposus – a possible element in the pathogenesis of low back pain. *Spine* **12**: 760–764.

Marchand, F., Ahmed, A.M. (1990) Investigation of the laminate structure of the lumbar disc annulus fibrosus. *Spine* **15**: 402–410.

Mixter, W.J., Barr, J.S. (1934) Rupture of the intervertebral disc with involvement of the spinal canal. *New England Journal of Medicine* **211**: 210–215.

Mooney, V., Robertson, J. (1976) The facet syndrome. *Clinical Orthopaedics and Related Research* **115**: 149–156.

Moridaira, K., Handa, H., Murakami, H. *et al.* (1994) Primary Hodgkin's disease of the bone presenting with an extradural tumour. *Acta Haematologica* **92**: 148–149.

Nachemson, A. (1966) The load on lumbar discs in different positions of the body. *Clinical Orthopaedics* **45**: 107–122.

Nachemson, A., Elfstrom, G. (1970) Intravital dynamic pressure measurements in lumbar discs, a study of common movements, manoeuvres and exercises. *Scandinavian Journal of Rehabilitation Medicine* (Suppl. 1) 1–38.

Norris, C.M. (1993) *Sports Injuries Diagnosis and Management for Physiotherapists.* Butterworth-Heinemann.

O'Flynn, K.J., Murphy, R., Thomas, D.G. (1992) Neurogenic bladder dysfunction in lumbar intervertebral disc prolapse. *British Journal of Urology* **69**: 38–40.

Oliver, J., Middleditch, A. (1991) *Functional Anatomy of the Spine.* Butterworth-Heinemann.

Oliver, M.J., Twomey, L.T. (1995) Extension creep in the lumbar spine. *Clinical Biomechanics* **10**: 363–368.

Ongley, M.J., Klein, R.G., Dorman, T.A. *et al.* (1987) A new approach to the treatment of chronic low back pain. *Lancet* **July**: 143–146.

Osborne, G. (1974) Spinal stenosis. *Physiotherapy* **60**: 7–9.

Osti, O.L., Cullum, D.E. (1994) Occupational low back pain and intervertebral disc degeneration – epidemiology, imaging and pathology. *Clinical Journal of Pain* **10**: 331–334.

Palma, L., Mariottini, A., Muzii, V.F. *et al.* (1994) Neurinoma of the cauda equina misdiagnosed as prolapsed lumbar disc. *Journal of Neurosurgical Sciences* **38**: 181–185.

Palmgren, T., Gronblad, M., Virri, J. *et al.* (1996) Immunohistochemical demonstration of sensory and autonomic nerve terminals in herniated lumbar disc tissue. *Spine* **21**: 1301–1306.

Parke, W.W., Schiff, D.C.M. (1971) The applied anatomy of the intervertebral disc. *Orthopedic Clinics of North America* **2**: 309–324.

Pople, I.K., Griffith, H.B. (1994) Prediction of an extruded fragment in lumbar disc patients from clinical presentations. *Spine* **19**: 156–158.

Porter, R.W. (1992) Spinal stenosis of the central and root canal. In: *The Lumbar Spine and Back Pain*, 4th edn (Jayson, M., ed.). Churchill Livingstone, pp. 313–332.

Porter, R.W. (1995) Pathology of symptomatic lumbar disc protrusion. *Journal of the Royal College of Surgeons of Edinburgh* **40**: 200–202.

Porter, R.W., Oakshot, G. (1994) Spinal stenosis and health status. *Spine* **19**: 901–903.

Porter, R.W., Hibbert, C.S., Wicks, M. (1978) The spinal canal in symptomatic lumbar disc lesions. *Journal of Bone and Joint Surgery* **60-B**: 485–487.

Rauschning, W. (1993) Pathoanatomy of lumbar disc degeneration and stenosis. *Acta Orthopaedica Scandinavica* **64**: (Suppl. 251): 3–12.

Roberts, S., Eisenstein, S.M., Menage, J. *et al.* (1995) Mechanoreceptors in the intervertebral discs, morphology, distribution and neuropeptides. *Spine* **20**: 2645–2651.

Rydevik, B., Olmarker, K. (1992) Pathogenesis of nerve root damage. In: *The Lumbar Spine and Back Pain*, 4th edn (Jayson, M., ed.). Churchill Livingstone, pp. 89–90.

Saal, J.S. (1995) The role of inflammation in lumbar pain. *Spine* **20**: 1821–1827.

Saal, J.A., Saal, J.S., Herzog, J. (1990) The natural history of lumbar intervertebral disc extrusions treated non-operatively. *Spine* **15**: 683–686.

Schwarzer, A.C., April, C.N., Derby, R. *et al.* (1994a) The relative contributions of the disc and zygapophyseal joint in chronic low back pain. *Spine* **19**: 801–806.

Schwarzer, A.C., April, C.N., Derby, R. *et al.* (1994b) Clinical features of patients with pain stemming from the lumbar zygopophyseal joints – is the lumbar facet syndrome a clinical entity? *Spine* **19**: 1132–1137.

Supik, L.F., Broom, M.J. (1994) Sciatic tension signs and lumbar disc herniations. *Spine* **19**: 1066–1068.

Swezey, R. (1993) Pathophysiology and treatment of intervertebral disk disease. *Rheumatic Disease Clinics of North America* **19**: 741–757.

Takahashi, H., Suguro, T., Okazima, Y. *et al.* (1996) Inflammatory cytokines in the herniated disc of the lumbar spine. *Spine* **21**: 218–224.

Taylor, J., Twomey, L. (1994) The lumbar spine from infancy to old age. In: *Clinics in Physical Therapy, Physical Therapy of the Low Back*, 2nd edn (Twomey, L., Taylor, J., eds). Churchill Livingstone, pp. 1–56.

Teplick, J.G., Haskin, M.E. (1985) Spontaneous regression of herniated nucleus pulposus. *American Journal of Roentgenology* **145**: 371–375.

Twomey, L.T. (1992) A rationale for the treatment of back pain and joint pain by manual therapy. *Physical Therapy* **72**: 885–892.

Twomey, L., Taylor, J. (1982) Flexion creep deformation and hysteresis in the lumbar vertebral column. *Spine* **7**: 116–122.

Twomey, L.T., Taylor, J. (1994) The lumbar spine: structure, function, age changes and physiotherapy. *Australian Physiotherapy Journal, 40th Jubilee Issue*, **72**: 19–30.

Umehara, S., Tadano, S., Abumi, K. *et al.* (1996) Effects of degeneration on the elastic modulus distribution in the lumbar intervertebral discs. *Spine* **21**: 811–820.

Vernon-Roberts, B. (1992) Age-related and degenerative pathology of intervertebral discs and apophyseal joints. In: *The Lumbar Spine and Back Pain*, 4th edn (Jayson, M., ed.). Churchill Livingstone, pp. 17–41.

Vucetic, N., Määttänen, H., Svensson, O. (1995) Pain and pathology in lumbar disc hernia. *Clinical Orthopaedics and Related Research* **320**: 65–72.

Waddell, G. (1992) Understanding the patient with backache. In: *The Lumbar Spine and Back Pain*, 4th edn (Jayson, M., ed.). Churchill Livingstone, pp. 469–485.

Waddell, G., McCulloch, J.A., Kummel, E., Venner, R.M. (1980) Nonorganic physical signs in low back pain. *Spine* **5**: 117–125.

Yamamoto, I., Panjabi, M.M., Oxland, T.R., Crisco, J.J. (1990) The role of the iliolumbar ligament in the lumbosacral junction. *Spine* **15**: 1138–1141.

Yamashita, T., Minaki, Y., Ozaktay, A.C. *et al.* (1996) A morphological study of the fibrous capsule of the human lumbar facet joint. *Spine* **21**: 538–543.

Zimmermann, M. (1992) Basic neurophysiological mechanisms of pain and pain therapy. In: *The Lumbar Spine and Back Pain*, 4th edn (Jayson, M., ed.). Churchill Livingstone, pp. 43–59.

14 The sacroiliac joint

Summary

Sacroiliac problems tend to be long-standing and are difficult to diagnose, often mimicking pain of lumbar origin. This chapter begins with a presentation of the anatomy of the joint and links it with possible pathology and methods of differential diagnosis of its mechanical and non-mechanical lesions.

Contraindications to treatment are few and emphasis is placed on assessment strategies on which to base treatment selection and appropriate exercise programmes.

Anatomy

The bony pelvis consists of the two innominate bones, articulating anteriorly at the symphysis pubis, and the sacrum which is suspended posteriorly between the innominate bones by its ligaments. The function of the bony pelvis is to support and transmit body weight from the trunk to the lower limbs, to protect and provide support for the viscera, and to provide attachment for ligaments and leverage for muscles.

The *sacrum* is a large triangular mass of bone formed by the fusion of the five sacral vertebrae (Fig. 14.1). The *sacral base* lies

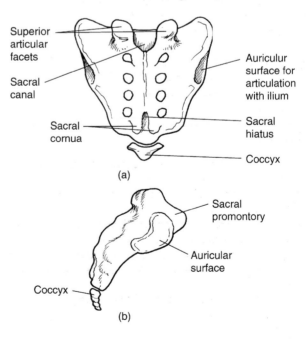

Fig. 14.1 (a, b) Sacrum, showing bony landmarks.

superiorly and is angulated upwards and forwards, articulating with the fifth lumbar vertebra to form the lumbosacral angle. Its anterior border is the *sacral promontory*. The apex of the sacrum lies inferiorly and articulates with the coccyx, a small triangular bone formed by the fusion of approximately four small vertebrae.

The pelvic surface of the sacrum is relatively smooth whilst its dorsal surface is roughened and displays three distinct crests. A *median crest* represents the fused spinous processes, an *intermediate crest* the fused articular processes and a *lateral crest* the fused transverse processes of the sacral vertebrae. The lateral crest provides attachment for the posterior sacroiliac ligaments.

The laminae and spinous processes of the fourth and fifth sacral vertebrae are absent, forming an opening known as the *sacral hiatus*. Anatomical anomalies are common here and elements of the other vertebrae may be missing, making this a variably sized opening (Trotter, 1947). The *sacral cornua* are the remnants of the articular processes of the fourth or fifth sacral vertebra projecting downwards on either side of the sacral hiatus. They provide palpable bony landmarks for the sacral hiatus which is clinically relevant in the placement of a caudal epidural injection.

The *sacral canal* is triangular in shape and formed by the fused sacral vertebral foramina. The dural sac usually terminates at the level of the lower border of the second sacral vertebra where it contracts into a filament and continues through the sacral canal to the coccyx, to become continuous with the periosteum (Trotter, 1947). Four pairs of sacral foramina provide exit for the sacral spinal nerves.

The lateral surface of the sacrum is expanded superiorly and provides an articulating surface for the sacroiliac joint. This surface bears an auricular (ear-like) surface anteriorly, which is shaped more like an L than an ear, and a pitted irregular surface posteriorly, for the attachment of the posterior and interosseous sacroiliac ligaments.

The *hip or innominate bone* is made up of the *ilium* above, the *pubis* in front and the *ischium* behind. The *acetabulum* is the cup-shaped hollow on its outer surface at the junction of the three component bones.

The ilium possesses several palpable bony landmarks. Those relevant here are:

- The iliac crest which gives an approximate indication of the level of the spinous process of L4.
- The anterior superior iliac spine (ASIS) which lies at the anterior end of the iliac crest.
- The anterior inferior iliac spine (AIIS) which lies below the superior spine and is not so readily palpable.
- The posterior superior iliac spine (PSIS), indicated by a dimple (dimple of Venus) approximately 4 cm lateral to the spinous process of S2.
- The posterior inferior iliac spine (PIIS) lying below the superior spine and difficult to palpate.

The *iliac fossa* lies medially, its posterior aspect thickened, roughened and marked by the iliac tubercle for the attachment of the posterior and interosseous sacroiliac ligaments. In front of the roughened area lies an auricular-shaped articular surface corresponding to the articular surface of the sacrum. Laterally the blade of the ilium provides attachment for the gluteal muscles.

The sacroiliac joint

The sacroiliac joint is essentially a synovial joint with its surfaces covered by articular cartilage, lined with synovial membrane and surrounded by a fibrous capsule, reinforced by ligaments. However, the presence of the sturdy *interosseous ligament* converts the sacroiliac joint into a part synovial joint and part syndesmosis.

The auricular-shaped articular facets on the ilium and the sacrum have reciprocal surfaces to provide the joint with great stability – a bump on one surface will articulate with a pit on the other. The joint surfaces are relatively plane in the young, but following puberty they develop irregularities, more so in the male sacroiliac joint, giving it inherent stability. The iliac auricular surface develops a central ridge lying between two shallow depressions, which fit into the central depression, bordered by two ridges, on the sacral surface. The way in which the joint surfaces interdigitate allows weight-bearing, but restricts movement, contributing to the stability of the joint. Major subluxation of the joint is not common, but the interdigitating articular surfaces make minor subluxation a possibility.

The suspension of the wedge-shaped sacrum between the two ilia provides it with a self-locking mechanism. Increasing weight applied to the sacral base will hold the sacrum more tightly *in situ* through tension in its ligaments (Fig. 14.2) (Kapandji, 1974). The fibrous capsule is reinforced by strong posterior ligaments and

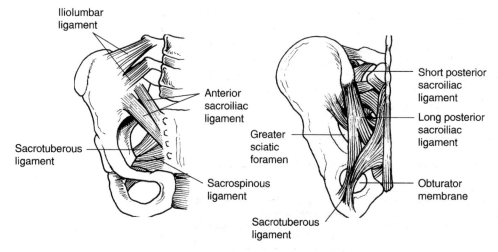

Fig. 14.2 The sacroiliac joint and ligaments. From Palastanga *et al.* (1994) with permission.

weaker anterior ligaments, whilst a set of accessory ligaments contributes a stabilizing effect on the joint. The *interosseous sacroiliac ligament* forms the main union between the sacrum and ilium.

The *posterior sacroiliac ligament* has long and short fibres covering the posterior aspect of the interosseous ligament. Short horizontal fibres are placed superiorly where they resist forwards movement of the sacral promontory. Longer vertical fibres are more superficial and resist a downwards movement of the sacrum relative to the ilium. The long posterior fibres are said to be tense under counternutation, an upwards, backward, nodding movement of the sacrum (Vleeming *et al.*, 1996) (see below).

Accessory ligaments exert a stabilizing effect on the joint: the *sacrotuberous ligament* attaches by a broad base from the posterior superior iliac spine, the side of the sacrum and the coccyx. Its fibres converge to pass downwards and laterally, twisting and broadening again at its attachment to the ischial tuberosity where it blends with the tendon of biceps femoris and the lower fibres of gluteus maximus.

The *sacrospinous ligament* is thinner and triangular, lying anterior to the sacrotuberous ligament. It passes from the lower part of the sacrum and coccyx to the spine of the ischium and its pelvic surface blends with the coccygeus muscle.

The sacrotuberous and sacrospinous ligaments lie below and lateral to the joint, preventing the tendency for the apex of the sacrum to tilt upwards as body weight is directed down on to the base of the sacrum. The *iliolumbar ligament* anchors the fifth lumbar vertebra to the ilium, stabilizing the lumbosacral junction against the tendency for the sacral promontory to move forwards under the influence of gravity and body weight.

Movement of the sacroiliac joint

Many strong muscles pass over the sacroiliac joint, but none directly affects it. There seems to be a general agreement that movement does occur at the sacroiliac joint, but how much and in which direction is still not certain. A little anteroposterior rotation combined with translation occurs (Williams *et al.*, 1989; Oliver and Middleditch, 1991). Kapandji (1974) referred to the movement as nutation and counternutation (Latin, *nutare* = to nod).

Nutation	Counternutation
Sacral base moves down and forwards	Sacral base moves up and back
Apex moves up	Apex moves down
Anteroposterior distance of the inlet decreases	Anteroposterior distance of the inlet increases
Anteroposterior distance of the outlet increases	Anteroposterior distance of the outlet decreases
Iliac bones approximate	Iliac bones move apart

In a study of healthy individuals between the ages of 20 and 50 years, the average total rotational movement in the sacroiliac joint between erect standing and standing on one leg was 2° (Jacob and Kissling, 1995). One subject, excluded from this analysis because of occasional symptoms, was found to have more than 6° of movement.

Functionally, movements at the sacroiliac joint occur in combination with the adjacent joints. Variations between the two joints and between individuals are common, making objective examination of these joints difficult. Generally, lumbar spinal flexion is accompanied by nutation and lumbar spinal extension is accompanied by counternutation.

Although the sacroiliac joints are relatively immobile and stable, they are susceptible to mechanical trauma. Joint sprain and minor subluxations occur and respond well to manipulation. As synovial joints they are subject to the various forms of arthritis and the degenerative changes associated with the ageing process. Reduced mobility seems to occur through a process of fibrous bands or fibrocartilaginous adhesion formation rather than bony ankylosis (Cassidy, 1992; Palastanga *et al.*, 1994).

Mechanical lesions are less common in the older age group as movements reduce. The ligaments of the female pelvis relax during and after pregnancy, increasing the range of movement and making the sacroiliac joint locking mechanism less effective. During this time the relative hypermobility of the sacroiliac joints makes them susceptible to strain and subluxation.

Nerve supply

The nerve supply is variable and differs between individuals and often between the two sacroiliac joints in the same person. The sacroiliac joint and its surrounding ligaments receive a supply derived from L3–S2 nerve roots (Lee, 1989; Oliver and Middleditch, 1991; Palastanga *et al.*, 1994). Some of the supply is directly from the sacral plexus and dorsal rami and some indirectly via the superior gluteal nerve and obturator nerve. This extensive segmental supply and variation means that pain patterns can be confusing and may mimic other conditions.

Differential diagnosis at the sacroiliac joint

Manipulative techniques are appropriate for mechanical lesions of the sacroiliac joint, i.e. minor subluxations and ligamentous strain. Assessment for displacement of the joint may be attempted through palpation tests but, in clinical practice, the small amount of movement at the sacroiliac joint makes this assessment difficult. Other means of applying compression, shear and distraction to the joints will be suggested, to incriminate the joint as a cause of pain. This section will discuss the differential diagnosis at the sacroiliac joint to distinguish mechanical lesions from other pathology.

Mechanical lesions of the sacroiliac joint

Diagnosis is made from the history, pain provocation tests and palpation for asymmetry. Diagnosis of sacroiliac joint sprain, with or without subluxation, usually responds well to manipulation. The indications, contraindications and treatment techniques will be described later in this chapter.

Other causes of sacroiliac pain and associated signs and symptoms

Arthritis can affect the sacroiliac joint since it is a mobile, weight-bearing part synovial joint and may develop the same problems as other synovial joints. Normally arthritis will manifest itself as the capsular pattern, but as movement at this joint occurs passively there is no recognizable capsular pattern. The joint undergoes degenerative changes, reducing the mobility of the joint still further, making mechanical lesions less likely in the older age group. Inflammatory arthritis, particularly ankylosing spondylitis, affects this joint.

Ankylosing spondylitis is a chronic seronegative inflammatory arthritis affecting the axial skeleton in particular (Kumar and Clark, 1994; Rai, 1995). It affects men more commonly than women, although it may exist subclinically in women. It has an insidious onset in men under the age of 40, who complain of back and buttock pain, persisting for several months. The symptoms are typical of an inflammatory condition, with the pain and early-morning stiffness eased by movement and exercise. Sacroiliac joints are often the first target for the disease and sacroiliitis may be seen on X-ray. The later stages involve the whole spine, when the X-ray appearance is of a 'bamboo' spine. The disease is related to the presence of factor human leukocyte antigen (HLA)-B27 and blood tests will usually confirm clinical diagnosis. On examination there is loss of the lumbar lordosis, increased thoracic kyphosis and decreased chest expansion. Sacroiliitis gives severe pain when the sacroiliac joints are stressed.

Reiter's syndrome is a form of seronegative reactive arthritis that can follow gastrointestinal or genital tract infections (Kumar and Clark, 1994; Keat, 1995). The arthritis affects the lower limb joints, more readily the knees and ankles, but can also affect the sacroiliac joints. Non-specific urethritis and conjunctivitis may accompany the condition.

Serious non-mechanical conditions can affect the sacroiliac joint and need to be excluded before manipulation is applied. Serious conditions of the pelvis may produce the 'sign of the buttock' (see Chapter 9) and the patient is unwell. Pain associated with the sacroiliac joint in the elderly should be viewed with suspicion until proven otherwise, since mechanical lesions are rare in the sacroiliac joints in this age group.

Infection, as in osteomyelitis in the pelvis or upper femur, produces severe pain felt in the pelvic region and the patient is unwell with a high fever and marked tenderness over the affected bone.

Septic arthritis, although uncommon in the sacroiliac joint, presents dramatically with pain, heat and swelling. The patient is unwell and febrile.

Fracture of the sacrum or pelvic bones is suspected if the patient presents with a history of trauma, severe pain and much bruising.

Malignant disease can involve the sacroiliac joint directly or indirectly (Silberstein *et al.*, 1992). Metastases may be a cause of pain in the pelvis of older patients.

Other musculoskeletal lesions can produce pain felt in the region of, or referred to, the sacroiliac joint. Differential diagnosis is difficult because the signs and symptoms overlap considerably.

Lumbar disc lesions produce pain felt in one or both buttocks. Distinguishing féatures of the history may help exclude it as a cause of pain, but lesions commonly coexist. Disc lesions are aggravated by posture and movement, eased by rest, and often better in the early morning. Dural involvement produces pain on coughing, sneezing and straining; radicular involvement produces objective neurological signs and sensory neurological symptoms.

Hip joint pathology refers pain to the L3 dermatome and may involve unilateral low back and upper buttock pain. Examination of the hip produces positive signs.

Gluteal bursitis may produce buttock pain and reveal a muddled set of signs on examination of the hip. Trigger points in the buttock area may be misleading.

Coccydynia is pain in the region of the coccyx which can arise following direct trauma such as a fall directly on to the bottom. The lumbar spine can also refer pain to the area of the coccyx.

Commentary on the examination

Observation

A general observation is made, including the patient's *face, posture and gait*. Serious conditions of the pelvis may produce severe pain, of which night pain is a feature and this may be evident in the face of the patient, who looks tired and drawn from lack of sleep. The posture and gait may show abnormalities and these need careful assessment to ascertain if they are relevant to the patient's presenting condition. Generally, a mechanical lesion of the sacroiliac joint rarely alters the gait pattern whilst sacroiliitis can be very painful, and the patient may not like to weight-bear on the affected side.

History (subjective examination)

A careful history is taken because the differential diagnosis of mechanical lesions, subluxation or strain of the sacroiliac joint is particularly reliant on features of the history.

The patient's *age* is relevant as mechanical lesions of all joints in this region tend to present as a condition of middle age. Caution is required in the elderly and the young who seemingly present with a mechanical sacroiliac joint lesion, as this is uncommon. Younger patients may show postural asymmetry which may need correction to avoid later problems.

Occupation, sports, hobbies and lifestyle may all have relevance to a sacroiliac mechanical lesion. Any occupation or sport that involves increased weight-bearing through one leg may place abnormal stresses on the sacroiliac joint, e.g. driving, ballet, hurdling.

Mechanical lesions of the sacroiliac joint affect both sexes, but it is more common in women. The irregularities in the articular surfaces are more predominant in the male sacroiliac joint, giving it a greater inherent stability. During pregnancy, the ligaments of the pelvis soften to allow more movement and the joints are more susceptible to injury and subluxation. If subluxation occurs during this time and is not reduced, the abnormality remains once the ligaments tighten in the postpartum phase and the patient may encounter long-term problems.

The nature of the nerve supply to the sacroiliac joint and its surrounding ligaments makes the *site and spread* of the pain difficult to relate to specific diagnosis. The site and spread could be equally indicative of lumbar spine or hip pathology or mimic other conditions. Commonly a localized buttock pain is present, often centred around the posterior superior iliac spine, that may also be tender to the touch. The spread of pain from the sacroiliac joint may be into the groin and front of the thigh, into the buttock and posterior thigh, and possibly into the calf. As the pelvis is a ring, abnormal mechanics can have a 'knock-on' effect on the other side and produce confusing signs in the so-called good leg.

Schwarzer *et al.* (1995) found no conventional predictive features of sacroiliac joint pain except for a strong association with groin pain. Fortin *et al.* (1994) looked at patterns of pain referral using provocative injections into the sacroiliac joint and established a variable response. All subjects felt pain locally, initially over the sacroiliac joint, with variable referral to the lateral aspect of the buttock, to the greater trochanter and into the upper lateral thigh. This variation in pain response is consistent with the variable and extensive nerve root supply to the sacroiliac joint.

The mode of *onset and duration* of the symptoms of sacroiliac mechanical lesions can be helpful. Sacroiliac subluxation may have a sudden onset, when it is usually associated with some form of trauma, e.g. a fall from a height, slipping down the stairs jarring the leg, or a motor vehicle accident, where the foot was placed heavily on the brake. A torsional strain is common and the mechanism of injury may involve straightening up from the stooped position (Leblanc, 1992).

A gradual strain of the sacroiliac joint may occur through repeated minor trauma which is often related to occupation, e.g. constant driving over rough ground or persistent pressure being exerted through one sacroiliac joint.

If female, the patient should be questioned about any significant events during pregnancy that may have provoked symptoms. Gynaecological surgery and obstetric delivery often require the use of the lithotomy position, when the woman is positioned lying on her back with her hips and knees flexed to 90° this tilts the pelvis posteriorly and may place undue stress on the sacroiliac joints.

The duration is also relevant. Patients have usually had their problem for a long time since it produces a dull ache, which may be tolerated more than the pain of acute onset, or severe sciatica, associated with lumbar pathology. The duration of symptoms also gives a prognostic indicator. Adaptive shortening occurs in chronic subluxation and the chance of correction using manipulative techniques after a long duration is slim. However, manipulation may help the pain even without correction of the deformity.

The *symptoms and behaviour* need to be considered. The behaviour of the pain indicates the nature of the condition and should distinguish it from a lumbar disc displacement or a hip joint problem. As an inflammatory ligamentous condition it behaves in a typical inflammatory way with early-morning stiffness and pain, relieved by movement and made worse with rest. Sleep can be disturbed as the pain wakes the patient when turning at night. The pain may also be worse when lying on the affected side. Twinges of pain are common, especially after a period of rest, when the patient takes time to get going again.

Patients may complain of other symptoms which are typical of mechanical sacroiliac pain and distinguish it from other lesions. They cannot sit still or stand for long periods and the joint likes to be moved and exercised. Sunbathing, for example, is extremely uncomfortable, since they do not like lying flat with legs outstretched and find it hard to lie prone whilst reading a book. They cannot balance very well on the affected leg.

The absence of certain symptoms is also relevant in distinguishing sacroiliac joint problems from pain of lumbar origin, particularly arising from nerve root compression. There should be no paraesthesia and no bladder or bowel symptoms. A cough and sneeze may provoke a little pain, but this should always be in the back and not in the leg.

Symptoms of serious pathology, such as night pain and sweats, fever, feeling generally unwell or unexplained recent weight loss, should be excluded.

Other joint involvement will alert the examiner to possible inflammatory arthritis. However, the initial presentation of ankylosing spondylitis in the sacroiliac joints is common, without other joint signs or symptoms.

Past medical history will give information concerning conditions that may be relevant to the patient's current complaint, always with the possible presence of serious illness in mind. An indication of the general health of the patient will indicate any systemic illness and it may be pertinent to take the patient's temperature. Recent pregnancy may be a less sinister element of medical history that could be relevant to sacroiliac joint problems.

A mechanical lesion of the sacroiliac joint is a common cause of pain in pregnancy, particularly in the later stages. The increase in weight, change in posture and release of the hormone relaxin all contribute to mechanical instability of the pelvis. Manipulation is indicated in these patients and the pregnancy is not a contraindication in itself (Golighty, 1982; Daly *et al.*, 1991).

The *medications* currently being taken by the patient should be listed. This may provide further indication of the patient's past medical history or alert the examiner to possible serious pathology and contraindications to treatment, e.g. tamoxifen, which is a chemotherapeutic drug to combat breast cancer. Anticoagulants and the use of long term steroids should also be considered.

Inspection

Position the patient in standing, undressed to underwear and in a good light. Assessment for **bony deformity** and overall posture is made with particular attention to:

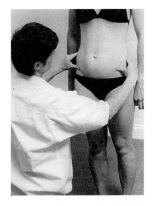

Fig. 14.3 Assessing level of iliac crests and anterior superior iliac spines.

- Level of iliac crests (Fig. 14.3).
- Level of ASIS (Fig. 14.3).
- Level of PSIS (Fig. 14.4).
- Leg length.
- General spinal curvatures.
- Increased or decreased lordosis.

The level of the posterior superior sacroiliac spines is particularly relevant to asymmetry in relation to sacroiliac subluxation. However, be aware that anomalies commonly exist and the presence or absence of obvious asymmetry without associated symptoms is not necessarily relevant to mechanical dysfunction of the sacroiliac joint.

Colour changes, muscle wasting and swelling are unusual unless there is a history of trauma. In sacroiliac strain or subluxation, an area of apparent swelling is sometimes present over the sacrum, usually associated with muscle spasm.

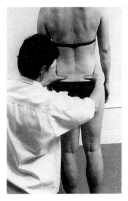

Fig. 14.4 Assessing level of posterior superior iliac spines.

State at rest

Before any movements are performed, the state at rest is established to provide a baseline for subsequent comparison.

The suggested sequence for the objective examination will now be given, followed by a commentary including the reasoning in performing the movements and the significance of the possible findings.

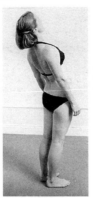

Fig. 14.5 Active lumbar extension.

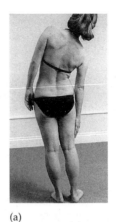
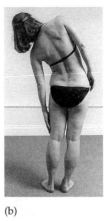

(a)   (b)

Fig. 14.6 Active lumbar side flexions.

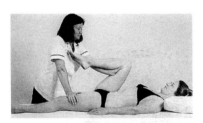

(a)

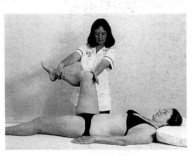

(b)

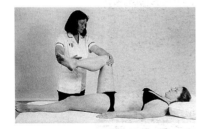

(c)

Fig. 14.8 Passive hip movements: (a) flexion; (b) medial; and (c) lateral rotation.

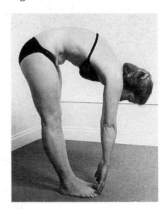

Fig. 14.7 Active lumbar flexion.

Examination by selective tension (objective examination)

Eliminate the lumbar spine:

- Active lumbar extension (Fig. 14.5)
- Active right lumbar side flexion (Fig. 14.6a)
- Active left lumbar side flexion (Fig. 14.6b
- Active lumbar flexion (Fig. 14.7)

Eliminate the hip:

- Passive hip flexion (Fig. 14.8a)
- Passive hip medial rotation (Fig. 14.8b)
- Passive hip lateral rotation (Fig. 14.8c)

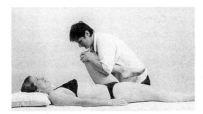

Fig. 14.9 Shear test with the femur pointing towards the ipsilateral shoulder.

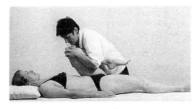

Fig. 14.10 Shear test with the femur pointing towards the contralateral shoulder.

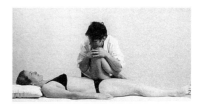

Fig. 14.11 Shear test with the femur pointing towards the contralateral hip.

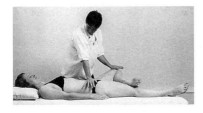

(a)

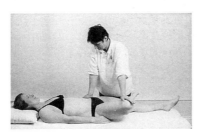

(b)

Fig. 14.12 (a, b) FABER or 4-test.

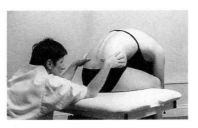

Fig. 14.13 Piedallu's sign.

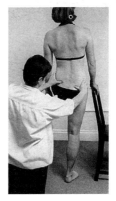

(a)

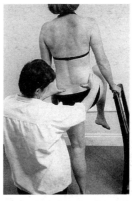

(b)

Fig. 14.14 (a, b) The 'walk' test.

Provocative shear tests for the posterior sacroiliac ligaments:

- Hip flexion towards the ipsilateral shoulder (Fig. 14.9)
- Hip flexion towards the contralateral shoulder (Fig. 14.10)
- Hip flexion towards the contralateral hip (Fig. 14.11)

Provocative test for the anterior sacroiliac ligaments:

- FABER test (Fig. 14.12a,b)

Palpation

- For tenderness

Palpation tests to determine treatment technique:

- Piedallu's sign (Fig. 14.13)
- The 'walk' test (Fig. 14.14)

Examination of the sacroiliac joint must include elimination of the lumbar spine and hip joint as possible alternative causes of pain. The active movements of the lumbar spine and passive hip movements are assessed for range of movement and provocation of pain. If the lesion lies in the sacroiliac joint, pain is usually felt at the end of range of theses movements, especially lumbar extension and passive hip lateral rotation. The gross limitation of lumbar range associated with disc lesions is not expected.

Shear tests are applied using the femur in hip flexion and adduction to assess principally the posterior ligaments. All three tests are performed on the painfree side first for subsequent comparison with the painful side. Place the patient in supine lying and flex the hip towards the ipsilateral shoulder. Grasp the patient's knee with linked hands and lean forwards to rest your forearms on either side of the thigh. Lean back a little to take the tension off the hip capsule and apply a thrust down through the line of the shaft of the femur to stress the posterior sacroiliac joint ligaments. Pain in the back on the affected side denotes a positive test.

Repeat the test twice, but using in turn hip flexion towards the contralateral shoulder and hip flexion towards the contralateral hip, as the starting positions. Take care to release some pressure from the hip joint before applying the downward thrust.

With knowledge of anatomy, one could deduce that the positions described selectively test the iliolumbar, sacrotuberous and sacrospinous ligaments respectively. However, for the purposes of the manipulative techniques, there is little clinical relevance in isolating the ligaments in this way. It is sufficient to establish whether or not the test is positive to incriminate the joint as a whole.

The *FABER test* assesses mainly the anterior ligaments and derives its name from the combination of movements applied, being *F*lexion, *AB*duction and *E*xternal *R*otation of the hip. It is also known as Patrick's test or the '4-test' because of the resultant position of the limb (4).

Perform the test on the painfree side first for subsequent comparison. With the patient in supine lying, the foot of one leg is placed on the knee of the other and the leg allowed to rest in lateral rotation and abduction. An assessment is made of the range of movement which is usually limited in sacroiliac joint problems. Pain reported at this stage is more likely to be indicative of hip joint pathology. Stabilise the opposite side of the pelvis and stress the sacroiliac joint by placing gentle downward pressure on the flexed knee. Pain now reported in the back incriminates the sacroiliac joint as a cause of symptoms (Hoppenfeld, 1976).

Palpation may be conducted for tenderness which is often located over the PSIS and surrounding area and is absent on the unaffected side. However, such tenderness is also often present in lumbar pathology and should not be taken by itself as a positive sign of sacroiliac joint involvement.

Diagnosis at the sacroiliac joint is confirmed by the history (subjective examination) and positive pain provocation tests. *Palpation tests* which assess symmetry and movement of the pelvis can then be applied to determine the choice of treatment.

Piedallu's sign (Fig. 14.6) is the presence of asymmetrical movement of the PSIS during trunk flexion (Grieve, 1981) Position the patient in sitting, crouching down if necessary, and assess the level of each PSIS from behind. The PSIS on the painful side may be lower than the other. Ask the patient to bend forwards and note the 'skyline' view. If positive, the previously lower PSIS will now rest higher with respect to the other since the subluxed sacro-iliac joint moves as a single unit with the sacrum, rather than demonstrating the normal independent 'shuffling' movement between the sacrum and the ilium.

The *'walk' test* (Fig. 14.5) may be applied. The patient stands using the wall or a chair to balance themselves. Crouch down so that you are at eye level with the sacrum and the PSISs. Tuck each thumb up and under the PSIS on either side to firmly locate their position. Ask the patient to flex alternate hips to 90°, without tilting the pelvis, and note the movement of one PSIS in relation to the other.

The test may provide a clue for the application of treatment techniques in that if the PSIS on the painful side appears to be 'high riding' in relation to the other, then a technique, and appropriate exercises, will be selected to produce a downward movement, and vice versa. No movement abnormality may be detected in which case more general treatments will be applied.

The *ipsilateral kinetic test* (Fowler, 1994) may also be applied to assess symmetry on movement. With the patient in standing, supported against a wall, place your right thumb on the right PSIS. Place your left thumb on the median sacral crest, keeping thumbs parallel. Ask the patient to flex the right hip and knee to 90°. The right innominate bone should rotate backwards on the fixed sacrum and the movement of the right thumb should be caudal. The test is positive and demonstrates hypomobility if the right thumb moves cranially instead of caudally as the patient hitches the right side of the pelvis. Repeat the test on the other side to compare.

Other pain provocation tests for the sacroiliac ligaments can be applied. It is not necessary to include all these tests. The choice is left to the reader as to which provide pertinent information for diagnosis and treatment selection.

The *distraction test* applies stress to both ASISs. With the patient in supine lying, cross your hands across the patient's pelvis before placing a hand directed laterally against each ASIS. Direct the stress posterolaterally to stretch the anterior sacroiliac joint ligaments. A positive test will produce pain in the patient's back in the area of the affected joint. This test can be most uncomfortable for the patient and care should be taken to apply a firm stretch rather than a cruel 'jab'. A painful squeeze or stretch of the anterior soft tissues does not constitute a positive test.

The *compression test* applies firm steady downward pressure over the ilium with the patient lying on their more comfortable side on a low couch. This test theoretically stresses the posterior sacroiliac joint ligaments and, if positive, pain will be produced in the region of the offending joint. The shape of the pelvis and the strength of the supporting ligaments make this a test which is hard to apply

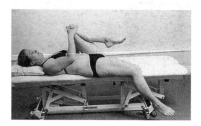

Fig. 14.15 Gaenslen's test.

effectively unless the operator possesses considerable strength and large hands. Those with lesser attributes would be advised to apply the tests described below.

The ***pelvic torsion test (Gaenslen's test)*** (Fig. 14.15) may be applied. Place the patient in supine lying with one hip and knee fully flexed to the chest and the other fully extended over the edge of the couch. This position applies opposing torsional stresses to the sacroiliac joints. Repeat the test by moving the patient to the other edge of the couch and reversing the position of the legs. A position which reproduces the patient's back pain may be a useful guide for the development of home exercises to achieve and maintain mobility (see below).

Reproduction of the patient's pain on the provocation tests constitutes a positive result. Laslett and Williams (1994) assessed the reliability of various provocation tests and found that the distraction, compression and pelvic torsion tests, listed above, have the greatest intertherapist reliability.

Having completed the examination, an hypothesis is established relating to the patient's signs and symptoms. If a diagnosis of a mechanical lesion of the sacroiliac joint is made, manipulation is the treatment of choice provided no contraindications exist.

Mechanical lesions of the sacroiliac joint

The choice of treatment technique depends on the findings on examination and the subsequent response to treatment. Progression of treatment is based on the process of constant re-examination.

As examination of the sacroiliac joint is not usually conducted in isolation, the recommended guidelines for safe practice of manipulation are the same as that covered in the lumbar spine (see Chapter 13). The practitioner must take all due care whilst applying the treatment techniques.

Indications for sacroiliac joint manipulation:

- History of a mechanical lesion of the sacroiliac joint, subluxation or sprain.
- Absence of signs in the lumbar spine and hip.
- Palpation tests indicate a pelvic rotation or asymmetry and may help with choice of treatment.
- At least one positive pain provocation test.

Contraindications for sacroiliac manipulation are few since there should be an absence of neurological signs and symptoms as well as an absence of signs of cauda equina compression or serious pathology associated with the lumbar spine.

> **Contraindications for sacroiliac joint manipulation**
>
> - History indicating anything other than a mechanical sacroiliac joint lesion with special reference to inflammatory conditions or serious pathology.
> - Anticoagulants and blood clotting disorders.

Sacroiliac manipulation procedure

It is recommended that a course in orthopaedic medicine is attended before the treatment techniques described are applied in clinical practice (see Appendix).

For all sacroiliac techniques, the height of the couch is a matter of personal choice. As a suggestion, placing the couch at the level of your mid-thigh gives you the opportunity to assist the technique by gapping of the joint.

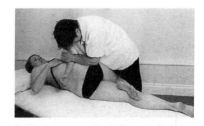

Fig. 14.16 Sacroiliac joint-gapping technique.

Sacroiliac joint-gapping technique

The indication for this technique is that there is no pelvic asymmetry or difference in movement of the PSIS during the palpation tests.

Position the patient in side lying, painful side uppermost, pulling the underneath shoulder well through to stabilize the patient. Flex the upper leg so that the hip and knee are at 90° with the pelvis rotated slightly forwards of the midline. Stand in front of and facing the patient and place your forearm closest to the patient's head, comfortably in the patient's waist under the ribs, to fix the lumbar spine. Place your other forearm on the blade of the ilium, to be at right angles with your forearm in the patient's waist. Rest your caudal knee on the patient's flexed knee and apply downwards pressure to gap the sacroiliac joint. Continue to take up the slack by drawing the forearm on the ilium towards you and apply a minimal-amplitude, high-velocity thrust at the end of range (Figs 14.16 and 14.17).

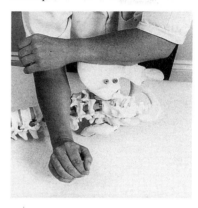

Fig. 14.17 Sacroiliac joint-gapping technique, demonstrating arm positions on skeleton.

Rotation of the pelvis down on the painful side

The indication for this technique is the palpation tests indicating that the PSIS is up on the painful side in relation to the other PSIS.

Position the patient as above and fix under the rib cage with the forearm as before. Place the flexed hip and knee towards more hip flexion to assist rotation of the pelvis downwards on the painful side. Place the medial epicondyle of your other elbow on the patient's ischial tuberosity and rest your caudal knee on the patient's flexed knee to apply downwards pressure, gapping the joint. Once all the slack has been taken up, by rotating your body and arms to pull the ischial tuberosity towards you, apply a minimal-amplitude, high-velocity thrust (Figs 14.18 and 14.19).

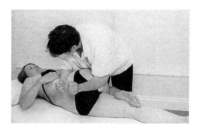

Fig. 14.18 Rotation of the pelvis down on the painful side.

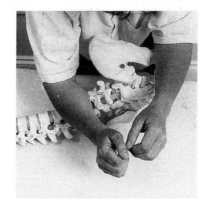

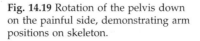

Fig. 14.19 Rotation of the pelvis down on the painful side, demonstrating arm positions on skeleton.

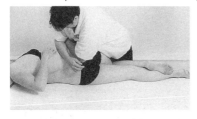

Fig. 14.20 Rotation of the pelvis up on the painful side.

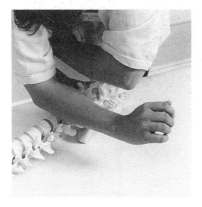

Fig. 14.21 Rotation of the pelvis up on the painful side, demonstrating arm positions on skeleton.

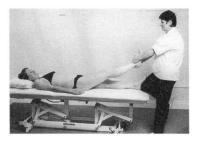

Fig. 14.22 Leg tug.

Rotation of the pelvis up on the painful side

The indication for this technique is the palpation tests indicating that the PSIS is down on the painful side in relation to the other PSIS.

Position the patient as above and fix under the rib cage with one forearm. Place the flexed hip and knee towards hip extension to assist rotation of the pelvis upwards on the painful side. Place the forearm of your other arm to apply pressure just behind the iliac crest, but keep your forearms parallel and in the same plane. Rest your caudal knee on the patient's flexed knee to apply downwards pressure, gapping the joint. Squeeze your arm on the iliac crest towards and under your other arm and, once all the slack has been taken up, apply a minimal-amplitude, high-velocity thrust (Figs 14.20 and 14.21).

Leg tug

The indication for this technique is any sacroiliac mechanical lesion; it is particularly useful during the later stages of pregnancy.

Position the patient comfortably in supine lying with the couch at about knee height. Hold the ankle and place your knee against the patient's foot on the good side, to prevent the patient slipping down the bed. Apply a degree of distraction together with a circumduction movement of the hip. Once the patient relaxes, apply a sharp caudal tug (Fig. 14.22).

Reducing a sacroiliac subluxation or relieving stress on the ligaments can be very successful. Following treatment, attention should be given to the prevention of recurrence. Discussions with the patient will allow advice to be given about lifestyle habits that may be contributing to the condition and any imbalances and postural problems can be addressed. Following reduction of subluxation in the later stages of pregnancy, a supportive brace may be helpful. The following exercises may be useful in a maintenance programme:

- Standing with one leg on a stool, ask the patient to make a lunging movement forwards, involving flexion at the hip and extension at the lumbar spine. Upwards movement of the PSIS is encouraged on the side of the standing, extended leg, and downwards movement of the PSIS is encouraged on the side of the flexed leg (Fig. 14.23a,b).
- This is the same position as that used for the pelvic torsion test (Gaenslen's test; see above). In supine lying, ask the patient to flex one knee to the chest whilst the other leg hangs over the edge of the couch. Movement of the PSIS upwards is encouraged in the extended leg and movement of the PSIS downwards in the flexed leg (Fig. 14.24).

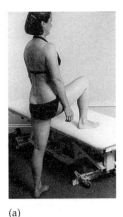

(a)

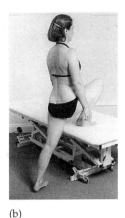

(b)

Fig. 14.23 (a, b) Exercise in standing, encouraging movement of the posterior superior iliac spine.

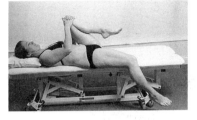

Fig. 14.24 Exercise in supine lying, encouraging movement of the posterior superior iliac spine.

Sacroiliac traction

The use of traction is not indicated with a sacroiliac joint problem. Where the differential diagnosis is uncertain between a lumbar or sacroiliac joint problem, the latter may be suspected if the application of traction makes the pain worse, since the position of the pelvic harness over the ilia applies stress through the sacroiliac joints when the traction is applied.

Sclerosant injections

In cases of extreme laxity of the sacroiliac joints, associated with frequent episodes of subluxation, sclerosant injections may be used to induce scarring in the ligaments, so tightening the tissues to support the joint (see Chapter 13). It is important that the subluxation is reduced before the injections are given.

Sclerosants would not be appropriate in pregnancy but, in any event, the ligamentous softening is likely to resolve spontaneously within 4–5 months of delivery.

References

Cassidy, J.D. (1992) The pathoanatomy and clinical significance of the sacro-iliac joints. *Journal of Manipulative and Physiological Therapeutics* **15**: 41–42.

Cibulka, M.T. (1992) The treatment of the sacro-iliac joint component to low back pain – a case report. *Physical Therapy* **72**: 917–922.

Daly, K.M., Frame, P.S., Rapaza, P.A. (1991) Sacro-iliac subluxation: a common, treatable cause of low back pain in pregnancy. *Family Practice Research Journal* **11**: 149–159.

Fortin, J.D., Dwyer, A.P., West, S., Pier, J. (1994) Sacro-iliac joint – pain referral maps upon applying a new injection/arthrography technique. Part II: clinical evaluation. *Spine* **19**: 1483–1489.

Fowler, C. (1994) Muscle energy techniques for pelvic dysfunction. In: *Grieve's Modern Manual Therapy*, 2nd edn (Boyling, J.D., Palastanga, N., eds). Churchill Livingstone, pp. 781–791.

Golighty, R. (1982) Pelvic arthropathy in pregnancy and the puerperium. *Physiotherapy* **68**: 216–220.

Grieve, G. (1981) *Common Vertebral Joint Problems*. Churchill Livingstone.

Hoppenfeld, S. (1976) *Physical Examination of the Spine and Extremities*. Appleton Centuary Crofts.

Jacob, H.A.C., Kissling, R.O. (1995) The mobility of the sacro-iliac joints in healthy volunteers between 10 and 50 years of age. *Clinical Biomechanics* **10**: 352–361.

Kapandji, I.A. (1974) *The Physiology of the Joints, the Trunk and the Vertebral Column*, vol. 3. Churchill Livingstone.

Keat, A. (1995) Reiter's syndrome and reactive arthritis. In: *Collected Reports on the Rheumatic Diseases*, pp. 61–64. Arthritis and Rheumatism Council for Research.

Kumar, P., Clark, M. (1994) *Clinical Medicine*, 3rd edn. Baillière Tindall.

Laslett, M., Williams, M. (1994) The reliability of selected pain provocation tests for sacro-iliac joint pathology. *Spine* **19**: 1243–1249.

Leblanc, K. (1992) Sacro-iliac sprain: an overlooked cause of back pain. *American Family Physician* **Nov**: 1459–1463.

Lee, D. (1989) *The Pelvic Girdle*. Churchill Livingstone.

Oliver, J., Middleditch, A. (1991) *Functional Anatomy of the Spine*. Butterworth-Heinemann.

Palastanga, N., Field, D., Soames, R. (1994) *Anatomy and Human Movement*. Butterworth-Heinemann.

Rai, A. (1995) Ankylosing spondylitis. In: *Collected Reports on the Rheumatic Diseases*. Arthritis and Rheumatism Council for Research, pp. 65–68.

Schwarzer, A.C., Aprill, C.N., Bogduk, N. (1995) The sacro-iliac joint in chronic low back pain. *Spine* **20**: 31–37.

Silberstein, M., Hennessy, O., Lau, L. (1992) Neoplastic involvement of the sacro-iliac joint – MR and CT features. *Australasian Radiology* **36**: 334–338.

Trotter, M. (1947) Variations of the sacral canal: their significance in the administration of caudal analgesia. *Anesthesia and Analgesia* **Sept/Oct**: 192–202.

Vleeming, A., Pool-Goudzwaard, L., Hammudoghlu, D. *et al.* (1996) The function of the long dorsal sacro-iliac ligament. *Spine* **21**: 556–562.

Williams, P.L, Warwick, R., Dyson, M., Bannister, L.H. (1989) *Gray's Anatomy*, 37th edn. Churchill Livingstone.

Wilson, D.J. (1989) Diagnosis and treatment of sacro-iliac joint dysfunction. *Physiotherapy* **75**: 500–501.

Appendix

Courses in orthopaedic medicine

Orthopaedic medicine courses, for physiotherapists and medical practitioners, are held at a variety of venues both nationally and internationally. The course design consists of distance learning packages, modular taught blocks, intermodular projects and a final practical and theoretical examination. The educational aims of the course include the development of clinical reasoning skills, critical analysis of outcomes and self-evaluation.

The course content includes clinical examination and diagnosis, applied anatomy, soft-tissue treatment techniques of manipulation and mobilization, and injection techniques. Much of the course is devoted to practical work in small groups with close supervision and feedback. The courses are supported by a comprehensive illustrated manual.

The basic course acts as an introduction to injection techniques for physiotherapists and, at the time of writing, plans are underway for the development of an advanced module to teach injection skills to physiotherapists.

For more details of the courses available please contact the following organizations:

Society of Orthopaedic Medicine (registered charity no 802164)

Course organizer

Mrs K.M. Kesson Dip Grad Phys MCSP SRP Cert Ed
1 The Mall
Faversham
Kent
ME13 8JL

Orthopaedic Medicine International

Course organizer

Mr R.J. Packham BSc (Hons) MCSP SRP
13 Mavisbank
Kinross
Perthshire
KY13 7QR

Details of the specific interest group, the Association of Chartered Physiotherapists in Orthopaedic Medicine (ACPOM), are available from:

The Chartered Society of Physiotherapy
14 Bedford Row
London WC1R 4ED

Glossary

Allodynia Pain produced by a stimulus which is not normally painful.

Anomalous cross-links An abnormal number of cross-links (adhesions), developing as a result of a stationary attitude of collagen fibres; responsible for the toughness and resilience of scar tissue.

Capsular pattern A limitation of movement in a specific pattern which is peculiar to each joint and indicates the presence of an arthritis.

Close-packed The position in which a joint is most stable, when the joint surfaces fit closely together and are maximally congruent.

Compression A squashing or pushing force resulting in the structure becoming shortened and broadened.

Corticosteroids Potent anti-inflammatory drugs. In orthopaedic medicine: injections used to treat chronic inflammatory soft-tissue lesions, acute episodes of degenerative osteoarthrosis and inflammatory arthritis.

Creep A property of viscoelastic structures which consists of a small, almost imperceptible movement, occurring when a constant stress is applied for a prolonged period of time.

Cross-links Either weak intramolecular hydrogen bonds connecting collagen molecules or stronger covalent intermolecular bonds connecting collagen fibrils and fibres. The links provide connective tissue structures with tensile strength and the greater the number of cross-links, the stronger the structure.

Deformation A change in length or shape due to the application of a stress, represented as strain on the stress–strain diagram.

Distraction/traction A force applied in opposite directions across a joint causing the joint surfaces to separate.

Dysaesthesia Damage to any of the senses, especially touch, but not to the point of total anaesthesia.

Elasticity The property of a material or a structure which allows it to deform when a force is applied. The change is temporary and the original form is restored when the deforming force is removed.

Elastic range Represented on the stress–strain diagram as the range of loading within which a material or structure remains elastic, i.e. it can resume its original form after the deforming force is removed.

End-feel A specific sensation imparted through the examiner's hands at the extreme of passive movement.

Enthesis The point at which a tendon inserts into bone.

Enthesopathy A lesion at the teno-osseous junction, e.g. tennis elbow at the common extensor origin.

Fatigue A process by which a structure fails when subjected to repetitive low loading cycles.

Force An action which produces movement by pushing or pulling, known as mechanical stress and expressed as the force per unit area.

Force couple The application of equal, but opposite, parallel forces.

Glycosaminoglycans (GAGs) Long-chain molecules, the building blocks for proteoglycans.

Grade A mobilization A passive, active or active/assisted mobilization performed within the patient's painfree range at peripheral joints.

Grade A movement A mid-range painfree movement applied to spinal joints.

Grade B mobilization A mobilization applied at the end of available range. A sustained stretching technique aimed to produce permanent lengthening of connective tissue structures.

Grade B movement Indicates the end of range at the spinal joints.

Grade C mobilization A manipulation involving a minimal-amplitude, high-velocity thrust applied at the end of range once all of the slack has been taken up. It can be applied to certain peripheral or spinal lesions.

Hysteresis A property of viscoelastic structures in which the resumption of its original length occurs more slowly than the deformation.

Load A general term describing the application of a force and/or moment (torque) to a structure.

Local anaesthetic A pain-inhibiting drug. In orthopaedic medicine injections, used for its diagnostic and therapeutic effects.

Macrofailure Occurs when there is rupture of a structure and it is unable to sustain further load. Represented by a rapid fall in the stress–strain curve.

Microfailure   Occurs when a structure reaches its elastic limit with progressive failure of cross-links and fibrils.

Moment   A force that produces bending or torque.

Motion segment   A functional spinal segment consisting of two adjacent vertebral bodies together with their joints and surrounding soft tissues.

Non-capsular pattern   A pattern of limited and/or painful movements which does not fit the capsular pattern of that particular joint.

Paraesthesia   Numbness, tingling, 'pins and needles'.

Plasticity   The property of a structure which permits it to undergo permanent deformation when the distorting force is large enough to load the structure beyond its elastic range.

Plastic range   Represented on the stress–strain diagram as the range of loading within which a material or structure cannot resume its original form once the deforming force is removed, i.e. the elastic limit of the structure is exceeded.

Pressure phenomenon   Pain and paraesthesia occurring as pressure is applied.

Proteoglycans   Protein–carbohydrate complex consisting of GAGs covalently bound to protein.

Release phenomenon   The sensation of deep painful paraesthesia occurring as pressure is released from a nerve trunk.

Selective tension   The application of appropriate stress to soft-tissue structures in order to test function.

Set   The difference between the original and final length or shape of a structure once the deforming force is removed.

Shear   A force applied parallel to the surface of the structure, causing angular deformation.

Sign of the buttock   Pain on straight leg raise which increases on flexing the knee and hip. It is a sign of serious pathology.

Stiffness   The resistance of a structure to the deforming force.

Strain   The deformation or change in dimension of a material or structure in response to an externally applied load or force.

Stress   The load or force applied to a structure resulting in strain or deformation.

Stress–strain curve   A diagrammatic representation of the mechanical behaviour of a material or structure. Stress is plotted on the y axis and represents the tensile, compressive, shear or torsional force applied. Strain is plotted on the x axis and represents the deformation or elongation of the material.

Tendinitis   Inflammation of a tendon.

Tendinosis   Degenerative tendon changes.

Tenosynovitis   Inflammation between a tendon and its sheath.

Tensile strength   The maximum stress or load sustained by a material.

Tension   A force of equal and opposite loads which results in lengthening and narrowing of the fibres of a material or structure.

Torsion   A combination of shear, tensile and compressive force or load applied to a structure causing it to rotate about an axis. The load is called the torque.

Traction/distraction   A force applied in opposite directions across a joint causing the joint surfaces to separate.

Translation   Parallel movement of two opposing surfaces causing them to slide across one another.

Transverse friction massage   A specific type of massage applied to connective tissue structures to produce therapeutic movement, traumatic hyperaemia, pain relief and improved function.

Viscoelasticity   The property of a material to change when under constant deformation.

Viscosity   The property of a fluid which resists flowing.

Wolff's law   A law that states that bone is laid down where it is needed along the lines of stress, and reabsorbed when not needed.

Yield point   The point of the stress–strain curve at which appreciable deformity occurs, without any appreciable increase in load.

Index